Acute Trauma Care in Developing Countries

This evidence-based manual highlights the early management of acutely injured trauma victims arriving in emergency triage areas. It caters to the needs of developing nations in pre-hospital as well as in-hospital emergency trauma care and provides clear practical guidelines for the management of victims of major trauma. The book covers basic principles for managing a crashing trauma patient, followed by effective treatment by different subspecialties. Input from experienced anaesthesiologists, intensivists, orthopaedics, vascular surgeons, plastic surgeons and radiologists make this book a gold standard for good practice for professionals.

Key features:

- Covers all aspects of acute trauma, including orthopaedics, vascular surgery, plastic surgery, neurosurgery, burns and radiology
- Elaborates on damage control resuscitation and management of initial and life-threatening injuries; useful for professionals dealing with trauma patients in the emergency area
- Guides in initial fluid therapy and pain control along with initial patient resuscitation

Acute Trauma Care in Developing Countries

A Practical Guide

Edited by
Chief Editors: Kajal Jain and Nidhi Bhatia

Associate Editors: Tanvir Samra and Vishal Kumar

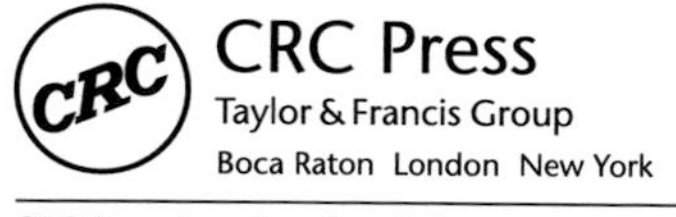

CRC Press is an imprint of the
Taylor & Francis Group, an **informa** business

First edition published 2023
by CRC Press
6000 Broken Sound Parkway NW, Suite 300, Boca Raton, FL 33487-2742

and by CRC Press
4 Park Square, Milton Park, Abingdon, Oxon, OX14 4RN

CRC Press is an imprint of Taylor & Francis Group, LLC

ISBN: 9781032271576 (hbk)
ISBN: 9781032271552 (pbk)
ISBN: 9781003291619 (ebk)

DOI: 10.1201/9781003291619

Typeset in Palatino
by Deanta Global Publishing Services, Chennai, India

Contents

Section II: Crashing Trauma Patient

Foreword

As per data from the Government of India, about 328 people died every day in 2022 due to trauma despite the fact that there were COVID-19 lockdowns. This number would be much higher during non-pandemic times, and some policy decisions for improvement of trauma care all over the country need to be made. Trauma care as a speciality is still in its nascent phase in India and much effort is required to improve care of such patients. In my opinion this book is one step forward in this regard. I must congratulate both the chief editors – Drs Kajal Jain and Nidhi Bhatia, who are young enthusiastic anaesthesiologists – for compiling a simple, easy-to-read and comprehensive book in which all the chapters have been written by clinicians directly involved in all aspects of trauma care for many years. All the authors work in the Advanced Trauma Centre located on the campus of the Post Graduate Institute of Medical Education and Research, Chandigarh, a testament to patient care in North India.

Care of such patients requires a thorough knowledge of issues such as management of airways, massive blood loss, coagulopathy, hypothermia, acidaemia, head injury and damage control surgery, among others. The content of this manual-sized book not only gives a review of all such important topics but also discusses the immediate care of such patients at the injury site and in the intensive care units.

There are separate chapters on management of trauma in pregnant patients and those with burns, topics that are usually overlooked in such books. A special chapter from the military perspective in managing such patients makes this book a "complete manual".

This book is meant for a wide readership that should include not only doctors of all age groups but also nurses and paramedical staff involved in trauma care. It is highly recommended that this manual of trauma care be made available – maybe free of cost – in all units that are taking care of patients with trauma.

Anjan Trikha MBBS, DA, MD, MNAMS, FICA, FAMS, FAOA
Professor, Department of Anaesthesiology, Pain Medicine and Critical Care
Incharge, Trauma Anaesthesia and Intensive Care
JPN Apex Trauma Centre
All India Institute of Medical Sciences
New Delhi, India

Foreword

It gives me immense pleasure to write the Foreword to this very practical book titled *Acute Trauma Care in Developing Countries: A Practical Guide*. I have been working as an anaesthesiologist at Ganga Medical Centre & Hospital, Coimbatore, India, a 650-bed tertiary care referral centre for trauma for the past 25 years, and I completely understand the value of this very important book. I congratulate the chief editors Dr Kajal Jain, Dr Nidhi Bhatia and the trauma team of the Post Graduate Institute, Chandigarh, for their efforts in making this book a reality. This book has come at a very crucial time for our nation, as we have an enormous increase in the incidence of trauma cases, especially due to road traffic accidents. The book is very comprehensive and has incorporated all the facets of trauma management. It is increasingly evident that quick and timely intervention considerably decreases morbidity and mortality and thus paves the way for very good outcomes. The first section of the book is very important and deals concisely with the principles of acute trauma care; this is a must-read for all medical and paramedical staff involved in the care of trauma victims. The second section of the book focuses on the crashing trauma patient. These chapters focus on the skill sets that must be acquired to aid in resuscitating a bleeding patient rapidly and effectively. The third section emphasizes the subspecialty areas of trauma care, including insights into subjects such as trauma in pregnancy and burns. This book will enrich all trauma care providers with current updates and evidence-based practice of trauma care. This book is a must-read for all anaesthesiologists, surgeons, intensivists, emergency care physicians, physician assistants and paramedical staff involved in trauma care.

J Balavenkatasubramanian, MD, DA
Senior Consultant and Academic Director
Department of Anaesthesia & Perioperative Care
Ganga Medical Centre & Hospital
Coimbatore, India

Foreword

It is a privilege, pleasure and pride to write the Foreword of a book that is edited by authors who have had extensive professional relations with me for the last few decades and several young authors of this book have been trained under me or at least mentored by me during their careers as trauma surgeons. The exceptional paradigm of this book is that it is authored by anesthesiologists, critical care physicians and trauma surgeons who have first-hand experience at the level I trauma center of one of the premier teaching institutes of the country – the Postgraduate Institute of Medical Education & Research, Chandigarh, India. I have yet to see a book of this kind that focuses and emphasizes exclusively on acute trauma care in the developing world, and this book will prove its worth by being a landmark work to reckon with in this field. Various difficult but common scenarios of clinical presentations referred to advanced trauma centers are very lucidly discussed in the relevant chapters of this book which will serve as guidelines for the management of similar cases presenting at different centers across the globe. The suggested readings mentioned at the end of each chapter will further help the readers in expanding their knowledge on the same subject. All the clinical case discussions in this book are real-life scenarios encountered by the concerned writers, and hence this book provides a scientific, rational, deliverable approach to managing such cases in resource-constrained settings as well.

I compliment the astute observations of the authors and congratulate the editors for their brilliant compendium *Acute Trauma Care in Developing Countries: A Practical Guide* and wish all of them the best and expect many more such compendiums in the future.

Dr (Prof.) Sameer Aggarwal
MBBS, MS (Ortho.), MAMS, FIMSA
Professor of Orthopaedics Surgery
Nodal Officer (Advanced Trauma Centre)
PGIMER, Chandigarh, India

Preface

Trauma represents one of the most serious threats to public health the world over. Trauma claims more lost quality of life than other diseases and sadly affects the younger population. Due to continued efforts of skilled trauma providers working in complex systems, we are able to mitigate the impact on those who have life-threatening injuries. Many advancements revolve around quality improvement in resuscitation, anaesthesia, advanced monitoring and timely surgical intervention. However, we (India) still lack accreditation of trauma systems conducive to our environment, and there is a strong need to develop trauma systems on par with international counterparts. At this time, this trauma manual will serve as a ready reference for all who provide care for trauma patients. We have chosen a wide range of topics aimed at all members of the trauma team (pre-hospital, trauma triage, intensive care and operating room). All the authors have likewise been chosen given their expertise from working in a high-volume tertiary trauma centre. The book is indispensable for those with an interest in care of the injured, which may range from a simple isolated fracture to a complex injury with multisystem involvement.

We would like to thank all the authors who have contributed chapters to this book as well as the publishers who have facilitated this journey. We are particularly grateful to Shivangi Pramanik and Himani Dwivedi for their tireless efforts and constant guidance. On behalf of all our authors, we hope this book enables all of you to provide the best of care to all trauma victims.

Kajal Jain and Nidhi Bhatia

About the Editors

Kajal Jain, MD, MAMS, FICA is a consultant anaesthetist at Post Graduate Institute of Medical Education and Research, Chandigarh. She is the programme director for a three-year academic postdoctoral doctorate of medicine course in trauma anaesthesia and acute care. She has represented the institute at national and international meetings to discuss trauma-related issues and research. She is actively engaged in the care of potential organ donors, hospital infection control and antibiotic stewardship programmes of the hospital. She has conducted numerous workshops dedicated to triage and disaster management. Her main areas of interest are trauma resuscitation on arrival and critical trauma care.

Nidhi Bhatia, MD, DNB, MAMS is a consultant anaesthetist in the Department of Anaesthesia and Intensive Care, Post Graduate Institute of Medical Education and Research, Chandigarh. She is part of the core faculty in a three-year academic postdoctoral doctorate of medicine course in trauma anaesthesia and acute care. She has a keen interest in the fields of acute trauma care, ultrasound-guided regional analgesia, obstetric anaesthesia and airway management. She has been a certified instructor for the American Heart Association–accredited BLS and ACLS courses since 2010. She is also an Advanced Trauma Life Support (ATLS) instructor; a founding member and treasurer of the Society of Trauma Anaesthesia and Critical Care; a member of the National Academy of Medical Sciences (NAMS) (Perioperative Medicine); special section editor for the *Journal of Anaesthesiology Clinical Pharmacology*; and an Executive Council member of the Indian Society for the Study of Pain (ISSP), Chandigarh chapter. She has 75 publications (international and national) and 11 book chapters to her credit. She has received ten best paper awards, including two international awards and the prestigious Obstetric Anaesthesia Society of Asia Oceania (OASAO) Gold Medal for "Best Research Paper".

Contributors

Kishore Abuji, MS
Senior Resident
Department of General Surgery
Post Graduate Institute of Medical Education and Research
Chandigarh, India

Ashish Aditya, MD
Assistant Professor
Department of Anaesthesia and Intensive Care
Post Graduate Institute of Medical Education and Research
Chandigarh, India

Chirag Kamal Ahuja, MD, DM
Associate Professor
Department of Radiodiagnosis
Post Graduate Institute of Medical Education and Research
Chandigarh, India

Aashima Arora, MD
Associate Professor
Department of Obstetrics and Gynaecology
Post Graduate Institute of Medical Education and Research
Chandigarh, India

Anjishnujit Bandyopadhyay, MD, DM
Senior Resident
Department of Anaesthesia and Intensive Care
Post Graduate Institute of Medical Education and Research
Chandigarh, India

Nidhi Bhatia, MD, DNB, MAMS, DM
Professor and Core Faculty
Department of Anaesthesia and Intensive Care
Post Graduate Institute of Medical Education and Research
Chandigarh, India

Anjuman Chander, MD
Senior Resident
Department of Anaesthesia and Intensive Care
Post Graduate Institute of Medical Education and Research
Chandigarh, India

Rajeev Chauhan, MD, DM
Associate Professor
Department of Anaesthesia and Intensive Care
Post Graduate Institute of Medical Education and Research
Chandigarh, India

Rajesh Chhabra, MS, MCh
Professor
Department of Neurosurgery
Post Graduate Institute of Medical Education and Research
Chandigarh, India

Devendra Kumar Chouhan, MS
Professor
Department of Orthopaedics
Post Graduate Institute of Medical Education and Research
Chandigarh, India

Narendra Chouhan
Anaesthesiologist and Critical Care Specialist
Abu Dhabi, United Arab Emirates

Sarvdeep Singh Dhatt, MS
Professor
Department of Orthopaedics
Post Graduate Institute of Medical Education and Research
Chandigarh, India

Komal A Gandhi, MD
Associate Professor
Department of Anaesthesia and Intensive Care
Post Graduate Institute of Medical Education and Research
Chandigarh, India

Chandrasekhar Gendle, MS, MCh
Assistant Professor
Department of Neurosurgery
Post Graduate Institute of Medical Education and Research
Chandigarh, India

Akash Kumar Ghosh, MS
Senior Resident
Department of Orthopaedics
Post Graduate Institute of Medical Education and Research
Chandigarh, India

Ujjwal Gorsi, MD
Associate Professor
Department of Radiodiagnosis
Post Graduate Institute of Medical Education and Research
Chandigarh, India

Sunil K Gupta, MS, MCh
Professor and Head
Department of Neurosurgery
Post Graduate Institute of Medical Education and Research
Chandigarh, India

Tarush Gupta, MS, MCh, DNB
Associate Professor
Department of Plastic Surgery
Post Graduate Institute of Medical Education and Research
Chandigarh, India

Amarjyoti Hazarika, MD
Associate Professor
Department of Anaesthesia and Intensive Care
Post Graduate Institute of Medical Education and Research
Chandigarh, India

Anudeep Jafra, MD
Associate Professor
Department of Anaesthesia and Intensive Care
Post Graduate Institute of Medical Education and Research
Chandigarh, India

Kajal Jain, MD, MAMS, DM
Professor and Course Coordinator
Department of Anaesthesia and Intensive Care
Post Graduate Institute of Medical Education and Research
Chandigarh, India

Narender Kaloria, MD, DM
Assistant Professor
Department of Anaesthesia and Intensive Care
Post Graduate Institute of Medical Education and Research
Chandigarh, India

Bisman Jeet Kaur, MD, DM
Senior Resident
Department of Anaesthesia and Intensive Care
Post Graduate Institute of Medical Education and Research
Chandigarh, India

Shahnawaz Khan, MS
Senior Resident
Department of Orthopaedics
Post Graduate Institute of Medical Education and Research
Chandigarh, India

Vishal Kumar, MS, FRCS
Associate Professor
Department of Orthopaedics
Post Graduate Institute of Medical Education and Research
Chandigarh, India

Ankur Luthra, MD, DM
Associate Professor
Department of Anaesthesia and Intensive Care
Post Graduate Institute of Medical Education and Research
Chandigarh, India

Karthigeyan M, MS, MCh
Associate Professor
Department of Neurosurgery
Post Graduate Institute of Medical Education and Research
Chandigarh, India

Shalvi Mahajan, MD, DM
Assistant Professor
Department of Anaesthesia and Intensive Care
Post Graduate Institute of Medical Education and Research
Chandigarh, India

Jeetinder Kaur Makkar, MD, DM, DNB, MNAMS, FRCRC
Fellow
Interventional Pain
University of Manitoba, Canada
Manitoba, Canada
and Professor
Department of Anaesthesia and Intensive Care
Post Graduate Institute of Medical Education and Research
Chandigarh, India

Shyam Charan Meena, MD
Associate Professor
Department of Anaesthesia and Intensive Care
Post Graduate Institute of Medical Education and Research
Chandigarh, India

Deepak Neradi, MS
Department of Orthopaedics
Post Graduate Institute of Medical Education and Research
Chandigarh, India

Sandeep Patel, MS, DNB
Assistant Professor
Department of Orthopaedics
Post Graduate Institute of Medical Education and Research
Chandigarh, India

Shamik Kr Paul, MD, DM
Reader/Instructor
Department of Anaesthesiology and Critical Care
Armed Forces Medical College, Pune
Pune, India

Sharad Prabhakar, MS
Professor
Department of Orthopaedics
Post Graduate Institute of Medical Education and Research
Chandigarh, India

Sushant K Sahoo, MS, MCh
Associate Professor
Department of Neurosurgery
Post Graduate Institute of Medical Education and Research
Chandigarh, India

Pravin Salunke, MS, MCh
Professor
Department of Neurosurgery
Post Graduate Institute of Medical Education and Research
Chandigarh, India

Tanvir Samra, MD
Associate Professor
Department of Anaesthesia and Intensive Care
Post Graduate Institute of Medical Education and Research
Chandigarh, India

Rashi Sarna, MD
Assistant Professor
Department of Anaesthesia and Intensive Care
Post Graduate Institute of Medical Education and Research
Chandigarh, India

Ajay Savlania, MS, MCh
Associate Professor
Department of General Surgery
Post Graduate Institute of Medical Education and Research
Chandigarh, India

Apinderpreet Singh, MS, MCh
Associate Professor
Department of Neurosurgery
Post Graduate Institute of Medical Education and Research
Chandigarh, India

Lakhvinder Singh, MD
Associate Professor
Department of Transfusion Medicine
Post Graduate Institute of Medical Education and Research
Chandigarh, India

Harshit Singla, MD
Senior Resident
Department of Anaesthesia and Intensive Care
Post Graduate Institute of Medical Education and Research
Chandigarh, India

Haneesh Thakur, MD, DM
Senior Resident
Department of Anaesthesia and Intensive Care
Post Graduate Institute of Medical Education and Research
Chandigarh, India

Mandeep Tundak, MD, DM
Senior Resident
Department of Anaesthesia and Intensive Care
Post Graduate Institute of Medical Education and Research
Chandigarh, India

Venkata Vineeth Vaddavalli, MS
Senior Resident
Department of General Surgery
Post Graduate Institute of Medical Education and Research
Chandigarh, India

Abbreviations

AAST	American Association for Surgery of Trauma
ABG	arterial blood gas
ACV	assist control ventilation
AHA	American Heart Association
AIIMS	All India Institute of Medical Sciences
ALS	Advanced Life Support
ANGELS	Active Network Group of Emergency Life Savers
AP	antero-posterior
ARDS	acute respiratory distress syndrome
ARF	acute renal failure
ASA	American Society of Anesthesiologists
ASB	assisted spontaneous breathing
ASIA	American Spinal Injury Association
ATLS	Advanced Trauma Life Support
ATLS-OE	Advanced Trauma Life Support – Operational Environment (or Operational Emphasis)
ATP	AIIMS Triage Protocol
ATS	Australasian Triage Scale
BAES	British Association of Accident and Emergency Medicine
BLS	Basic Life Support
CAT	Combat Application Tourniquet
CATS	Centralised Accident and Trauma Services
CCR	Canadian C-Spine Rule
CCS	central cord syndrome
cmH_2O	centimetre of water
COVID-19	coronavirus disease 2019
CPR	cardiopulmonary resuscitation
CRBSI	catheter-related blood stream infection
CSF	cerebrospinal fluid
CSI	cervical spine injury
CT	computed tomography
CTAS	Canadian Triage and Acuity Scale
CUF	Care Under Fire
CVC	central venous catheter/catheterization
DAI	diffuse axonal injury
DCR	damage control resuscitation
DCS	damage control surgery
DIC	disseminated intravascular coagulation
DPL	diagnostic peritoneal lavage
DVT	deep vein thrombosis
ECG	electrocardiogram
ECMO	extracorporeal membrane oxygenation
ED	emergency department
EDH	extradural haemorrhage
EMRI	Emergency Medical Research Institute
EMS	emergency medical services
EMT	emergency and military tourniquet
EMTS	emergency medicine and trauma services
ERC	emergency response centre
ERCP	endoscopic retrograde cholangiopancreatography
ESI	Emergency Severity Index
ESR	erythrocyte sedimentation rate
$EtCO_2$	end-tidal carbon dioxide
ETT	endotracheal tube
FAST	focused assessment with sonography for trauma
FES	fat embolism syndrome
FFP	fresh frozen plasma
FiO_2	fraction of inspired oxygen
FLACC scale	Face, Legs, Activity, Cry, Consolability Scale
Fr	French
FSC	forward surgical centre
FV	femoral vein
GCS	Glasgow Coma Scale
GI	gastrointestinal
HFNC	high-flow nasal cannula
HI	head injury
HMEs	heat moisture exchangers
HR	heart rate
HRQoL	health-related quality of life
ICP	intracranial pressure
ICU	intensive care unit
IHT	intrahospital transport
IJV	internal jugular vein
IO	intraosseous
IV	intravenous
LMWH	low molecular weight heparin
LOX	liquid oxygen
MARCHE	massive haemorrhage, airway management, respiration/breathing, circulation, hypothermia prevention and everything else
MESS	Mangled Extremity Severity Score
MRI	magnetic resonance imaging
MTS	Manchester Triage System
NEXUS	The National Emergency X-Radiography Utilization Study
NICE	National Institute for Health and Care Excellence
NMDA	N-methyl-D-aspartic acid
NRS	Numerical Rating Scale

NSAID non-steroidal anti-inflammatory drugs
OIS Organ Injury Scale
OT operation theatre
OTFC oral transmucosal fentanyl citrate
P-ACV pressure assist/control ventilation
PCV pressure-controlled ventilation
PE pulmonary embolism
PEA pulseless electrical activity
PEEP positive end expiratory pressure
PIV peripheral intravenous
POCUS point-of-care ultrasound
PRBC packed red blood cells
PSV pressure support ventilation
PTU patient transfer unit
PTV pressure-targeted ventilation
RDP random donor platelets
REBOA resuscitative endovascular balloon occlusion of the aorta
RM recruitment manoeuvre
RR respiratory rate
SAH subarachnoid haemorrhage
SAVE Secondary Assessment of Victim Endpoint
SBP systolic blood pressure
SCM sternocleidomastoid
SCV subclavian vein
SDAP single-donor apheresis platelets
SDH subdural haemorrhage
SIMV synchronized intermittent mandatory ventilation
SJT SAM Junctional Tourniquet
SOFTT Special Operations Forces Tactical Tourniquet
SOV superior ophthalmic vein
SpO2 oxygen saturation
START Simple Triage and Rapid Treatment
T2RF type 2 respiratory failure
TACEVAC Tactical Evacuation Care
TBI traumatic brain injury
TCA traumatic cardiac arrest
TCCC Tactical Combat Casualty Care
TCDs target compression devices
Td tetanus diphtheria
Tdap tetanus diphtheria acellular pertussis
TFC Tactical Field Care
Ti inspiratory time
TIC trauma-induced coagulopathy
TIG tetanus immunoglobulin
TV tidal volume
USG ultrasonography/ultrasonogram
V-ACV volume assist/control ventilation
VAP ventilator associated pneumonia
VAS visual analogue scale
VCV volume-controlled ventilation
VHA viscoelastic haemostatic assays
VILLI ventilator-induced lung injury
VTV volume-targeted ventilation
WBC white blood cell
WDMET Wound Data and Munitions Effectiveness Team
WL window level
WW window width
XABCDE exsanguinating haemorrhage, airway, breathing, circulation, disability, exposure

SECTION I

PRINCIPLES OF ACUTE TRAUMA CARE

1 Pre-hospital Care of Trauma Victims and Triaging on Arrival

Ashish Aditya, Tanvir Samra, Anjuman Chander and Harshit Singla

LEARNING OBJECTIVES

The healthcare system in India is overburdened by its large population and does not have an "organized" pre-hospital and post-discharge rehabilitative service. However, some form of "first aid" is provided to the trauma victim by bystanders or police personnel. Thus, the aim of this chapter is to highlight:

- The existing literature on onsite care in India
- Types of pre-hospital care
- Types of triage

PRE-HOSPITAL CARE OF TRAUMA VICTIMS IN INDIA

Trauma-related morbidity in India contributes to one-fifth of the global burden of injuries. The outcome for trauma victims is time dependent, and therefore countries lacking organized pre-hospital care services report high mortality. This "preventable cause" of low survival needs urgent attention.

A study conducted in the early 1990s in the national capital (New Delhi) on patients with head injuries reported no pre-hospital/first aid management in 65% of cases. Till 2006, 80% of trauma victims in India could not get medical access within the "first golden hour". A study from South India reported a marginal improvement over a 10-year interval in availability of onsite care by paramedical personnel (0.75% in 2000–2001 to 12% in 2010–2011). In a study conducted in 2014, an interesting observation was that the figures from semi-urban/rural areas were comparable; onsite first aid was done to 18.5% of injured patients received.

Transport Facilities

Transport facilities for trauma victims in India were practically non-existent in the early 1990s; only 0.5% of trauma patients were brought to the hospital in ambulances. Even in 2000–2001, autorickshaws played a pivotal role in transporting trauma victims to the hospital (55% of cases). The situation has improved gradually, and now 44.5% of injured patients are transported by ambulances. But ambulance services are non-existent in semi-urban/rural areas; in 2014 only 7.5% of individuals were transported to the hospital in ambulances. Another issue is that the majority (80%) of ambulances lack an attending doctor or paramedic staff.

There is no central emergency medical system, and most ambulances are privately owned or are hospital-based. However, now there are two ambulance services – 108 and 1298 – in public–private partnership with respective state governments (Figure 1.1). Most patients are transported to an appropriate healthcare facility, which may be a few kilometres or many hundreds of kilometres away to cater to the need of the patient.

Thus, we summarize the available ambulance services:

- Dial 108 is a free, not-for-profit emergency service operated by GVK EMRI (Emergency Medical Research Institute). GVK EMRI is currently operational in 17 states and union territories of India.
- Similarly, 1298 is another emergency medical service provider run by Ziqitza Healthcare Limited; however, it is a paid service.
- Centralized Accident and Trauma Services (CATS), launched in Delhi in 1991, was the first pre-hospital system of its kind. CATS is run by the Delhi government in coordination with All India Institute of Medical Sciences (AIIMS) and receives calls from the toll-free numbers 102 and 1099.
- Active Network Group of Emergency Life Savers (ANGELS) is another non-profitable organization functioning in a few districts in the Indian state of Kerala.

Types of Pre-hospital Care

Globally, three types of pre-hospital care exist, namely first responder care, basic pre-hospital care and advanced pre-hospital trauma care (Table 1.1).

Emergency service personnel typically perform low threshold interventions prior to transfer to hospital (Figure 1.2). Some of them are enumerated next:

1. Placement of cervical collar/stabilization of cervical spine (if cervical spine trauma is suspected based on primary survey or mechanism of injury)
2. Oxygen support or airway protection (in case of altered sensorium or respiratory distress)
3. Bleeding control with pressure bandage or placement of tourniquets

DOI: 10.1201/9781003291619-2

Dial 108 and 1298 are similar in its operational aspects.

"Communication Officer"

(Receives the call, collects facts about the emergency, transfers this information further)

"Dispatch Officer"

Identifies the closest Global Positioning System – enabled ambulance and activate it to the scene of emergency.

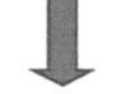

Ambulance

Has an Emergency Medical Technician (EMT), monitoring system and life support measures.

EMTs are formally trained individuals with skills of BLS (Basic Life Support)/ALS (Advanced Life Support).

Figure 1.1 Pre-hospital ambulance service flow chart

Table 1.1: Types of Pre-hospital Care

First Responder Care	Basic Pre-hospital Trauma Care	Advanced Pre-hospital Trauma Care
• Who are first responders? Any member of the community present at the scene of trauma. • Role of first responder care: Important in countries where no pre-hospital care system exists. • How is it established? By teaching general public basic first-aid techniques, recognition of emergencies and their management until formally trained healthcare personnel arrive to give additional care.	• Involves people who have been formally trained in principles of basic pre-hospital care (basic life support). • The provider is given extensive training in scene management, rescue, stabilization and transport of injured people.	• It includes a regional call management centre or a control room with a highly integrated communication network which helps to mobilize advanced care aid at the site of trauma. • A sufficient number of advanced ground or air ambulances equipped with a sophisticated monitoring system and professional skilful healthcare personnel.

4. Administration of intravenous fluids if haemorrhage or shock suspected
5. Administration of analgesia

TRIAGE

Triage comes from the French verb *trier*, meaning "to sort". Triage is the process of determining the priority of a patient's treatment based on the severity of injury or condition, or likelihood of recovery with or without treatment. Triage is an important tool where resources are limited, be it supplies or healthcare staff in developing countries such as India. Also, triage plays an important role in managing mass causalities, including natural disasters, explosions, accidents and similar events where a large number of injured victims congregate at a single or a few healthcare facilities.

Types of Triage

- Pre-hospital triage/primary triage/field triage

  Field triage is practised in disaster scenarios, usually done by rescuers, and the objective is to do the greatest good to the greatest number of patients. Simple Triage and Rapid Treatment (START) followed by Secondary Assessment of Victim Endpoint (SAVE) is done in such scenarios.

- Intra-hospital triage or secondary triage or emergency department triage

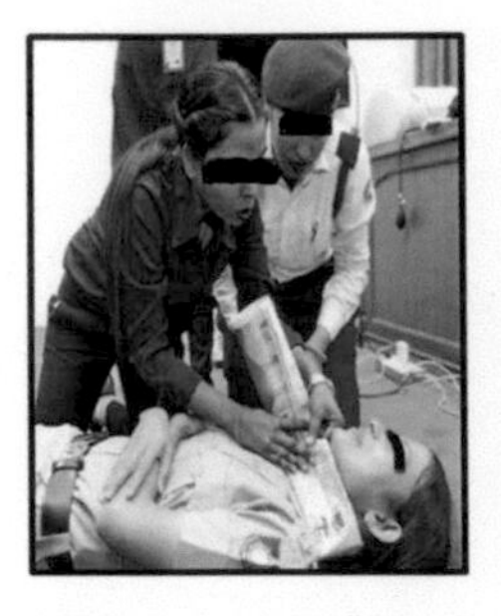

Stabilization of cervical spine

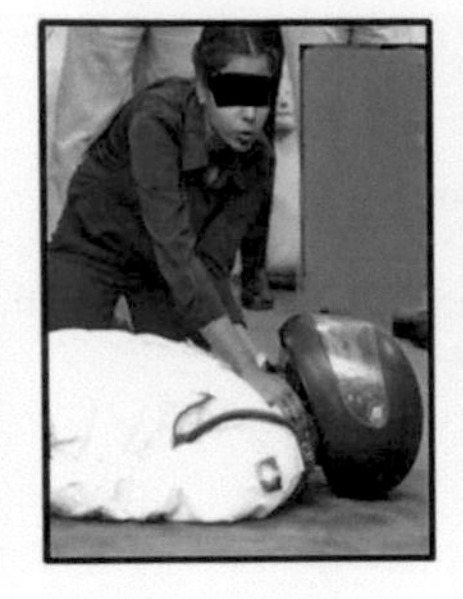

Helmet removal

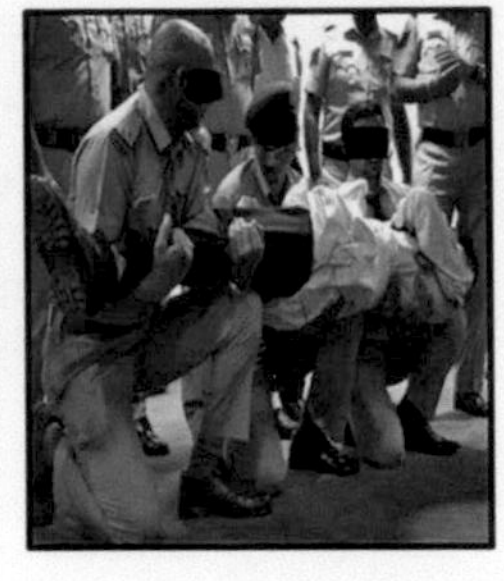

Mobilization and log rolling

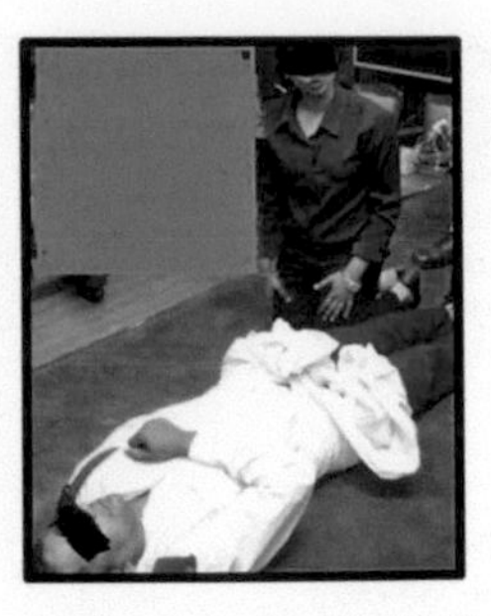

Application of pelvic binder

Figure 1.2 Pre-hospital care

Table 1.2: Five-Tier Triage and Their Colour Codes

Red: Life-threatening injuries requiring immediate medical or surgical intervention. Good chances of recovery with minimum resources and staff.

Yellow: Requires intermediate intervention within two to four hours, where such delay may not change the outcome.

Green: Minor injuries requiring medical or surgical intervention; however, this can safely be delayed.

Blue: Injuries requiring extensive treatment, and in a resource-limited setting, efforts are considered futile.

Black: Label given to dead. Resuscitation will not be provided. Prevents unnecessary expenditure of resources and time.

Triage in the emergency department (ED) requires an emergency physician/nurse or any other healthcare worker. The idea is to provide the best care for each individual.

- Specialist triage or tertiary triage

Specialists do tertiary triage after initial resuscitation and stabilization in the emergency department by an emergency physician. The idea is to assess the need of special care like surgery, intensive care unit admission, specialist medical care and area allocation accordingly to decrease the burden on the ED.

Emergency Department Triage

Trauma triage/ED triage is done using various trauma assessment tools, which are mainly based on the ABCDE resuscitation system: A, airway; B, breathing; C, circulation; and D, disability/neurological status assessment. This is followed by E, a complete exposure of the patient (undressing the patient) for assessment of secondary injuries.

Different hospitals use different triage systems, including the Emergency Severity Index (ESI), Canadian Triage and Acuity Scale (CTAS), Manchester Triage System (MTS), and Australasian Triage Scale (ATS). These are five-level triage systems with five different categories. Patients are colour coded red, yellow, green, blue or black, in decreasing order of severity of injury (Table 1.2).

Priority is given to the most saveable patient with the most urgent conditions. In India it is difficult to use any of the aforementioned internationally accepted five-tier complex algorithm-based triage systems because of India's large population, limited trained emergency physicians and unavailability of trained personnel for triage. Patients in the ED triage area in our centre are triaged into traffic-colour-coded categories: red, yellow and green (Table 1.3).

Once triage is done, a colour-coded tag/band/card is attached to the patient. Documentation is important with date and time of triage, chief presenting complaint, brief history, initial assessment, initial triage category allocated, and any diagnostic or treatment measures initiated. Re-triage is important if the patient's condition changes while waiting for treatment.

The three-tier triage system for ED triage in our centre is in line with the in-hospital AIIMS Triage Protocol (ATP), which has been used and validated in previous studies and has been reported to reduce over-triage and under-triage.

Comparing all the existing international triage systems with the AIIMS Triage Protocol,

Table 1.3: Three-Tier Triage in India

Red	Yellow	Green
Patients who need immediate care defined by the presence of any altered physiological parameters, any time-sensitive conditions or conditions with increased urgency.	Those who have no red criteria but have semi-urgent conditions needing admission for monitoring, evaluation and treatment.	Patients are given minor treatment and discharged.

Table 1.4: Comparison of Triage Systems

ESI 1 ESI 2	CTAS I CTAS II CTAS III	MTS 1 MTS 2	ATS 1 ATS 2 ATS 3	Red
ESI 3 ESI 4	CTAS IV	MTS 3	ATS 4	Yellow
ESI 5	CTAS V	MTS 4	ATS 5	Green

Emergency Severity Index (ESI), Canadian Triage and Acuity Scale (CTAS), Manchester Triage System (MTS) and Australasian Triage Scale (ATS).

we found that the ESI 1 and 2; CTAS I, II and III; MTS 1 and 2; and ATS 1, 2 and 3 partially match with the red category.

The yellow cadre of ATP is somewhat similar to ESI 3 and 4, CTAS IV, MTS 3 and ATS 4.

The ATP green category matches with MTS 4 and category 5 of all systems (Table 1.4).

PITFALLS OF ED TRIAGE

- Failure to recognize and acknowledge high-risk chief complaints like chest pain, abdominal pain or severe headache.
- Failure to observe vital signs. Each patient's temperature must be taken and repeated if it does not match the clinical condition; respiratory rates must be carefully counted.
- Failure to document the triage observations. Appropriate documentation is an important part of the medical record. These records must be available for review by the physician who later sees the patient.
- Failure to re-triage.

CONCLUSION

For greatest good to the greatest number of people in a disaster, an organized and clear triage system must be in place to properly prioritize treatment and management. The system must be recognized by the parties involved and simple enough to provide vital information when limited time and resources are available. Key to performing triage in a disaster setting is performing mock drills at regular intervals.

SUGGESTED READING

1. Colohan AR, Alves WM, Gross CR, et al. Head injury mortality in two centres with different emergency medical services and intensive care. *J Neurosurg.* 1989;71:202–7. doi: 10.3171/jns.1989.71.2.0202.
2. Florance B, Das Adhikari D, David SS. Comparative study of the practice of first aid and effectiveness of pre-hospital care over a period of 10 years in trauma patients admitted to the emergency department. *Natl J Emerg Med.* 2015;3:117–20.
3. Fitzgerald M, Dewan Y, O'Reilly G, Mathew J, McKenna C. India and the management of road crashes: towards a national trauma system. *Indian J Surg.* 2006; 68:226–32.
4. Shrivastava SR, Pandian P, Shrivastava PS. Pre-hospital care among victims of road traffic accident in a rural area of Tamil Nadu: a cross-sectional descriptive study. *J Neurosci Rural Pract.* 2014 Nov;5(Suppl 1):S33–8. doi: 10.4103/0976-3147.145198. PMID: 25540536; PMCID: PMC4271379.
5. Sharma M, Brandler ES. Emergency medical services in India: the present and future. *Prehosp Disaster Med.* 2014;29:307–10. doi: 10.1017/S1049023X14000296. Epub 2014 Apr 10. PMID: 24721137.

6. Sahu AK, Bhoi S, Galwankar S, et al. All India Institute of Medical Sciences triage protocol (ATP): ATP of a busy emergency department. *J Emerg Trauma Shock*. 2020;13:107–9. doi: 10.4103/JETS.JETS_137_19.
7. Kumar R, Bhoi S, Chauhan S, et al. (A264) Does the implementation of START triage criteria in the emergency department reduce over-and under-triage of patients? *Prehosp Disaster Med*. 2011;26:72–3. doi: 10.1017/S1049023X11002482.

2 Primary and Secondary Surveys

Sharad Prabhakar

LEARNING OBJECTIVES

- Steps of the primary and secondary surveys
- Identify life-threatening injuries
- Adjuncts of the primary and secondary survey

PRIMARY SURVEY WITH CONCOMITANT RESUSCITATION

The primary survey involves assessment of life-threatening conditions in trauma care by adhering to the following sequence (ABCDE):

- Airway maintenance with cervical spine control/immobilization
- Breathing and ventilation
- Circulation (identification and control of haemorrhage)
- Disability (assessment of neurologic status)
- Exposure/environmental control

The aim of the primary survey is to identify life-threatening conditions and treat them in a prioritized sequence, because initially it may not be possible to identify specific anatomic injuries.

In a clinical scenario, a trauma clinician can quickly assess ABC and D (10-second assessment) by asking the patient his or her name and asking what happened. An appropriate response by the patient suggests the following:

- The ability of the patient to speak clearly implies no major airway compromise.
- The ability to generate air movement for speech indicates breathing is not severely compromised.
- If the patient is alert enough to describe what happened, this indicates the level of consciousness is not markedly decreased.

Airway Maintenance with Cervical Spine Control/Immobilization

Upon initial evaluation of a trauma patient, the airway is secured first.

- Look for foreign bodies obstructing the airway. Be wary of facial, mandibular, tracheal or laryngeal fractures which can result in airway obstruction. Suction to clear blood and secretions. Secure the neck in a hard cervical collar. Assume that a cervical spine injury exists unless proven otherwise.
- Establish a definitive airway if there is any doubt about the patient's ability to maintain airway patency. This is especially true for patients with head trauma and a Glasgow Coma Scale (GCS) of 8 or lower; initially the jaw-thrust or chin-lift manoeuvre is carried out. If the patient is unconscious or has no gag reflex, an oropharyngeal airway may be temporarily placed, as arrangements are being made to intubate the patient. While intubating, the cervical collar is opened and a team member manually restricts cervical spine motion.
- Frequently re-evaluate airway patency. Progressive airway loss may occur in a deteriorating patient.
- Establish an airway surgically if intubation is contraindicated or cannot be carried out.

Breathing and Ventilation

Ventilation or adequate gas exchange requires adequate function of the lungs, chest wall and diaphragm.

- The aim is to identify life-threatening injuries like tension pneumothorax, massive haemothorax, open pneumothorax, and tracheal or bronchial injuries.
- Expose the patient's neck and chest. Assess the tracheal position, jugular venous distension and chest wall movement. Auscultate to ensure both sides are being ventilated. Percussion may be difficult in a restless, noisy patient.
- Every trauma patient requires supplemental oxygen. Always monitor oxygen saturation.
- Intubation followed by positive pressure ventilation may convert a simple pneumothorax to a tension pneumothorax. Ensure the chest tube is placed before positive pressure ventilation.

Circulation (Haemorrhage Control)

- Haemorrhage is an important cause of preventable death after injury. Once tension pneumothorax has been excluded as a cause

DOI: 10.1201/9781003291619-3

for ongoing shock, assume that hypotension is due to blood loss.

- Impaired circulating blood volume may also be suspected in a patient with an altered level of consciousness (possible decreased cerebral perfusion), ashen grey facial skin with pale extremities and a rapid thready pulse.
- Vascular access with two large-bore peripheral venous cannulas is established, and blood samples for baseline tests and cross match are obtained, including a pregnancy test for all females of childbearing age. Other tests include blood gases and lactate levels. Consider a cut down or central line in case peripheral access is not available.
- Identify and control external sources of haemorrhage. Judicious use of a tourniquet may be required. A surgeon's help to identify and clamp bleeding vessels may be needed. Blind clamping can cause further damage.
- Major areas of internal haemorrhage, especially the chest, abdomen, retroperitoneum, pelvis and long bones, may be identified by appropriate examination and imaging [e.g. chest X-ray, pelvic X-ray, diagnostic peritoneal lavage (DPL) or focused assessment with sonography for trauma (FAST)]. Early intervention in the form of pelvic binders or clamps, or extremity splints helps limit internal haemorrhage.
- Definitive haemorrhage control is essential along with appropriate replacement of intravascular volume. Aggressive volume resuscitation is not a substitute for haemorrhage control. Use warm crystalloids to initiate fluid resuscitation (98.6°F to 104°F).
- Be aware of coagulopathy in severely injured trauma patients. Tranexamic acid administration can be considered within 3 hours of injury.

Disability (Neurologic Evaluation)

The aim of a neurologic examination is to establish the patient's level of consciousness, determine pupillary size and reaction, identify lateralizing signs and to look for a spinal cord injury level.

- The GCS score is the go-to score for objectively monitoring patient consciousness.
- Be wary of drug and alcohol intoxication. Consult a neurosurgeon once brain injury is identified.

Exposure and Environmental Control

- Be wary of hypothermia as a potentially lethal complication. After initial assessment, keep the patient covered with warm blankets, administer warm saline and keep patient warmers on.

Adjuncts

- Physiological parameters including pulse rate, blood pressure, pulse pressure, body temperature, ABG levels and urinary output are assessed to ensure adequacy of resuscitation.
- Periodic re-evaluation is required in a dynamically worsening patient.

SECONDARY SURVEY

- Begins only after the primary survey is completed, patient resuscitation is underway and improvement in the patient's vitals has been demonstrated.
- Must not interfere with the primary survey.
- It involves a detailed head-to-toe evaluation of the trauma patient, with each region of the body being examined.
- A complete history should be taken, with emphasis on allergies, medications, past illness or pregnancy, last meal and events/environment related to the injury.
- Assessment of mechanism of trauma as blunt trauma, penetrating or thermal trauma to determine injury patterns to vital structures.
- Sequential physical examination from head to toe, including maxillofacial injuries, cervical spine and neck, chest, abdomen and pelvis, perineum/rectum/vagina, musculoskeletal system, and neurological symptoms are evaluated. Do not forget to turn the patient over to assess the spine and back.
- Be wary of common pitfalls; for example, facial oedema in patients with massive facial injury precludes a complete eye examination, or compartment syndrome can develop in long bone fractures with rapidly evolving swelling.
- Adjuncts to the secondary survey include radiological investigations like X-rays, CT scans and ultrasound. No unstable patient is to be shifted for a CT scan or X-rays unless accompanied by a clinician.

- Adequate record-keeping and legal considerations. It is important to accurately document the patient's condition and resuscitative procedures performed to avoid legal challenges later.
- Teamwork with a team leader is the established way of managing trauma patients.

SUMMARY

The sequence of treatment of a polytrauma patient thus runs as follows:

- Triage
- Primary survey with resuscitation
- Adjuncts to the primary survey and resuscitation
- Secondary survey
- Adjuncts to the secondary survey
- Re-evaluation
- Definitive care

CONCLUSION

The steps of the primary and secondary surveys underline a methodical life-saving approach in a trauma scenario, combining optimization with continued intervention so as not to miss life-threatening injuries.

SUGGESTED READING

1. Sasser SM, Hunt RC, Faul M, et al. Guidelines for field triage of injured patients: recommendations of the national expert panel on field triage, 2011. *MMWR Recomm Rep.* 2012;61(RR-1):1–20.

2. Teixeira PG, Inaba K, Hadjizacharia P, et al. Preventable or potentially preventable mortality at a mature trauma center. *J Trauma.* 2007;63:1338.

3. Neugebauer EAM, Waydhas C, Lendemans S, et al. Clinical practice guideline: the treatment of patients with severe and multiple traumatic injuries. *Dtsch Arztebl Int.* 2012;109:102–8.

4. Leeper WR, Leepr TJ, Yogt K, et al. The role of trauma team leaders in missed injuries: does specialty matter? *J Trauma.* 2013;75:387–90.

5. American College of Surgeons. Committee on Trauma. *Advanced Trauma Life Support: Student Course Manual.* Ninth Edition. Chicago, IL: American College of Surgeons; 2018.

3 Clearing the Cervical Spine

Apinderpreet Singh, Rajesh Chhabra and Pravin Salunke

LEARNING OBJECTIVES

- Understand spinal stability and its biomechanics
- Know the mechanism of cervical spine injury (CSI) and classify the extent of injury as per neurological status
- Define the high-risk and low-risk patients for harbouring CSI
- Choosing the right investigation tool for timely diagnosis of CSI
- Learn difference in adult and paediatric C-Spine injuries

INTRODUCTION

The incidence of cervical spine injury (CSI) in polytrauma patients is 3.7%. While it can be seen in approximately 3% of conscious patients, the incidence rises to 8% in comatose and unconscious ones. Henceforth, early identification and management of cervical spine injuries in the ER is very important. A fixed protocol and clearance protocol needs to be established for defining patients as high risk and low risk for harbouring CSI. This protocol will not only help in triaging and ensuring appropriate management of patients with CSI, but will also identify patients who can be cleared, thus preventing prolonged C-Spine immobilization, related complications, unnecessary investigations and radiation exposure. Therefore, C-Spine clearance attains an important role in decreasing the morbidity and mortality associated with cervical spine injury as well as improving health-related quality of life (HRQoL).

Acute spinal cord injury in children, on the other hand, is sometimes overlooked and missed due to many confounding factors. The difference in the anatomy and biomechanics of the spine makes diagnosis difficult and challenging. In the scenario of multiple injuries, non-cooperation for clinical examination and synchondroses confusing as fractures, the question of whether the child has a spine injury becomes important. To alleviate the confusion, various studies have attempted to formulate guidelines for spine injury diagnosis and management.

Before we discuss the diagnostic dilemmas of cervical spine injury, we should be well versed with the contributing factors for spinal stability as well as the anatomical and physiological difference in the spinal framework of adults and children.

SPINAL STABILITY

Spinal stability may be defined as the ability of the spine to resist displacement of vertebral structures under physiological conditions, so as to prevent damage or irritation to neural structures, as well as to prevent incapacitating deformity or pain. Spinal stability is achieved with the contribution of three systems:

(1) Vertebrae providing the bony frame

(2) Apophyseal joints, intervertebral discs and ligaments contributing to the dynamics

(3) Muscles under the control of neural elements

Disruption of any of these systems individually or in combination leads to spinal instability.

Spinal Framework in Children: How It Is Different from Adults

The paediatric cervical spine differs from adults anatomically as well as radiologically. As a child grows older, the spine undergoes significant changes in structure and physiology. Because of these developmental variations, the changes have been divided into three broad categories according to the age:

1) 0–2 years of age – This age group of patients differs significantly from adults. The head size is larger with a higher head:body ratio, the supporting ligaments are elastic, neck muscles are weak, vertebrae and the end plates are non-ossified and are wedge shaped, epiphysis is present, and the intervertebral disc space is larger. In this age group, the C2–3 facet joints are more horizontally located, giving the appearance of C2–3 dislocation, which is actually nothing but a physiological variation.

2) 2–10 years of age – As a child grows older, the spine and supporting framework tend to approach the adult form. The head:body ratio starts normalising, the supporting ligaments becomes less elastic, neck muscles become stronger, vertebrae are more calcified and facets are stronger. The vertebral bodies (though more calcified) are still wedge shaped, the intervertebral disc space is still wider than the adult counterpart, and epiphysis is still not fused.

 DOI: 10.1201/9781003291619-4

3) 10–16 years of age – The spine at this age almost matches those of adults. The head:body ratio normalises, ligament elasticity is less than adults, the vertebral body height is almost as adults, and the epiphysis is fused.

CLINICAL FEATURES SUGGESTING CSI

Neck pain is usually the most common presenting symptom of CSI. Other important features which should alarm the attending physician of the suspicion of CSI are motor and sensory loss, torticollis, respiratory depression with reversed respiratory pattern, unexplained hypotension and bradycardia (spinal shock), and sometimes altered mental status (because of hypotension and hypoxia). The American Spinal Injury Association has developed a grading system, named ASIA grading, to quantify the extent of neurological injury:

- Grade A – Complete paralysis with no sensory or motor function.
- Grade B – Sensory incomplete. Only sensory function is present, but no motor function is preserved more than three levels below the motor level on either side of the body.
- Grade C – Motor incomplete. Motor function has some preservation of function more than three levels below the ipsilateral motor level. Less than half of key muscle functions below the neurological level have a muscle grade ≥3.
- Grade D – Motor incomplete. At least half of key muscle functions below the neurological level have a muscle grade ≥3.
- Grade E – Normal. Motor and sensory functions are preserved.

SPINE INJURY SYNDROMES IN INCOMPLETE SPINAL CORD INJURY

A complete injury is defined as one with complete motor and sensory loss below the neurological level of injury. Any partial preservation of sensory or motor functions below the level of injury is called incomplete SCI. Traditionally incomplete SCI have been classified into seven categories: central cord syndrome, Brown Séquard syndrome, anterior cord syndrome, conus medullaris syndrome, cauda equina syndrome, posterior cord syndrome and mixed syndrome. The three most common are:

Central cord syndrome – This particular form of injury occurs almost exclusively in the cervical spine region and more commonly in old age groups where the canal diameter is compromised due to degenerative changes already present. Even a trivial trauma can cause central cord syndrome in such cases. There is greater weakness in the upper limbs than in the lower limbs with sacral sparing. This is because the corticospinal tracts are lying medial to lateral as we go downwards from the cervical region. The sacral fibres lie most lateral, hence causing sacral sparing.

Brown-Séquard syndrome – Classically called the hemisection of cord, it is seen in sharp injuries. There will be relatively greater ipsilateral posterior column and motor loss, associated with contralateral loss of sensitivity to pain and temperature.

Anterior cord syndrome – This type of lesion involves the anterior horn cells. Vascular insult is one common cause, producing variable loss of motor function and of sensitivity to pain and temperature while preserving proprioception.

WHEN TO SUSPECT CSI

The cervical spine injury in presence of obvious findings should instigate the treating team for further investigations and management. However, the chances of missing a CSI are high in doubtful cases. It is advisable to keep a high index of suspicion so as to not miss any significant injury; but a set-criteria needs to be framed too, to avoid unnecessary investigations. For the adult population, certain tools have been developed to define high and low risk patients for CSI. The National Emergency X-Radiography Utilization Study (NEXUS) and Canadian C-Spine Rule (CCR) are the two tools most commonly used primarily for determining when radiography should be utilized in patients with suspected C-Spine injury. These criteria have been followed for pediatric population too by some centres. Taking both the tools into consideration, the following recommendations can be drawn:

Patients at High Risk for CSI

The following group of patients should always be suspected of a CSI requiring further investigations: a dangerous trauma mechanism like a fall from a height of >3 feet or 5 stairs; a high-speed motor vehicular collision (>100 km/h); an accident with sudden acceleration and deceleration or rollover; accidents involving axial loading like falling heavy objects or diving from a height; the presence of tingling, numbness or any neurological deficit; the presence of other significant injury suggesting dangerous trauma.

Patients at Low Risk for CSI

NEXUS Criteria

Patients who are conscious and alert without any evidence of intoxication, with no focal neurological deficits, with absence of any painful distracting injuries, or demonstrating no posterior midline cervical tenderness are at low risk of sustaining a CSI, and unnecessary radiology for cervical spine screening can be avoided. While all the low-risk clinical features are easily identifiable by focused history and examination, a painful distracting injury needs further elaboration. It may be defined as the presence of any significant pain elsewhere in the body which might render the patient to ignore his neck pain. Long bone fractures, degloving injuries, crush injuries, chest and abdominal injuries and burns are a few examples. In adults it might be easier to classify such entities, but in children the differentiation might not be simple, as the injury need not to be significant enough to cause distraction from cervical pain because their response is variable to even minor painful stimuli. The clinician needs to be extra cautious while examining children.

Canadian C-Spine Rule (CCR)

As per the CCR guidelines, any patient who has a simple rear-end motor vehicular accident, is either sitting or ambulatory, doesn't have a midline cervical tenderness, has delayed onset neck pain, and is able to actively rotate his neck to 45° to either side is a low-risk candidate for CSI and doesn't need further radiological investigation. In patients meeting low-risk criteria, the cervical collar can be removed and patients can be followed clinically. They should be further investigated only if any new symptoms indicative of CSI are noticed.

A flow chart for management of CSI as per NEXUS Criteria and the Canadian C-Spine Rule is shown in Figure 3.1.

CERVICAL SPINAL INJURY IN CHILDREN

Blunt trauma is usually the major cause of CSI in children. Though motor vehicular accidents and falls remain the most common cause of CSI

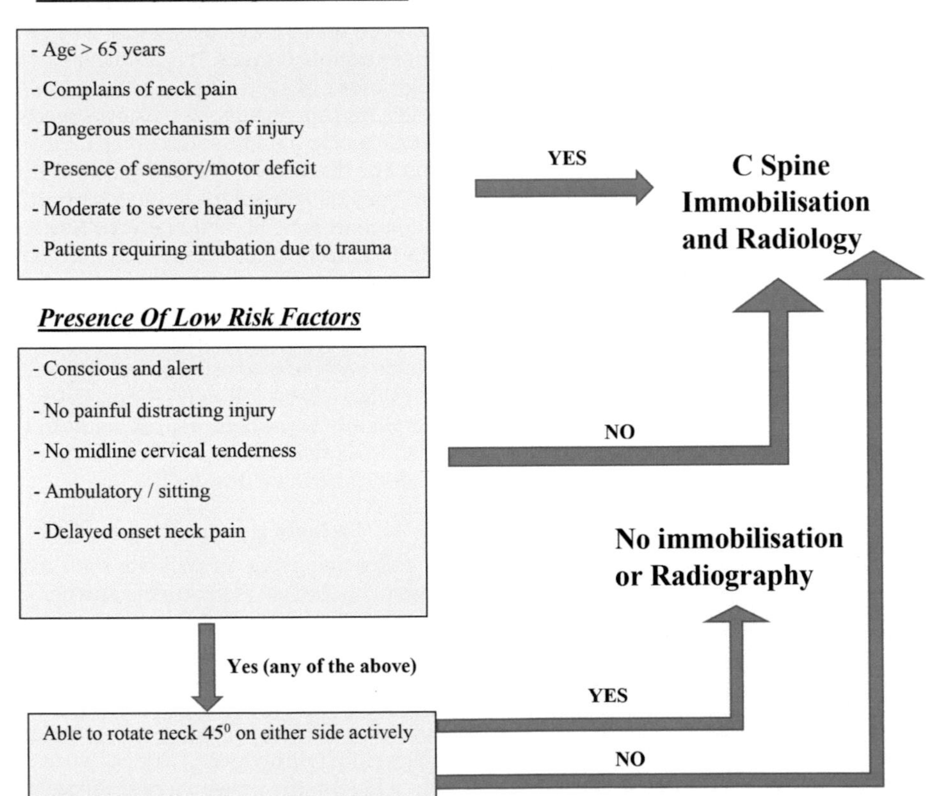

Figure 3.1 Flow chart for management of cervical spine injury as per NEXUS Criteria and the Canadian C-Spine Rule

in children, in younger children, inflicted injuries and pedestrian injuries contribute majorly, while in older children, recreational and sports activities are the predominant contributors. Because of the unique anatomical variation, younger children tend to have upper cervical spine injuries (C1–C2), while the older ones tend to sustain sub-axial cervical spine injuries (C3–C7), just like adults.

IDEAL RADIOLOGICAL INVESTIGATIONS

X-ray

Plain radiograph of the cervical spine in lateral and anteroposterior view always remains the first-line investigation. An additional open mouth odontoid (OMO) view can also be obtained for adults and children above 9 years of age. OMO view provides no further information for younger children and can be avoided. The clinician should be cautious so as to not confuse fractures with synchondroses, particularly in younger age groups.

CT Scan

Several authorities have defined criteria for performing a CT scan in addition to the X-ray of C-Spine, including any patient with moderate to severe head injury; any patient requiring intubation because of trauma; a patient with neurological deficits; evidence of fractures on X-ray; where X-ray is non-contributory or technically difficult to perform; strong suspicion of CSI in spite of normal X-ray.

MRI

An MRI is not recommended as a first-line investigation in case of CSI. Equivocal plain radiography and CT scan, with suspicion of neurological or ligament injury, without evidence of any bony injury [previously grouped under SCIWORA (spinal cord injury without radiographic abnormality)] are a few indications for getting an MRI done.

CONCLUSION

Cervical spine injury is a serious entity which might cause permanent neurological deficits, severe morbidity and even death. Prompt diagnosis and management henceforth become important. Children, in particular, pose a significant diagnostic challenge for the reasons discussed. In a tertiary care and high-volume centre, focused history and examination and triaging the patients into high-risk and low-risk groups will help clinicians to avoid unnecessary investigations and will decrease the chances of missing a cervical spine injury particularly in equivocal conditions.

SUGGESTED READING

1. White AA, 3rd, Johnson RM, Panjabi MM, Southwick WO. Biomechanical analysis of clinical stability in the cervical spine. *Clin Orthop Relat Res*. 1975;109:85–96.
2. Panjabi MM. The stabilizing system of the spine. Part 1. Function, dysfunction, adaptation and enhancement. *J Spin Disord Tech*. 1992;5:383–9.
3. Hoffman JR, Wolfson AB, Todd K, Mower WR. Selective cervical spine radiography in blunt trauma: methodology of the National Emergency X-Radiography Utilization Study (NEXUS). *Ann Emerg Med*. 1998;32:461–9.
4. Stiell IG, Wells GA, Vandemheen KL, et al. The Canadian C-Spine rule for radiography in alert and stable trauma patients. *JAMA*. 2001;286:1841–8.
5. Slaar A, Fockens MM, Wang J, et al. Triage tools for detecting cervical spine injury in pediatric trauma patients. *Cochrane Database Syst Rev*. 2017;12.:CD011686. doi:10.1002/14651858.CD011686.pub2.
6. Rozzelle CJ, Aarabi B, Dhall SS, et al. Management of pediatric cervical spine and spinal cord injuries. *Neurosurgery*. 2013;72(Suppl 2):205–26.
7. Parent S, Mac-Thiong JM, Roy-Beaudry M, et al. Spinal cord injury in the pediatric population: a systematic review of the literature. *J Neurotrauma*. 2011;28:1515–24.
8. Chung S, Mikrogianakis A, Wales PW, et al. Trauma association of Canada pediatric subcommittee national pediatric cervical spine evaluation pathway: consensus guidelines. *J Trauma*. 2011;70:873–84.
9. National Institute for Health and Care Excellence. Triage, assessment, investigation and early management of head injury in children, young people and adults. www.nice.org.uk/Guidance/CG176/Evidence 2011 (accessed 5th November 2017).
10. Schuld C, Franz S, Bruggemann K, et al. International standards for neurological classification of spinal cord injury: Impact of the revised worksheet on classification performance. *J Spinal Cord Med*. 2016;39(5):504–12.

11. Garg B, Ahuja K. C-Spine clearance in poly-trauma patients: a narrative review. *J Clin Orthop Trauma*. 2021;12(1):66–71, ISSN 0976-5662. doi:10.1016/j.jcot.2020.10.020.

12. Maynard FM Jr, Bracken MB, Creasey G, et al. International standards for neurological and functional classification of spinal cord injury. American Spinal Injury Association. *Spinal Cord*. 1997;35:266–74. doi:10.1038/sj.sc.3100432.

4 Oxygen Therapy in Trauma

Shyam Charan Meena, Rajeev Chauhan and Ankur Luthra

LEARNING OBJECTIVES

- To assist healthcare providers in recognizing the best way to use oxygen while taking care of trauma triage emergencies
- To promote evidence-based oxygen therapy in trauma and acute care settings
- To raise awareness of the importance of oxygen, because too little or too much oxygen is dangerous
- To promote oxygen-saving strategies for optimum utilization of oxygen
- To know when to escalate and when to de-escalate oxygen therapy

INTRODUCTION

Trauma is considered as the number one killer of adult patients in developing countries, including India, and the cost of managing trauma is a major economic burden. The initial treatment of trauma patients is essential for the further course and should be based on guidelines. But the available literature in this area is very scanty because the research in these situations is difficult due to various limitations.

Oxygen is a frequently used medication in preclinical, trauma and emergency settings. Oxygen is cheap and easy to manage, without much risk for injury, especially when used for short periods. In the Advanced Trauma Life Support (ATLS) guidelines and pre-hospital trauma support guidelines, supplemental oxygen therapy is recommended internationally. This often leads to a notion of "predetermined" administration of oxygen even without any indication. However, the additional oxygen supply to patients carries the risk of hyperoxaemia, which can lead to damage to the lungs, and increased morbidity and mortality in both patients of acute illness (stroke, myocardial infarction, cardiac arrest) as well as surgical patients.

WHY DO WE NEED "EMERGENCY OXYGEN THERAPY GUIDELINES"?

- Thirty-four per cent of patients transported in ambulance and 15%–17% of hospitalized patients receive oxygen. Until 2008, there were no recommendations for the safe use of oxygen in emergency and trauma settings.
- It is believed that in the absence of hypoxaemia, supplemental oxygen will reduce shortness of breath. There is no evidence that oxygen is beneficial for patients with normoxia (normal arterial oxygen concentration) or very mild hypoxaemia. In addition to cardiovascular disease, there are many causes for shortness of breath, including anxiety, pain and metabolic acidosis. In these cases, oxygen therapy is not always required.
- The risk of hyperoxaemia is now widely recognized.
- Hyperoxaemia can narrow the coronary arteries due to vasoconstriction. Paradoxically, excessive oxygen supplementation during an acute heart attack can impair the oxygen supply to the heart muscle. The high-flow oxygen use leads to reperfusion injury, increase in size of infarct and mortality due to myocardial infarction.
- Hyperoxaemia has a similar effect on cerebral blood flow. A randomized controlled study showed that oxygen management in mild to moderate strokes is associated with increased mortality as compared to air.
- Critical care studies have shown that hyperoxaemia is associated with worse outcomes than normoxaemia in cardiac arrest survivors and in intensive care patients.
- Inadequate oxygen supply in patients at high risk for type 2 respiratory failure can lead to life-threatening hypercapnia (high arterial carbon dioxide), respiratory acidosis, organ dysfunction, coma and death.
- In 2010, the UK National Patient Safety Agency noted nine deaths which were directly related to improper oxygen treatment. Among them four patients died directly because of oxygen overload.
- Oxygen is a used as a medicine, but it is not correctly prescribed. Most hospitals do not conduct an oxygen audit and other safe oxygen treatment strategies.

In 2008, the British Thoracic Society issued the first official guidelines for emergency oxygen use. Table 4.1 enumerates the recommendations suggested as per existing guidelines for oxygen use in emergency, trauma and acute care settings.

DOI: 10.1201/9781003291619-5

As we have recently faced an oxygen crisis during the COVID-19 pandemic, it is wise to implement the oxygen-saving strategies (Table 4.2) in all hospital areas.

OXYGEN DELIVERY SYSTEMS

The selection of oxygen delivery devices depends upon:

1. Oxygen concentration required by the patient
2. Maximum oxygen concentration achieved by the delivery devices
3. Accuracy of the delivery devices
4. Patient comfort and mobility

Table 4.3 shows the approximate concentration of oxygen and required flow rates of commonly available oxygen delivery devices in trauma and acute care settings.

ESCALATION OF OXYGEN THERAPY

If SpO_2 <94%, then supplement O_2 via nasal prongs at 2–5 L/min or via a Venturi mask at 2–15 L/min. Then check for the SpO_2 and respiratory rate (continue same oxygen therapy if SpO_2 ≥94%; RR <30). A non-rebreather mask (NRM @ 10–15 L/min) should be commenced if SpO_2 <94%; RR >30.

DE-ESCALATION OF OXYGEN THERAPY

This is equally important (as much as escalation of oxygen therapy).

Step 1: If the patient is on NRM @ 15 L/min and has SpO_2 ≥94%, then reduce the flows to 12 L/min, then 10 L/min, then 8 L/min, then 6 L/min.

Table 4.1: Recommendations for Oxygen Use in Emergency, Trauma and Acute Care Settings

1. Oxygen is a medicine that must be prescribed and monitored by trained personnel.
2. Oxygen is the method to treat hypoxaemia only.
3. The majority of trauma victims have difficulty breathing and don't have hypoxaemia. Instead of prolonged oxygen therapy, they must be treated with adequate analgesia, appropriate monitoring and effective resuscitation in terms of intravenous warm fluids including blood components.
4. Oxygen is an important part of resuscitation and stabilization of critically injured patients. But once stabilized, the inspiratory concentration and flow rate of the oxygen must be titrated.
5. For all patients with acute symptoms who are not at risk of type 2 respiratory failure (T2RF), the recommended saturation range is 94%–98%.
6. For patients at risk of T2RF, the recommended saturation range is 88%–92%.
7. If the patient has an oxygen alert card due to previous T2RF, the desired oxygen range must be specified separately for the patient.
8. In critically injured trauma patients, treat the underlying aetiology instead of putting patients on high-flow oxygen therapy.
9. The oxygen audit should be conducted at regular time intervals in all hospital areas including emergency and trauma triage departments.
10. Oxygen-saving strategies should be followed in day-to-day practice.

Table 4.2: Oxygen-Saving Strategies

1. Early detection and repair of potential sources of oxygen leaks should be done on an urgent basis (e.g. breaks/cracks in flowmeters, pipelines, cylinders and humidification chambers).
2. Ensure adequate attachment of wall-mounted oxygen flowmeters.
3. For nebulization, air-driven nebulizers instead of oxygen-driven nebulization is preferred.
4. Make sure to switch off the oxygen flows when oxygen therapy is not being delivered.
5. Train all healthcare personnel working in trauma triage, ICU, operation theatres and recovery wards regarding the optimum use of oxygen and delivery devices.
6. Use of oxygen concentrators is preferred in mild cases.
7. Ensure adequate insertion of the oxygen delivery devices (e.g. nasal prongs, high-flow nasal cannula) inside the nostrils.
8. Ensure that the oxygen flow rate is in accordance with the FiO_2 requirement of the needy patient.
9. Deep-breathing exercises and chest physiotherapy along with adequate pain management should be practised, as these therapies help in rapid de-escalation of oxygen.
10. Counselling of patients and their attendants have their own role for optimally utilizing oxygen in trauma settings.

Table 4.3: Oxygen Delivery Devices

Oxygen Delivery Devices	Flow Rate Ranges	FiO_2	Way of Titration	Specific Comments
Nasal prongs	2–6 LPM	24%–40%	Should titrate according to flow rates	Best device for trauma victims who have adequate tidal volumes and normal breathing rate
Face mask	6–12 LPM	35%–60%	Should titrate according to flow rates	Ideally at least 6 LPM is required to prevent rebreathing of CO_2
Venturi mask	Fixed performance with appropriate adapter	Adapters of 24%, 28%, 31%, 35%, 40%, 60%	Can't titrate the flow rate, only FiO_2 can be titrated as per selected adapter	These adapters entrain a fixed amount of ambient air to deliver a fixed percentage of oxygen
Non-rebreather mask	10–15 LPM	60% to 91% can be effectively delivered	Can't titrate	Only advised for short duration or bridge therapy
High-flow nasal cannula (HFNC)	Up to 60 LPM	30%–100% FiO_2 can be provided	Both flow rate and FiO_2 can be titrated	Added PEEP is beneficial for the needy patients at high flow

LPM, litres per minute; FiO_2, fraction of inspired oxygen; CO_2, carbon dioxide; PEEP, positive end expiratory pressure.

Step 2: If the patient is maintaining $SpO_2 \geq 92\%$, then use Venturi mask at 10 L/min and reduce the flow rate gradually by 8 L/min, then 6 L/min, then 4 L/min, then 2 L/min.

Step 3: If the patient has $SpO_2 \geq 92\%$ and RR <25/min, then use nasal prongs at 2–5 L/min.

Step 4: If patient is maintaining $SpO_2 \geq 92\%$ and RR <25/min with nasal prongs at the lowest flow, then a room air trial should be given.

Hospitals typically rely on large liquid oxygen (LOX) supplies as their primary oxygen source. One litre of LOX provides approximately 860 L of gaseous oxygen, making this the most efficient system for oxygen storage and transportation. Alternate sources for oxygen in the hospital setting consist of compressed gas cylinders, usually of the E and H sizes. E-type cylinders are of smaller size and contain approximately 680 L of oxygen. Due to their relatively low volume of gas, these cylinders are typically used for transport of ventilated and non-ventilated patients and for very short periods to avoid disruption of the main LOX system. H-type cylinders are larger and heavier, contain approximately 6900 L of gas, require a wheeled cart for moving, and are used as the main backup for the LOX system in case of longer periods of disruption.

The appropriate selection of oxygen devices and delivery systems depends on the degree of hypoxaemia, existing evidence of the patient's underlying diagnosis and patient preference. The floor resident and other involved healthcare professionals should have a consolidated knowledge of all devices and systems so as to properly manage individualized patient-based plans for oxygen therapy.

The manifold department should have an exhaustive arrangement and long-term plan to resolve impending crises as seen during the COVID-19 pandemic. The manifold department should be able to readily provide answers to the following:

1. What if there is a sudden disruption in LOX conveyances?
2. How long will the present LOX supply last?
3. What amount of vaporous oxygen in chambers is accessible?
4. What size chambers are available, and how might they be circulated?
5. What should be done when there is a larger number of patients than oxygen outlets?
6. What is the refill plan?

These are amongst some of the significant inquiries that should be considered while making arrangements for encountering a calamity.

SUGGESTED READING

1. Kane B, Decalmer S, O'Driscoll B. Emergency oxygen therapy: from guideline to implementation. *Breathe*. 2013;9:246–53.

2. Taher A, Pilehvari Z, Poorolajal J, et al. Effects of normobaric hyperoxia in traumatic brain injury: a randomized controlled clinical trial. *Trauma Mon*. 2016;21: e26772.
3. Barzilay E, Lev A, Ibrahim M, et al. Traumatic respiratory insufficiency: comparison of conventional mechanical ventilation to high-frequency positive pressure with low-rate ventilation. *Crit Care Med*. 1987;15:118–21.
4. Eastwood G, Bellomo R, Bailey M, et al. Arterial oxygen tension and mortality in mechanically ventilated patients. *Intensive Care Med*. 2012;38:91–8.
5. Kilgannon JH, Jone AE, Shapiro NI, et al. Association between arterial hyperoxia following resuscitation from cardiac arrest and in-hospital mortality. *JAMA*. 2010;303:2165–71.
6. de Jonge E, Peelen L, Keijzers P, et al. Association between administered oxygen, arterial partial oxygen pressure and mortality in mechanically ventilated Intensive Care Unit patients. *Crit Care*. 2008;12:R156.

5 Early Analgesia on Arrival

Rashi Sarna and Nidhi Bhatia

LEARNING OBJECTIVES

- To classify trauma triage and familiarize with general clinical scenarios seen in secondary triage
- To do quick pain assessment and formulate an analgesia plan for the first 24 hours
- Pain monitoring standards and how to look for red-flag signs
- Role of regional analgesia in trauma triage

INTRODUCTION

Traumatic injuries are a global public health crisis and economic burden. India faces the highest cases of trauma with greater incidence of death due to road accidents compared to other nations worldwide. Evidence suggests that acute pain inflicted by trauma accounts for the highest percentage of severe pain in the emergency department (ED) as well as before hospitalization, and trauma subjects frequently feel moderate to severe pain more so when the injuries are multiple.

In addition to relieving suffering, early pain management carries advantages including reduction of the emotional (e.g. anxiety) and functional consequences of uncontrolled severe pain as well as reduced risk of infection and chronic pain development. This in turn optimizes patient satisfaction and recovery time. Although a vital component of emergency triage care, meagre standards of managing and assessing acute pain, especially in trauma situations, remains a matter of concern globally.

Two alternative approaches to analgesia can be equipotent, so it is important to act early rather than waiting for what is "assumed" to be the right resources and appropriate environment. Techniques in analgesia, especially regional analgesia and non-pharmacologic methods, can be beneficial, as they reduce the systemic delivery of agents which may have undue adverse effects. This chapter provides a brief overview of management of severe traumatic pain in an emergency triage setting. While it is not meant to be exhaustive, this chapter will provide an evidence-based assessment of concerns pertaining to this subject.

Management of Pain in ED Is Distinct

- The emergency medical field experiences severe pain predominantly.
- Patients present with highly emotional experiences of trauma, and this psychological aspect of pain must be considered while providing analgesia.
- Pain management often involves guardians who are undergoing equivalent stress as the patient himself.
- Unmanaged pain can itself complicate the hemodynamic continuum apart from the trauma itself. This increases the post-traumatic course of injury and hence needs as much attention as other components of trauma.

PATIENT CARE OBJECTIVES IN PAIN MANAGEMENT

- Individualized approach to assessment, planning and intervention for pain relief.
- Inclusive utilization of psycho-cognitive, non-pharmacological and pharmacological methods for analgesia.
- To render satisfactory pain relief to the subjects.
- Pain management is a combined effort from the trauma team which includes recognizing the status of pain in each subject at all times of review. Hence, it is important to train all professionals in healthcare in acquiring skills to management and assessment of pain successfully.

ETHICS OF PAIN CONTROL

- Pain must be addressed as a fifth vital sign.
- Treating "total" pain, including the emotional and cognitive aspects of pain.
- Pain is overall subjective and cannot be objectified. Hence, treating it requires empathy.
- Anticipate and treat pain pre-emptively rather than relieving pain.
- Let the patient understand and help the treating physician in controlling their own pain for personal satisfaction.
- Multimodal pain therapy is superior to individual therapies.
- Use a multidisciplinary approach in difficult cases.

DOI: 10.1201/9781003291619-6

COMPONENTS OF PAIN MANAGEMENT

- Grieving family and friends of the patient are also influencing factors in "total" pain management and must be counselled.
- Non-pharmacological methods include rendering an icepack, wheelchair, splints, sling, bandaging and dressing.
- Psychological counselling: An observant and empathetic attitude of paying attention and politely suggesting manoeuvres to cope with the pain using relaxation or distraction techniques.
- Reassurance: Consoling the patient and advising them to be brave and addressing their fears and concerns.
- Pharmacological: Titrated and individualized.

PAIN MANAGEMENT AREAS IN EMERGENCY

Triage

a. Primary triage
b. Secondary triage
   - Non-critical/green zone
   - Semi-critical/yellow zone
   - Critical/red zone
   - Observation ward
   - Procedural rooms

Different Phases of Emergency Medicine and Trauma Services (EMTS)

The patient is taken through various environments in the emergency department and transferred to and from while waiting for their turn to be seen by a doctor. Complete emergency care of the patient involves paramedics who are well trained for managing acute pain. For instance, in Australia a nurse is employed to implement the pain management. Hence the frontliners need to be well prepared on the management and assessment of pain so as to deliver suitable care.

Pain Supervision in Triage

All trauma subjects who come to ED should have their pain documented, diagnosed and given importance. This not only reduces morbidity and mortality but also helps the patient to forget the traumatic experience faster without any lasting distress. The British Association of Accident and Emergency Medicine (BAEM) in 2005, which provided strategies for managing pain in the ED, stated that analgesia should be rendered within 20 min of reaching triage in subjects with an acute pain score of 7–10. Those subjects with moderate pain, a pain score of 4–6, should be rendered with analgesia at triage.

Primary Triage

Primary triage is the initial triage rendered to all subjects who come to the ED. Pain assessment should start once the subject has arrived in front of the ED. A short history of pain should be recorded. At this time, the management of pain should be through non-pharmacological strategies like rendering trolleys or wheelchairs, walking sticks, or whatever is suitable to the patient. Ice packs, bandages, arm suspenders, cervical collars or immobilization must be rendered if necessary. Subjects must be rechecked thoroughly before they are sent to secondary triage.

Secondary Triage

This is the second phase of triage where patients are evaluated objectively and subjectively.

The purpose is to approve, to triage/prioritize, to grade and to manage pain. Again, a short history of pain is recorded to avoid any missing information. Objectively, all the vital signs, which includes pain scores like Numerical Rating Scale (NRS), visual analogue scale (VAS), Wong–Baker or FLACC scores for newborns, are recorded. The pain score must be registered in the pain comment chart. The emotive and intellectual facets of pain should be identified and managed (Figure 5.1).

Following secondary triaging, patients should be divided into green, yellow and red zones, depending on the severity of their pain and managed accordingly (Figure 5.2). Subjects with extreme or acute pain must be advanced to yellow and red zones correspondingly for modification of the analgesia strategy. The selection of analgesic should be based on the main assessment score and the World Health Organization (WHO) pain ladder. The WHO pain ladder, initially developed as a conceptual model to guide the management of cancer pain, is now accepted worldwide for the medical management of pain coupled with serious illness, including traumatic pain. Multimodal analgesia is critical for provision of adequate analgesia to the acutely injured patient; however, patient haemodynamics, respiratory and mental status must all affect the choice of pharmacologic interventions (Table 5.1).

With the advent of ultrasound, regional blocks have gained utmost importance for combating pain in the pre- as well as perioperative period. They decrease the need for sedatives and opioid

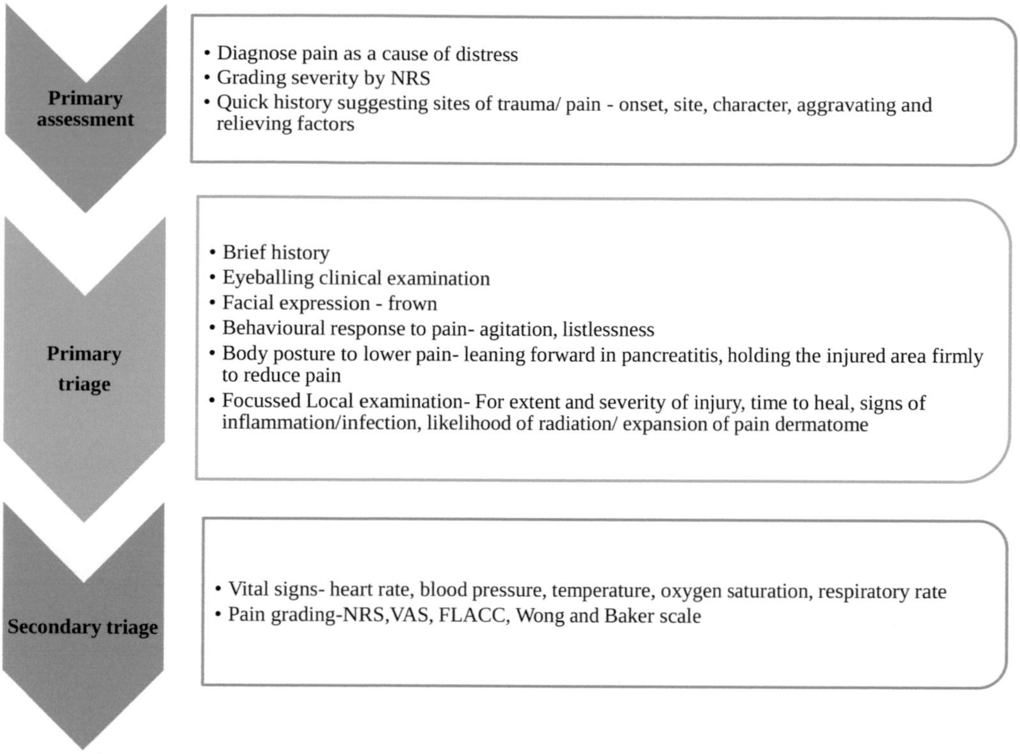

Primary assessment
• Diagnose pain as a cause of distress
• Grading severity by NRS
• Quick history suggesting sites of trauma/ pain - onset, site, character, aggravating and relieving factors
Primary triage
• Brief history
• Eyeballing clinical examination
• Facial expression - frown
• Behavioural response to pain- agitation, listlessness
• Body posture to lower pain- leaning forward in pancreatitis, holding the injured area firmly to reduce pain
• Focussed Local examination- For extent and severity of injury, time to heal, signs of inflammation/infection, likelihood of radiation/ expansion of pain dermatome
Secondary triage
• Vital signs- heart rate, blood pressure, temperature, oxygen saturation, respiratory rate
• Pain grading-NRS,VAS, FLACC, Wong and Baker scale

Figure 5.1 Pain supervision in triage

GREEN ZONE
NRS < 4 (Mild pain)
Oral PCM 1gm QID
or/and
NSAIDS /COX-2 inhibitor
YELLOW ZONE
NRS = 4-7(Moderate Pain)
Oral PCM 1gm QID
or/and
NSAIDS /COX-2 inhibitor
or/and
oral or iv tramadol 50-100mg TDS (weak opioid)
RED ZONE
NRS >7(Severe Pain)
Initiate IV Morphine at 0.1mg/kg
followed by
IV Morphine 5-10mg 4 hourly
Along with potent NSAIDS like ketorolac or diclofenac
Other drugs
IV Ketamine 0.5-1mg/kg boluses
If pain is still uncontrolled, refer to Emergency team or acute pain specialists (For PCA/Epidural / regional nerve blocks)

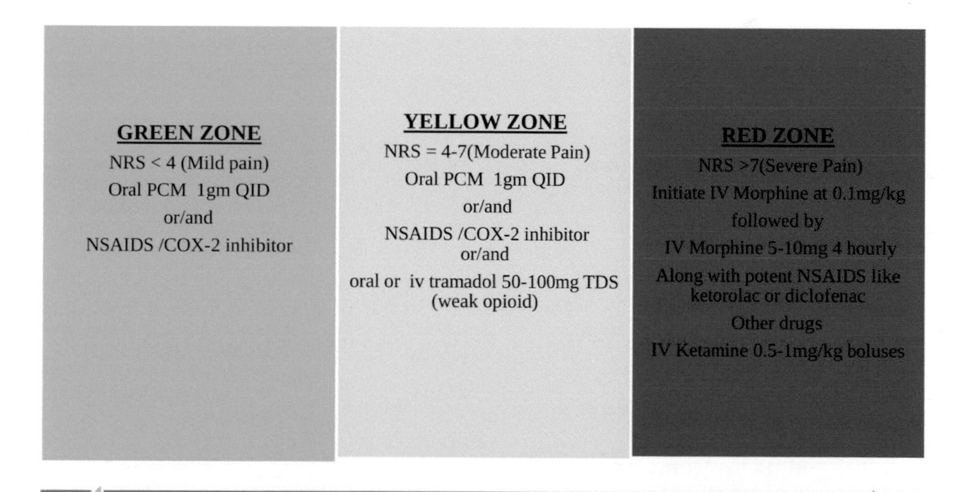

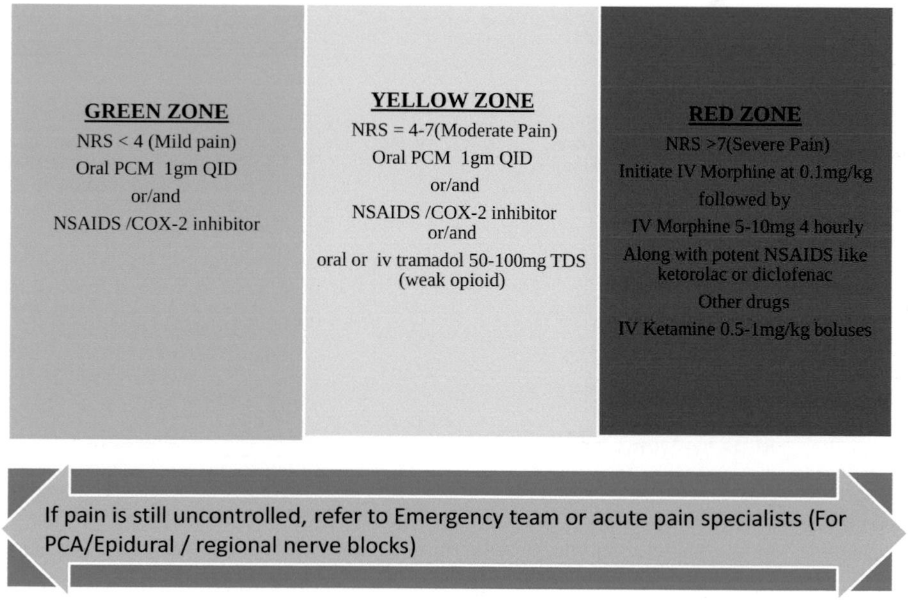

Figure 5.2 Patient division based on pain severity

Table 5.1: Pharmacological Analgesia in Trauma Patients

Drugs	Dosing	Route of Administration	Comments
Non-steroidal Anti-inflammatory Drugs			
Ibuprofen	400 mg 6 hrly (max 2400 mg/day)	PO	Contraindicated in • Gastrointestinal bleeding • Cardiac history Selective COX-2 NSAIDs reduce risk of major and upper GI bleeding
Ketorolac	10 mg 6 hrly for no more than 5 days	PO, IV	
Celecoxib	100 mg 12 hrly (400 mg/day)	PO	
Acetaminophen			
Paracetamol	15–20 mg/kg (max dose 4 g/day)	PO, PR, IV	To be used cautiously in liver disorders
Skeletal Muscle Relaxants			
Cyclobenzaprine	5 mg 8 hrly	PO	Have sedative effects; to be avoided in head injury patients
Methocarbamol	1 g 8 hrly	PO, IV	
Diazepam	2 mg 6 hrly (max dose 40 mg/day)	PO, IV	
Serotonin/Norepinephrine Reuptake Inhibitors			
Duloxetine	30–60 mg/day	PO	• Consider for neuropathic pain • Have sedative effect • Use cautiously in hepatic/renal dysfunction
Venlafaxine	225 mg/day	PO	
Anticonvulsants			
Pregabalin	150 mg BD (max 600 mg/day)	PO	• Consider for neuropathic pain • Have sedative effect • Use cautiously in elderly/renal dysfunction
Gabapentin	300 mg TDS	PO	
α2-Receptor Antagonists			
Clonidine	0.1 mg 8 hrly	PO	• Can cause hypotension and bradycardia • Sedative effect
Dexmedetomidine	1 mcg/kg bolus followed by 0.4–0.7 mcg/kg/hr	IV	
NMDA Antagonists			
Magnesium	30–50 mg/kg	IV	Contraindicated in myocardial damage
Ketamine	0.3 mg/kg bolus followed by 0.1 mg/kg/hr infusion	IV, IM	• Contraindicated in acute psychosis, cerebrovascular accident and cardiac decompensation • Dependence potential
Opioids			
Fentanyl	25–50 mcg every 30–60 min	IV	• Risk of addiction and opioid dependence • Watch for respiratory depression, delirium, constipation, nausea, vomiting
Morphine	IV: 2 mg 3 hrly	PO, IV	
Tramadol	50 mg 4 hrly (max dose 400 mg/day)	PO, IV	
Hydromorphone	PO: 2 mg 4 hrly IV: 0.4 mg 3 hrly	PO, IV	
Oxycodone	5 mg 4 hrly	PO	
Local Anaesthetics			
Lidocaine	5% patch for 24 hr 1.5 mg/kg IV bolus	Topical/IV	• Contraindicated in heart block • Watch for local anaesthetic toxicity

PO, per oral; IV, intravenous; IM, intramuscular; PR, per rectal.

Table 5.2: Regional Analgesia in Trauma Patients

Blocks	Indications	Patient Position	Comments
Thoracic/lumbar epidurals	Chest pain (rib fractures) Abdominal wall pain	Lateral/sitting	Contraindicated in hypovolemia, coagulopathy, septic patients, head/spine injury
Brachial plexus blocks (interscalene, supraclavicular, costoclavicular)	Shoulder dislocations, upper limb fractures, deformities	Supine	• Analgesia can be prolonged by placing catheters • Interscalene block can cause phrenic nerve palsy and Horner's syndrome
Femoral nerve block	Hip, femur, knee joint trauma	Supine	• Provides preoperative and postoperative analgesia • Less patient discomfort during positioning for spinal block
Fascia iliaca block	Hip/proximal femur fracture	Supine	• In comparison to femoral nerve block, provides more medial and lateral coverage • Provides preoperative and postoperative analgesia • Less patient discomfort during positioning for spinal block
Paravertebral blocks	• Chest or abdominal wall pain • Rib fractures	Sitting or lateral	• Can be given in patients in which epidural is contraindicated • Limited dermatomal spread compared to epidural
Serratus anterior block	Chest wall trauma (flail chest, fractured ribs)	Supine/lateral	• Superior analgesia • Facilitate extubation

Table 5.3: Analgesic Medications in Procedure Rooms

Drugs	Dosages
Fentanyl	1–2 mcg/kg followed by 0.5–1 mcg/kg IV
Ketamine	0.5–1 mg/kg followed by 0.25–0.5 mg/kg IV
Midazolam	0.02–0.03 mg/kg followed by 0.01–0.02 mg/kg IV
Propofol	0.5–1 mg/kg over 1 min followed by increments of 0.5 mg/kg IV

IV, intravenous.

requirements, improved patient comfort as well as transportation, and have been shown to significantly reduce length of stay in the ED. Some of the regional blocks that can be used in trauma patients are summarized in Table 5.2.

Follow-Up

Every trauma patient should be reassessed after 30–60 minutes of providing analgesia and again re-channelized to green, yellow or red zones based on the severity of pain. If the pain is still severe, the patient should be referred to the primary team for admission or adequate supply of analgesics.

Procedure Rooms

Several procedures achieved in the ED have grown exponentially over the last few decades. Executing such measures (both diagnostic and therapeutic) yield pain to the subjects and should be given attention appropriately by the healthcare workers. One must provide appropriate positioning, distraction, relaxation and coping strategies along with local anaesthesia. Various analgesic/sedation options are also available. Perhaps, there is no universal use of a single or combination of agents that can be advised in individual subjects. Hence, the clinicians must pander to the needs of the subject in minimizing pain and reducing the possible risk (Table 5.3).

SUGGESTED READING

1. Ahmadi A, Bazargan-Hejazi S, Heidari Zadie Z, et al. Pain management in trauma: a review study. *J Inj Violence Res*. 2016;8:89–98.DOI: 10.5249/jivr.v8i2.707.

2. Hennes H, Kim MK. Prehospital pain management: current status and future direction. *Clin Pediatr Emerg Med*. 2006;7:25–30.DOI: 10.1080/10903120590891705.

3. Cohen SP, Christo PJ, Moroz L. Pain management in trauma patients. *Am J Phys Med Rehabil.* 2004;83:142–61. DOI: 10.1097/01.PHM.0000107499.24698.CA.

4. Todd KH, Ducharme J, Choiniere M, et al. Pain in the emergency department: results of the pain and emergency medicine initiative (PEMI) multicenter study. *J Pain.* 2007;8: 460–6. DOI: 10.1016/j.jpain.2006.12.005.

5. Kelly AM. A process approach to improving pain management in the emergency department: development and evaluation. *J Accid Emerg Med.* 2000;17:185–7. DOI: 10.1136/emj.17.3.185.

6 Role of Intercostal Drainage Tube in Chest Trauma

Ajay Savlania

LEARNING OBJECTIVES

- Anatomical basis of chest tube insertion
- Indications and contraindications of intercostal drainage tube insertion
- Role of intercostal drainage tube in chest trauma
- Knowledge of complications associated with chest tube insertion

INTRODUCTION

It is almost impossible to imagine surgical residency without the memories of the learning process and insertions on intercostal drainage tubes. Chest trauma is second only to head trauma as a cause of traumatic deaths. The most common thoracic injury is a rib fracture accounting for 48.7% of cases, with 20.4% presenting with pneumothorax. Intercostal drainage is an important tool in the management in these patients. The dramatic clinical improvement following its insertion in pneumothorax and in drainage of collections makes it an important workhorse procedure in the hands of surgeons. Like any procedure in medicine there are common dos and don'ts that define this procedure.

HISTORY OF THE PROCEDURE

The idea of draining collections in the chest cavity has been present for thousands of years. The oldest known reference of thoracic drainage dates back to 5th century BC by Hippocrates. The first description of tube thoracostomy technique was by Wolfram von Eschenbach in his work *Parzival*. In his description:

> There lay a man pierced through,
> with his blood rushing inward …
> "I could keep this knight from dying
> and I feel sure I could save him
> if I had a reed,
> You would soon see him and hear
> him in health, because
> he is not mortally wounded.
> The blood is only pressing on his heart."
> He grasped a branch of the linden tree,
> slipped the bark off like a tube –
> he was no fool in the matter of wounds –
> and inserted it into the body through the wound.
> Then he bade the woman suck on it
> until blood flowed toward her.
> The hero's strength revived so that he could speak and talk again.

The first description of a water-seal chest drainage system may be attributed to Playfair in 1873 in the treatment of a child with thoracic empyema. Despite four aspirations the effusion recurred. Ultimately, he placed a gum rubber tube with one end in a container filled with water. This allowed the drainage of pus, and the symptoms improved. The modern three-chamber thoracic drainage system was first described by Howe in 1952. Tube thoracostomy was finally accepted as the standard of care at the time of the Vietnam War.

THE ANATOMICAL BASIS OF TUBE PLACEMENT

Though the intercostal drainage tube is commonly used, approximately 4%–5% of intercostal drainage tube placements have complications. To prevent these complications, good anatomical knowledge and appropriate sizing of tubes and accurate placement are necessary. The intercostal space is filled with intercostal muscles with the intercostal neurovascular bundle commonly present in the groove of the superior rib. Newer research shows the ideal spot is 50%–70% of the way down the interspace.

The British Thoracic Society has recommended the triangle of safety as the site for intercostal drainage tube insertion (Figure 6.1). The area is bordered by the anterior border of latissimus dorsi, the lateral border of the pectoralis major and a line along the fifth intercostal space. The midaxillary line is the most commonly advocated position because the innermost layer of the intercostal muscles are poorly developed and the long thoracic nerve is posterior to the midaxillary line along the fibres of the serratus anterior. The apex of the lung is intimately related with the cervical ganglion and separated only by a thin layer of fascia. It is important to be at least 2–3 cm from the apex to avoid any Horner's syndrome, to be 2–3 cm lateral to the vertebrae, especially

DOI: 10.1201/9781003291619-7

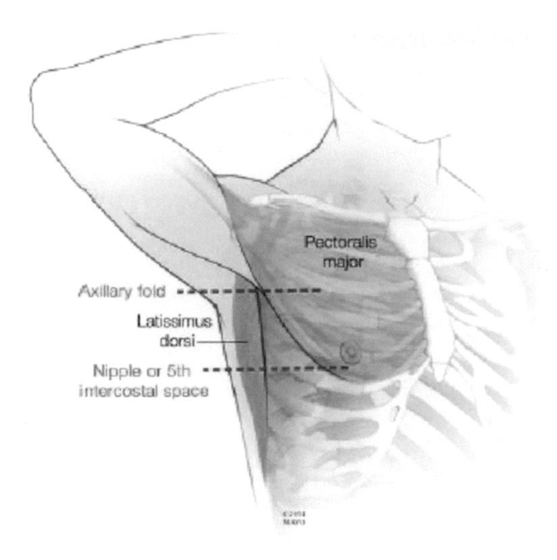

Figure 6.1 British Thoracic Society's Triangle of Safety detailing anatomic borders for placement of tube thoracostomy (TT) Reprinted with permission from Hernandez, M.C. et al., *The Journal of Trauma and Acute Care Surgery*, 81(2), 366–370, 2016

in children, to avoid the phrenic nerve and to avoid the mediastinum.

INDICATIONS

The most common indication for tube thoracostomy is pneumothorax and the second is hemithorax. The indications are multiple and commonly divided into emergent and non-emergent. The emergent indications are commonly seen in trauma patients. The indications include:

1. Pneumothorax in the setting of mechanical ventilation or trauma
2. A large pneumothorax
3. Pneumothorax in a clinically unstable patient
4. Tension pneumothorax after needle decompression
5. Hemopneumothorax and haemothorax
6. Oesophageal rupture with evidence of leak into pleural space

CONTRAINDICATIONS

Most contraindications like the presence of large bullae or coagulopathy are relative in the setting of trauma. The contraindications are decided by weighing the risk–benefit and proceeding.

ROLE OF INTERCOSTAL DRAINAGE TUBE IN THORACIC TRAUMA

The initial management of all thoracic trauma follows the ABCDE principle (airway, breathing, circulation, disability, exposure) of the Advanced Trauma Life Support (ATLS) guidelines.

1. Haemothorax: As per recent literature, a small volume (<300 ml) haemothorax can be conservatively managed. Although this is from small studies, most established guidelines recommend drainage of all haemothoraces irrespective of volume. As per the Eastern Association for the Surgery of Trauma (EAST) guidelines, all haemothoraces should be drained, and the initial approach should be with the use of an intercostal drainage tube, preferably large bore, commonly greater than 30 French in adults. The tube should be placed posteriorly as to allow dependent drainage. The presence of residual collection should always be addressed, not with a second chest tube but rather with video-assisted thoracoscopic surgery (VATS) (level 1 evidence). The timing of the surgery is also important, and VATS should be done preferably in the first 3 to 7 days (level 2 evidence). Unnecessary delay results in an increased rate of development of infections, necessitating thoracotomy and prolonged stay. The output also acts like a guide in the initial phase of the need to change intervention.

   Commonly, an unstable penetrating chest trauma patient is taken up for surgery or occasionally a resuscitative thoracotomy. In a hemodynamically stable patient, the indications for thoracotomy are:

   - More than 1500 ml of blood immediately evacuated by tube thoracostomy
   - Persistent bleeding from the chest, defined as 150 ml/h to 200 ml/h for 2 hr to 4 hr
   - Requirement of persistent blood transfusion to maintain hemodynamic stability

2. Pneumothorax: Blunt trauma or penetrating injury to the chest wall cause pneumothorax. Traumatic pneumothorax can be seen in blast injury patients without coexisting evidence of chest injuries. From the pathophysiological point of view, three types of pneumothoraxes have been described:

   - Closed pneumothorax: Occurs when there is no communication between the outside of the thorax and pleural space. The amount of air is usually small and absorbs spontaneously. Intercostal drainage tube insertion is needed if the pneumothorax is large or if the patient needs to be mechanically ventilated.

- Open pneumothorax: Presence of an open communication between the pleural cavity and area outside of the chest. The hole through which air enters is usually along the chest wall. This needs to be managed with airtight dressing on three sides to allow the flutter wall mechanism with an additional chest tube from a clean site as required.
- Tension pneumothorax: An emergency situation when the air enters the chest cavity but does not exit. It causes rapid patient deterioration. Immediate needle decompression followed by chest tube placement is required.

3. Massive air leak: It is a rare injury found in 2.5%–8% of blunt trauma patients. Subcutaneous emphysema, a large persistent air leak after tube thoracostomy and continued pneumothorax could signify a major tracheobronchial injury. These patients need to be managed with an emergency thoracotomy.
4. Occult pneumothorax: Occult pneumothoraces are injuries that are detected on CT scan but missed on X-ray. These are commonly located anteriorly. There is controversy regarding the management of these injuries, as about 20%–30% do not progress.

COMPLICATIONS

There are primarily two methods of intercostal drainage tube injury: the blunt dissection technique and the trocar technique. The trocar technique has a slightly higher rate of intrathoracic organ injury. It is best to avoid complications. A thorough knowledge of anatomy is needed for the correct recommended placement in the triangle of safety and preferably in the midaxillary line. The complications commonly seen with intercostal drainage tube insertion are as follows:

1. Tube malposition: It is the commonest complication of tube thoracostomy and commonly seen when the tube is inserted in suboptimal conditions and is more commonly observed with the trocar method. CT scan is confirmatory, and management is dictated based on the location. Intraparenchymal chest tube placement occurs more likely in the presence of pleural adhesions or pre-existing pulmonary diseases. Other malpositions include chest wall placement, fissure tube placement, mediastinal tube placement and abdominal placement.
2. Blocked drain: Non-functional drains due to kinking, angulation, clot formation or debris in the tube. The cardinal sign of a blocked tube is the failure of fluid within the tube to fluctuate with coughing or respiration.
3. Re-expansion pulmonary oedema: An uncommon but dangerous complication with a mortality rate of up to 20%. This occurs following drainage of long-standing large pleural effusions and occasionally due to pneumothorax. The important pathophysiological mechanism has been postulated due to increased endothelial permeability and loss of integrity of the alveolar capillaries leading to exudation of protein-rich fluid. Treatment is mainly supportive.
4. Infectious complications: Closed tube thoracostomy is classified as a clean contaminated procedure with a risk of infection between 4% and 8%. Empyema occurs more commonly after pleural effusion, as this allows nosocomial contamination.
5. Intercostal artery injury and chest wall arteriovenous fistula: The cause of haemorrhage during insertion of chest tube is due to injury to intercostal arteries. Classical teaching states that the dissection be done at the superior border of the lower rib. The safest zone to perform tube thoracostomy should be between 50% and 70% of the way down the interspace to avoid the variably positioned intercostal neurovascular bundle and inferior collateral artery.
6. Residual pneumothorax: This can be secondary to an air leak. It can be avoided during the removal of the chest tube by maintaining a sustained Valsalva manoeuvre.
7. Air leak: Most air leaks are minor and occur due to underlying disease rather than trauma. Most of them improve with prolonged intercostal tube drainage as they are minor. American College of Chest Physicians (ACCP) guidelines recommend drainage for at least 4 days. Prolonged drainage or high-volume air leaks warrant operative intervention.

REMOVAL OF INTERCOSTAL DRAINAGE TUBE

There is no ideal time for chest tube removal. Various criteria have included volume of output or radiographic resolution. In a single centre study done by Younes et al., the authors compared rates of reinsertion and complications based on various drain volumes for removal. They found that even at varying drain outputs of 50 ml, 100 ml or 200 ml there were no real differences in the rate of reintervention. This data needs to be interpreted with caution, especially because retained haemothorax can lead to the formation of an empyema complicating the course of these patients.

The common teaching in most textbooks without any high quality of evidence is:

- Stable clinical condition
- Wide-open lung on chest X-ray
- Discharge of less than 200 cc in 24 hr (institutional protocols may vary)
- No air leak (24 hr vs 48 hr is a common controversy as to the minimum duration passed after cessation of air leak)

Due to the varied practices and a brief review of the evidence available at present, ultimately clinical decision-making is based on the patient's characteristics and treating doctor's discretion. Common issues faced with removal of the chest tube include the following:

1. *Is it necessary to clamp the tube prior to removal?* A common practice in our institution is to have a period of clamping prior to removal of the chest tube. Becker et al. in their retrospective cohort study evaluated the effect of clamping trials on the need for subsequent pleural drainage in trauma patients. They followed 4 hr clamping trials prior to removal, and any clinical or radiographic deterioration would mean abandoning the planned removal. In their study, 214 patients were given the clamping trial and 285 patients were in the control group. Clamping trials were associated with fewer pleural drainage procedures [13 (6%) vs 33 (12%); adjusted OR 0.41 (95% CI 0.20 to 0.84)].
2. *Is a radiograph necessary after removal of the chest tube?* A common practice after removal of the intercostal drainage tube is a chest X-ray. In retrospective studies done by Johnson et al. and Cunningham et al., the authors found that routine X-rays do not change management but symptom-based use of X-ray is indicated. But it has been argued that routine X-ray is needed especially in patients with a history of air leaks or in those patients who, after discharge, do not have access to surgical care.

Based on these studies, the approach for removal needs to be a tailored approach based on patient characteristics.

CONCLUSION

Tube thoracostomy is an important part in the management of traumatic chest injuries. Good planning and placement technique is essential to avoid complications. They are the primary management of haemothorax and pneumothorax, with good clinical judgement being essential for planning their timely removal.

SUGGESTED READING

1. Locicero J, Feins RH, Colson YL, Rocco G. *Shields General Thoracic Surgery.* Eighth edition. USA: Wolters Kluwer, 2019.
2. Kulshrestha P, Munshi I, Wait R. Profile of chest trauma in a level I trauma center. *J Trauma.* 2004 Sep;57(3):576–81. DOI: 10.1097/01.ta.0000091107.00699.c7. PMID: 15454805.
3. Hughes J. Battlefield medicine in Wolfram's Parzival. *J Medieval Mil Hist.* 2010:8,119–30.
4. Von Eschenbach W (Mustard H, Passage C, trans.). *Parzival.* New York: Random House, 1961.
5. Kesieme EB, Dongo A, Ezemba N, et al. Tube thoracostomy: complications and its management. *Pulm Med.* 2012;2012:256878. DOI: 10.1155/2012/256878 PMID: 22028963.
6. Hernandez MC, Laan DV, Zimmerman S, et al. Tube thoracostomy: increased angle of insertion is associated with complications. *J Trauma Acute Care Surg.* 2016;81:366. DOI: 10.1097/TA.0000000000001098 PMID: 27120327.
7. American College of Surgeons. Committee on Trauma. *Advanced Trauma Life Support: Student Course Manual.* Tenth edition. Chicago, IL: American College of Surgeons; 2018.
8. Pohnán R, Blazkova S, Hytych V, et al. Treatment of hemothorax in the era of minimally invasive surgery. *Mil Med Sci Lett.* 2019 Dec 6;88:1–8.DOI: 10.1097/MCP.0000000000000062. PMID: 24852328.
9. Mowery NT, Gunter OL, Collier BR, et al. Practice management guidelines for management of hemothorax and occult pneumothorax. *J Trauma Acute Care Surg.* 2011;70:510–8. DOI: 10.1097/TA.0b013e31820b5c31. PMID: 21307755.
10. Younes RN, Gross JL, Aguiar S, Haddad FJ, Deheinzelin D. When to remove a chest tube? A randomized study with subsequent

prospective consecutive validation. *J Am Coll Surg.* 2002 Nov;195:658–62. DOI: 10.1016/s1072-7515(02)01332-7. PMID: 12437253.

11. Paydar S, Ghahramani Z, Ghoddusi Johari, et al. Tube thoracostomy (chest tube) removal in traumatic patients: what do we know? What can we do? *Bull Emergency Trauma.* 2015;3:37–40. PMID: 27162900.

12. Becker JC, Zakaluzny SA, Keller BA, et al. Clamping trials prior to thoracostomy tube removal and the need for subsequent invasive pleural drainage. *Am J Surg.* 2020;220:476–81. DOI: 10.1016/j.amjsurg.2020.01.007. Epub 2020 Jan 8. PMID: 31948700.

13. Johnson B, Rylander M, Beres AL. Do X-rays after chest tube removal change patient management? *J Pediatr Surg.* 2017;52:813–5. DOI: 10.1016/j.jpedsurg.2017.01.047. PMID: 28189452.

14. Cunningham JP, Knott EM, Gasior AC, et al. Is routine chest radiograph necessary after chest tube removal? *J Pediatr Surg.* 2014;49:1493–5. DOI: 10.1016/j.jpedsurg.2017.01.047. PMID: 28189452.

7 Intrahospital Transport of Trauma Patients

Amarjyoti Hazarika

LEARNING OBJECTIVES

- Decisions that need to be made before transporting a patient
- Learn about the complications that might occur during transportation
- Knowledge of the checklist that should be followed during intrahospital patient transport
- Learn the best way to transport patients while at the same time preventing complications

INTRODUCTION

Trauma patients need to be transferred from the emergency or triage areas for examination, or to their respective wards/operation theatres/procedural room/intensive care settings for further management/care. Transporting a trauma patient, whether hemodynamically stable or unstable, brings about risks and problems at several levels. Patients who are transferred are often unwell. The simple physical movement of some injuries, such as major unstable pelvic fractures, can precipitate bleeding. Movement with multiple IV infusions, invasive devices and ventilators increase the complexity of the transfer and effects morbidity and mortality. Problems to recognize and ameliorate during a transfer include inadvertent loss of an IV line, kinking and/or blockage of tracheal or intercostal tubes, and equipment failure.

DECISIONS TO BE MADE BEFORE TRANSPORTATION

1. It is important to decide whether the patient is fit to be moved and transportation would not further harm the patient.
2. Identify if the need for intervention/screening, requiring transportation, outweighs the potential risks of patient transport. Unstable patients should not be transferred for intervention if such care will not alter their outcome.
3. Confirm that all resources, equipment and manpower are adequately present to transport such patients (Figure 7.1).

THINGS THAT MIGHT GO WRONG DURING PATIENT TRANSFER

Complications Related to Airway Management

- Airway displacement, malposition or dislodgement.
- Equipment failure to support ventilation, such as disconnection of circuits and battery failure.
- Unawareness of steps of manual ventilation (complication increases when compared to mechanical ventilation).
- Odds of developing symptomatic pneumothorax, atelectasis and deep vein thrombosis are increased.

Haemodynamic Complications

- Alterations in haemodynamics during transport are always a reason for concern calling for strict vigilance.
- Decrease in blood pressure sometimes in substantial values leading to cardiac arrest.
- Increase in heart rate leading to arrhythmias and subsequent arrest.

Risk of Infection

- Risk of infection is increased in both the patient being transported and the healthcare workers who are transporting.
- Increased incidence of ventilator-associated pneumonia.

Interruption of Therapies

- Probability of interruption in vital infusions (e.g. sedatives, analgesics, vasopressors, inotropes).
- Potential interruption of therapies like continuous renal replacement therapy.
- Loss of intravenous access is a serious problem.
- Glucose dysregulation due to probable discontinuation of insulin pumps and changes in intravenous fluid infusions during transport.
- Disturbances in systemic acid-base balance.

DOI: 10.1201/9781003291619-8

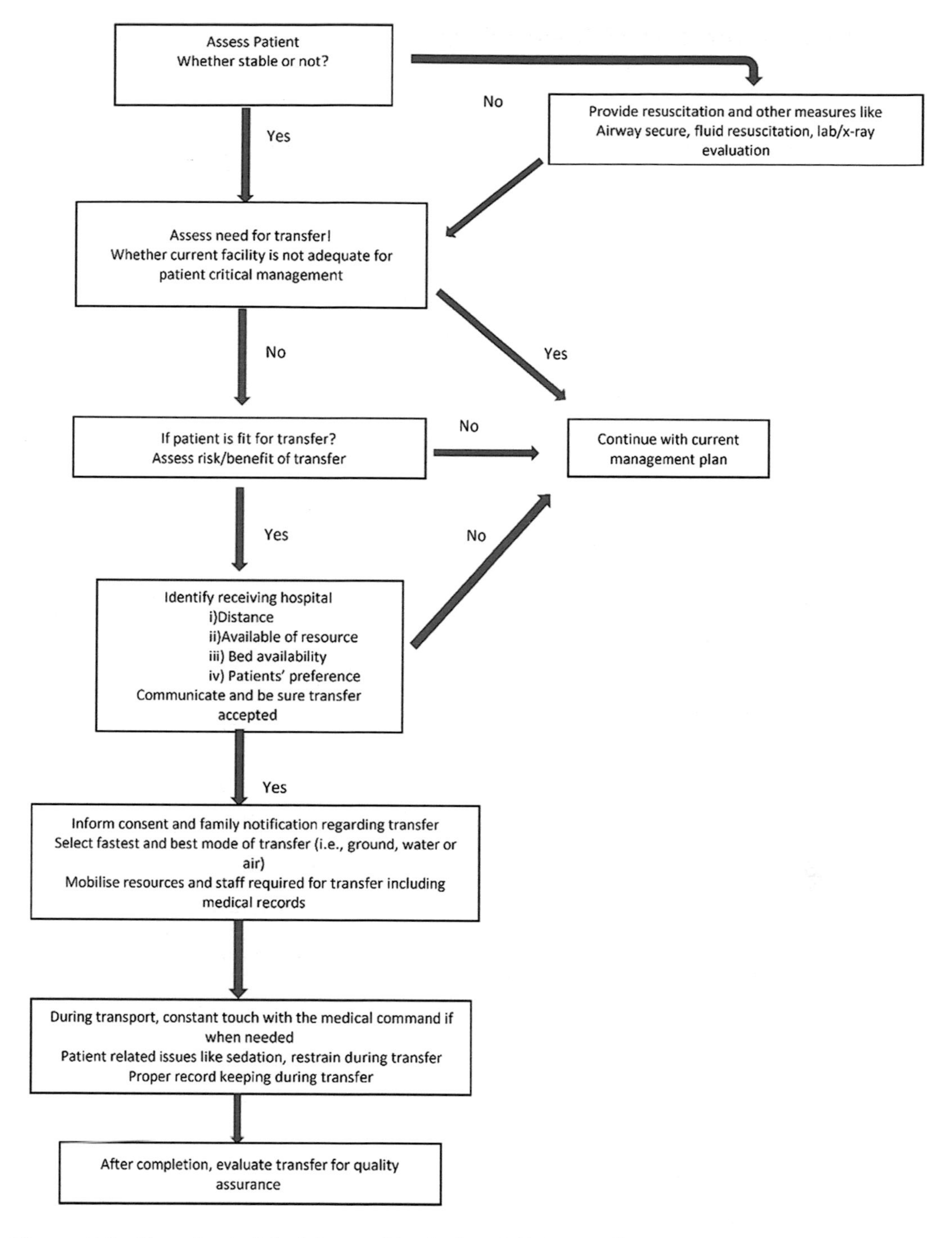

Figure 7.1 Flow chart of decision making before shifting a patient

Fractures

- Fractures are liable to get secondary injury via distraction, misalignment, neurovascular damage or other types of soft tissue injury even after traction or splint is applied.
- Spinal injury, one of the most critical injuries, can occur or get aggravated during transport, damaging vital neurologic and vascular structures.

Factors contributing to these complications are enumerated in Figure 7.2.

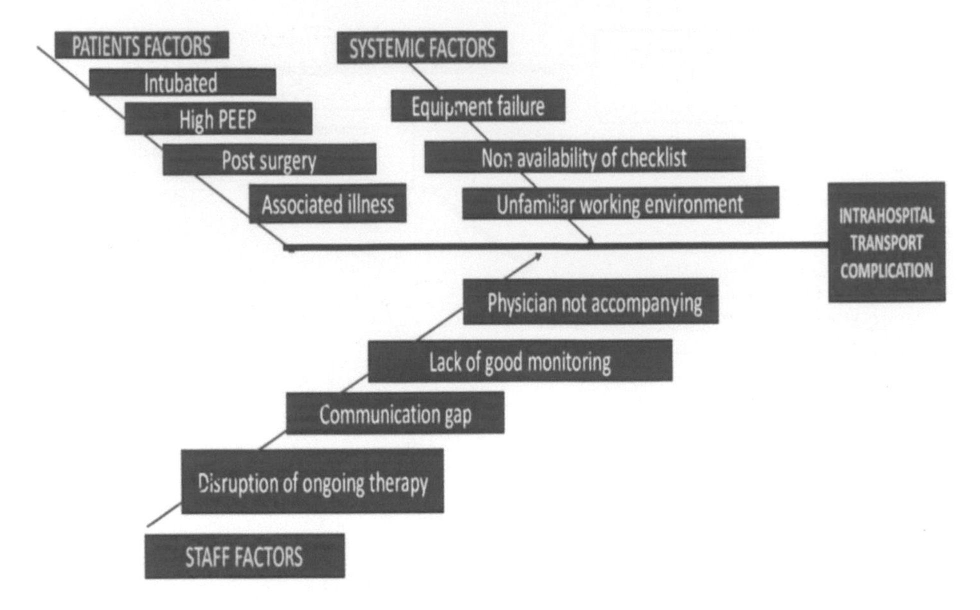

Figure 7.2 Factors contributing to complications during intrahospital transport

CHECKLIST FOR INTRAHOSPITAL TRANSPORT (IHT)

1. Adequate resuscitation targeting stable haemodynamics should be achieved before transport.
2. A proper checklist as per transfer protocol should be there for proper monitoring and audit of each IHT.
3. Confirm first whether the location to which the patient is being sent has the necessary set-up to take care of the patient, like oxygen and its device support, monitors, infusion pumps, ambulance, etc.
4. Every patient should have a blood pressure monitor, pulse oximetry and equipment for emergency airway management in addition to an oxygen source during transport.
5. The minimal requirements in destination locations include a suction device, an oxygen source, accessible electric connections, monitoring devices and an available crash cart.
6. Adequate manpower and equipment should be in place to carry out the transport.
7. Trolleys which are used for IHT must be able to enter lifts and pass through all doorways en route to the destination.
8. Counter check that all equipment and accessories are in working condition to carry out IHT.
9. Adequate resources at the disposal along with coordination and communications should be in place to tackle emergencies occurring during IHT (e.g. ventilator break down, power off).
10. In critically ill patients on mechanical ventilation, mechanical ventilation equipment should be available for transport and at the receiving location as mentioned earlier.
11. There should be designated medical staff available to overview the transfer in case of a critical event during transport.

HOW TO TRANSPORT THE PATIENT

1. All trauma patients should be ideally transported with a rigid collar, more so mandatory in patients with head and truncal injury (Figure 7.3).
2. If a collar is not available, use rolls made of cloth/towels/drapes on both sides of the neck to stabilize the neck in a neutral position (Figure 7.4).
3. Make sure all IV lines and devices like oxygen support, cylinder and vital monitors are attached to the patient and are in working condition with sufficient reserves to meet transportation requirements.
4. Vital monitors, infusion pumps and/or ventilators must be secured with straps to the trolleys or trolley poles so that they do not fall on the patient.
5. The physician or medical personnel shifting the patient should be at the head end, and the monitors should be placed in the direction facing the personnel.

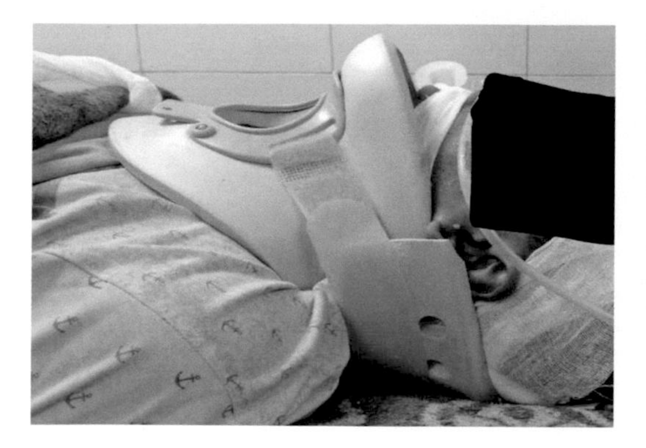

Figure 7.3 Transporting patient with rigid collar

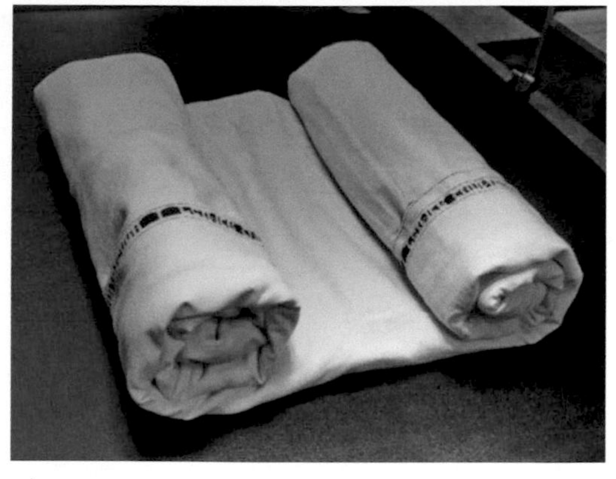

Figure 7.4 Cloth rolls for stabilizing the neck

Table 7.1: Important Checklist for Intrahospital Transport

Before	During	After
Staff involved with transport should be relieved of other tasks	Follow fastest and best route (i.e. elevators should be stationed to avoid delays)	Admission of the patient in the destination department
Stabilization of patient	Ongoing communication with destination	Reassess patient condition before handover
Check monitors and equipment	Continuous monitoring of the patient and recording them	Detail update to receiving team; transport team should not leave the area unless receiving team is fully satisfied with the patient information provided
Monitors attached to patient	Checking the status of the equipment being used	Recording of all events during transport
Safe transfer on the stretcher	Scope of immediate intervention if required	
Plan for the best and fastest route		
Communication between sending and receiving person		

6. When the patient is shifted from bed to trolley and vice versa during the process of IHT, one should use patient shifting rollers or combine the technique of logrolling.
7. Drainage bags, if present, should be emptied before IHT. Intercostal and other drains should be checked and clamped wherever required.
8. The transport team must give a thorough summary of the patient's medical record and relevant laboratory and radiographic copies to the receiving facility.
9. The transport staff must remain with the patient until the receiving team is fully ready to take over.
10. The transfer team and equipment should return to the place of origin (Table 7.1).

SUGGESTED READING

1. Warren J, et al. American College of Critical Care Medicine. Guidelines for the inter- and intrahospital transport of critically ill patients. *Critical Care Medicine*. 2004;32:256–62. doi: 10.1097/01.CCM.0000104917.39204.0A.
2. Knight PH, et al. Complications during intrahospital transport of critically ill patients: focus on risk identification and prevention. *International Journal of Critical Illness & Injury Science*. 2015;5:256–64. doi: 10.4103/2229-5151.170840.
3. Despoina A. Intrahospital transport policies: the contribution of the nurse. *Health Science Journal* [Internet]. 2014 [cited 2021 Jun 15];8(2). Available from: https://www.hsj.gr/medicine/intrahospital-transport-policies-the-contribution-of-the-nurse.php?aid=2749.

8 Care of Intubated Patients in Triage

Shalvi Mahajan and Komal A Gandhi

LEARNING OBJECTIVES

- Knowledge of the basic components of postintubation care such as monitoring, endotracheal tube care, analgesia, sedation, prevention of complications related to intubation and mechanical ventilation
- Development and implementation of system-appropriate protocol for the same

INTRODUCTION

Endotracheal intubation is a life-saving advanced airway procedure carried out in a triage area. Due to limited hospital capacity, intubated patients may spend critically important time in triage before being transferred to the appropriate area. A majority of urgent care during this period is provided by the trauma triage team. Therefore, a postintubation holistic management is essential even in the triage area for better outcomes.

Continuous haemodynamic monitoring, endotracheal tube care, provision of adequate analgesia/sedation, continued resuscitation and secondary survey, proceeding towards a definitive treatment plan and transfer to an intensive care unit, and early preventive measures to avoid associated complications should be ensured. Additionally, family counselling regarding the patient's clinical situation is an important component but is given the least importance by the treating team.

Important points to be taken care of in the postintubation period are described as a checklist (Table 8.1).

PATIENT POSITIONING

The patient should be propped up (30–45 degrees) unless contraindicated with a neutral neck position. It helps in decreasing intracranial pressure in the head injury position, allows movement of the diaphragm and decreases chances of aspiration of gastric contents.

MONITORING

Vital monitoring includes heart rate, ECG (electrocardiogram), blood pressure (non-invasive), oxygen saturation (SpO_2) by pulse oximetry and temperature. End-tidal carbon dioxide ($EtCO_2$) values with real-time waveform capnography are of paramount importance, especially in intubated patients, to confirm the placement of a tracheal tube in the airway and effective ventilation.

Temperature monitoring is often overlooked, although hypothermia is an important component of the lethal triad of shock. An acutely ill traumatic patient has a harder time regulating their body temperature due to exposure to a cold environment and massive volume resuscitation protocol.

Clinical monitoring of the Glasgow Coma Scale (GSC) and pupillary reactions should be interpreted in the background of sedation and analgesics administered.

ENDOTRACHEAL TUBE (ETT) CARE

ETT care is a broad entity that encompasses multiple arrays of activities. This includes confirmation of its position, prevention of accidental extubation and preventive measures for intubation-related complications.

Endotracheal Tube Position Confirmation

Once intubated, it is important to confirm the ETT position in the trachea. Clinical signs of tracheal intubation are the presence of bilateral air entry on auscultation, fog or mist in the ETT and visible chest rise. The best confirmatory sign is the detection of $EtCO_2$ in capnography. A postintubation chest radiograph, if available, allows confirmation of the ETT tip position. Moreover, it helps in the detection of upper lobe collapse, pneumothorax and associated rib fractures.

Point-of-care ultrasound (POCUS) can also help confirm the ETT position. With a linear ultrasound (US) probe kept horizontally in the suprasternal notch, the trachea is identified as a hyperechoic structure (air-mucosal interface) with comet tail artefacts. Successful ETT placement demonstrates an increase in artefacts and posterior shadowing (bullet sign). The oesophagus is situated posterolateral to the trachea. The presence of one or more hyperechoic linear structure with comet tail artefacts in the posterolateral (double tract sign) area marks oesophageal intubation. In addition, pleural sliding sign and diaphragmatic movements can reveal lung ventilation.

Routine Care

- Secure the ETT. Adhesive tapes and non-adhesive bandages are generally used in triage. With a beard or moustache, it is difficult

DOI: 10.1201/9781003291619-9

Table 8.1: Postintubation Care Protocol

	Postintubation Intervention
1	**Head up position** (30–45 degrees)
2	**Continuous vital monitoring** • HR, ECG, NIBP, SpO_2, $ETCO_2$, temperature • Clinical: GCS, pupils
3	**Oxygenation and ventilation monitoring** • SpO_2 • $ETCO_2$ • Arterial blood gas (ABG), $PaO_2/PaCO_2$ • Clinical parameters: colour of skin, mucosa, auscultation/bilateral air entry • Chest X-ray • Ultrasound
4	**Endotracheal tube care** • Documentation of ETT fixation position at lips, rule out endobronchial placement • ETT tie: firm fixation/loose fixation, dry/wet due to any secretions • ETT cuff pressure between 20 and 30 cmH_2O • ETT suctioning as per the requirement with aseptic techniques • Humidification of inspired gases, passive or active • Ventilator-associated pneumonia prevention bundle
5	**Investigations (whichever indicated)** ABG, lactates, blood sugar, routine lab investigations, haemogram, coagulogram, biochemistry, POCUS, FAST, CT scans, doppler studies
6	**Other (FAST HUGS BID)** • **F**eeding/fluids • **A**nalgesia • **S**edation • **T**hromboprophylaxis (graduated compression stockings or intermittent pneumatic compression devices or heparin), **t**emperature • **H**ead up • **U**lcer prophylaxis, **u**rine output • **G**lycaemic control • **S**ore prevention (pressure) – regular position change or use of alpha beds • **B**owel movement • **I**ndwelling catheters – need of catheters, days of insertion, any signs of infection (catheter-related blood stream infections, CLABSI; urinary tract infections), and early removal if not required • **D**rugs/**d**elirium

to use adhesive taping; here bandages or umbilical tape is used.

- Humidification of inhaled gases. Following intubation, the upper airway is bypassed, which provides 75% of humidification to inhaled air. Dry air predisposes to disruption of airway epithelium, inspissation of secretions, bronchospasm, atelectasis, etc. Hence, humidification of inspired gases is advised in intubated patients. In the triage area, either passive (heat moisture exchangers, HMEs) or active humidification is used. Passive humidifiers need not be changed daily unless copious secretions are present or if resistance to flow has increased. They can be safely changed after 48 hours. During nebulization, HMEs should be removed from the circuit.
- Suctioning of tracheal secretions. Suctioning is an application of negative pressure to the trachea through the distal part of the ETT to clear excess or abnormal secretions with the help of a suction catheter with or without disconnecting the ETT from the mechanical ventilator circuit (open or closed suctioning, respectively).

Suctioning steps

1. Suctioning should be done only when indicated (auscultate chest/any visible secretions).
2. Monitor vitals – Oxygen saturation, heart rate (HR), respiratory rate (RR), blood pressure (BP), $EtCO_2$, ventilator parameters (mode of ventilation, tidal volume, flow, pressure) and inspired oxygen percentage (FiO_2).
3. Prerequisites – Functional suction apparatus (wall mounted or portable). Suction pressure should be set at 100–120 mmHg (should not exceed 200 mmHg). Use the appropriate size suction catheter. One method to calculate the French (Fr) suction catheter size is Fr = [ETT size (mm) – 1] × 2. Use a suction catheter with an atraumatic tip if available, and lubricate the suction catheter.

4. Procedure – Use sterile gloves for open suctioning and clean gloves for closed suctioning. Set the FiO_2 to 100% for at least 60 seconds. Administer drugs to prevent hemodynamic response such as xylocaine 1.5 mg/kg 90 seconds before suction. The duration of suction should not exceed 15 to 20 seconds to prevent hypoxemia and atelectasis. Normal saline instillation is not preferred.
5. Documentation – Document the timings of suctioning, amount and characteristics of secretions, suction tolerance and any significant event during suctioning.

- ETT cuff pressure. It should be kept between 20 and 30 cmH_2O while sealing the trachea. It should be monitored and adjusted at least in every shift, after suctioning, after repositioning of the tube or if any audible leak is heard. Monitoring is to be done with a handheld cuff manometer. The palpatory method is not advised.

Prevention of Accidental Extubation

Securing the ETT after confirmation is an integral part of intubation. Inadequate sedation, agitation, perspiration, excessive oral secretions/bleeding and loose fixation can cause accidental or spontaneous movement of the ETT out of the trachea. Hence, adequate sedation and proper ETT fixation is required to prevent inadvertent extubation (in triage as well as during intrahospital transport). The combination of adhesive tape around the ETT along with a suture through the ETT offers resistance to removal.

Preventive Measures for Intubation-Related Complications

- Ventilator associated pneumonia (VAP). It is defined as pneumonia following endotracheal intubation and mechanical ventilation of at least 48 hours. Since patients can spend many hours in triage, implementation of a VAP prevention bundle is important.

  The VAP prevention bundle includes five main interventions: (1) head end elevation between 30 and 45 degrees, (2) daily oral care with chlorhexidine mouthwash at least twice a day, (3) deep venous thrombosis prophylaxis, (4) stress peptic ulcer prophylaxis and (5) daily sedative interruption and assessing readiness to extubate.

  In addition, the ETT with in-line suction and subglottic suctioning, maintenance of the ETT cuff pressures between 20 and 30 cmH_2O, and strict hand hygiene are other important elements of the VAP care bundle.
- Tracheal mucosal injury. If the ETT cuff pressures are kept above 30 mmHg, it produces ischaemia of tracheal mucosa.

VENTILATION MANAGEMENT

Once intubated, ventilation can be supported manually with an Ambu bag connected to oxygen or mechanically through a ventilator. Manual ventilation has drawbacks: an inability to control the tidal volume delivered and respiratory rate leading to hyper- or hypoventilation, overinflation of lungs, displacement of the ETT and manual exhaustion. Controlling oxygenation and ventilation, together with continuous monitoring of airway pressures and lung compliance, will be possible with the mechanical ventilator. A lung-protective strategy for ventilation should be adopted. Subsequently, frequent re-evaluation of clinical condition and arterial blood gas sampling can guide ventilator settings.

ANALGESIA AND SEDATION

Intubated patients experience pain and anxiety due to trauma, inability to speak (ETT in situ), airway suctioning, blood sampling, invasive catheterization, surgical procedures and intrahospital transportation. Sedatives are frequently required to manage anxiety/agitation; however, they lack analgesic properties. Undertreated pain has adverse impacts such as cardiac instability, respiratory compromise and immunosuppression. Thus, assessment and treatment of pain before giving sedatives, often termed *analgesia-first sedation*, is favoured. Hence, *multimodal analgesia* – site-appropriate regional analgesia (e.g. US-guided femoral blocks), systemic opioids (e.g. fentanyl, morphine) and nonopioid agents (acetaminophen, ketamine and non-steroidal anti-inflammatory drugs) – can be selected. Light sedation is a rule, except if only neuromuscular agents are administered where deep sedation or amnesia is required to avoid awakening a paralyzed patient until the effect of the medication is expected to have worn off. Currently, nonbenzodiazepine sedatives (propofol and dexmedetomidine) are preferred over benzodiazepine-based sedatives.

CIRCULATION

Monitoring of circulation focuses on *systemic blood pressure, intravascular volume and tissue perfusion*. Systemic blood pressure, one of the simplest means of monitoring global circulation and the target mean blood pressure should be

65 mmHg or above. Intravascular volume and fluid status can be assessed (a) non-invasively using real-time US-guided inferior vena cava diameter or two-dimensional echocardiography; or (b) invasively using invasive arterial blood pressure monitoring (systolic and pulse pressure variation parameters). Central venous pressure is also used, but it is an unreliable method. The simplest way to assess tissue perfusion is by measurement of urine output (target > 0.5 ml/kg) and lactate levels (< 2 mmol/L) in trauma cases.

Normal spontaneous negative pressure ventilation is converted into positive pressure ventilation after intubation. This will increase pressure in the central vessels and will reduce the pressure gradient. Consequently, a reduction of blood flow to the heart leads to a drop in cardiac output and lowering of blood pressures. Thus, patients may require hemodynamic support. Circulation can be maintained via fluids, vasopressor agents and blood/blood products depending on clinical parameters.

OTHER PRECAUTIONS

1. After intubation, before leaving the head end of the patient, a gastric tube should be inserted.
2. In addition, urinary catheterization should not be forgotten in intubated patients. The distended bladder can trigger unbalanced sympathetic activity, resulting in an uncontrolled hypertensive crisis.
3. Care of pressure points and use of an alpha mattress for prevention of bed sores is important.

INVESTIGATIONS

Arterial blood gas monitoring, fever workup, sugar monitoring as well as routine investigations should be done as and when required.

CONCLUSION

Acutely ill trauma patients spend critically important time in triage. The postintubation period is an indispensable component of airway management. Postintubation care aims to provide physiological stability to the patients while waiting for transfer to an adequate level of care in the hospital.

SUGGESTED READING

1. Abhishek C, Munta K, Rao SM, Chandrasekhar CN. End-tidal capnography and upper airway ultrasonography in the rapid confirmation of endotracheal tube placement in the patients requiring intubation for general anesthesia. *Indian J Anaesth*. 2017;61:486–9. doi: 10.4103 /ija.IJA _544_16.
2. Restrepo RD, Walsh BK. Humidification during invasive and noninvasive mechanical ventilation. *Respir Care*. 2012;57(5):782–8. doi: 10.4187/respcare.01766.
3. Sole ML, Su X, Talbert S, et al. Evaluation of an intervention to maintain endotracheal tube cuff pressure within therapeutic range. *Am J Crit Care*. 2011;20:109–17. doi: 10.4037/ajcc2011661.
4. Kallet RH. Ventilator bundles in transition: from prevention of ventilator-associated pneumonia to prevention of ventilator-associated events. *Respir Care*. 2019;64:994–1006. doi: 10.4187/respcare.06966.
5. Grap MJ, Munro CL, Unoki T, Hamilton VA, Ward KR. Ventilator-associated pneumonia: the potential critical role of emergency medicine in prevention. *J Emerg Med*. 2012;42:353–62. doi: 10.1016/j.jemermed.2010.05.042.

SECTION II

CRASHING TRAUMA PATIENT

9 Code Crimson in Trauma Triage

Haneesh Thakur and Kajal Jain

LEARNING OBJECTIVES

- What is Code Crimson
- Identifying patients requiring Code Crimson activation
- Criteria for activation of Code Crimson in trauma emergency
- Learning the steps and adjuncts to Code Crimson
- Knowledge of post-code management

INTRODUCTION

A code is a concise, shortest possible alarm in an emergency. Trauma "Code Crimson" is used to manage a patient with life-threatening haemorrhage who is unresponsive to resuscitation. It is activation of a streamlined process in the aforementioned scenario which includes the following: transfusion support to maintain vitals, supportive treatment and definitive intervention with surgical or radiological intervention to stop loss and prevent an unreversible injury and mortality.

The important aspects of trauma Code Crimson are:

- Identification of the massively bleeding patient unresponsive to initial fluid and blood therapy at the prehospital or trauma bay level
- Activating Code Crimson – process of activating personnel, resources and likely interventional procedures for salvaging the patient

IDENTIFYING PATIENTS REQUIRING CODE CRIMSON ACTIVATION IN TRAUMA EMERGENCY

1. Mechanism of injury: blunt trauma chest, abdomen, pelvis with hemodynamic instability
2. Blunt trauma patient with clinical signs of shock or systolic blood pressure < 90 mm Hg at any point, unresponsive to initial fluid resuscitation
3. Blunt trauma injuries to the head, neck or torso with positive eFAST, suggestive of massive haemothorax, pericardial tamponade, or abdominal or pelvic haemorrhage
4. Blunt or open fracture of multiple extremities with hemodynamic instability
5. Traumatic amputation of extremities
6. Penetrating trauma to the neck with vascular injuries
7. Penetrating trauma to chest or abdomen
8. Massively bleeding faciomaxillary trauma
9. Visible exsanguination from any part

CRITERIA FOR ACTIVATION

Activate trauma Code Crimson when an at-risk trauma patient is identified with signs of grade III or grade IV haemorrhage and unresponsive to initial fluid therapy or blood transfusion. According to the classification of haemorrhage by the American College of Surgeons, hypotension develops when the subject has already lost or exsanguinated beyond 30% of the circulating blood volume and is categorized under class/grade III or IV haemorrhage. For example, an adult with 60 kg of weight has a blood volume of 70 ml/kg, i.e. 4200 ml of blood. Loss of 30% of the blood (1260 ml) will initiate hypotension in this patient. This loss along with ongoing bleeding needs immediate support and definitive control. Cut-offs of systolic BP (for hypotension) and heart rate for the paediatric population is given in Table 9.1.

Proceed with CABCDE:

- Compression of exsanguinating site (for compressible haemorrhage).
- Protect airway, secure with an endotracheal tube and stabilize cervical spine.
- Check breathing and ventilation. Exclude and resolve life-threatening causes of obstructive shock or hypotension, i.e. tension pneumothorax, massive haemothorax.
- Start two wide-bore cannulas, rush one litre of crystalloid. Send blood samples for crossmatch as well as baseline investigations including blood gas analysis. Remember to exclude cardiac tamponade.

On activation of Code Crimson:

1. Call and confirm
2. Control bleeding
3. Charge Code Crimson pack
4. Conserve temperature

DOI: 10.1201/9781003291619-11

Table 9.1: Haemodynamic Cut-Offs for Trauma Code Crimson Activation

Age	SBP (mm Hg)	HR (rate per minute)
0–12 months	< 70	< 80 or > 180
12–24 months	< 75	< 70 or > 180
2–6 years	< 80	< 70 or > 180
> 6 years	< 90	< 60 or > 160

SBP, systolic blood pressure; HR, heart rate.

5. Check coagulopathy
6. Catch up on targets
7. Call off code
8. Management of complications

Call and Confirm

1. Call for help for additional hands.
2. Inform blood bank activating massive transfusion protocol.
3. Confirm a designated runner who runs to the blood bank and awaits blood products.
4. Inform trauma surgeon.
5. Inform radiologist for radiology and intervention.
6. Confirm readiness of the operating room and radiology suite with staff availability.

Control Bleeding

An exsanguinating patient will not become stable until the bleeding has been stopped, which depends upon the control of the bleeding as well as treatment of coagulopathy. The history, mechanism of trauma and imaging are very decisive in the management of the source. There are two types of haemorrhage: compressible and non-compressible. Compressible occurs when the haemorrhage is in an accessible area to allow pressure application, whereas non-compressible is not accessible to direct pressure. Apply pressure to the compressible bleeding site, while looking for non-compressible haemorrhage. Perform extended focused assessment sonography for trauma (eFAST) for evaluation of potential spaces of haemorrhage, such as pleural, pericardial, abdominal and pelvic space. The trauma surgeon should rapidly decide (less than 10 min) regarding the further disposition for definitive control of bleeding (operating theatre, interventional radiology, computed tomography).

Charge Code Crimson Pack

- Code Crimson Pack A
  - Request Code Crimson Pack A (4 units RBC, 4 units FFP); transfuse 2 units RBC and 2 units plasma preoperatively.
  - Start with Code Crimson A initially.
- Code Crimson Pack B
  - If the bleeding continues, ask for Code Crimson Pack B (6 units RBC, 6 units FFP, 2 cryoprecipitates, 1 pool platelets).
  - Use O negative RBC units in females or O positive RBC units in males.
  - Use group-specific blood as soon as possible.

A complete crossmatching process takes 45 minutes to 1 hour. It is sometimes very difficult to wait in emergencies where type-specific blood can be requested with informed consent and it is a life-saving measure. However, in emergency situations like Code Crimson, uncrossed matched packs are asked for.

The adjuncts are continued along with preparedness and can be remembered by mnemonic, as mentioned in Table 9.2.

Conserve Temperature

Prevention of hypothermia is always better than treating hypothermia, as it takes considerable time to increase body temperature with passive and active external methods. Ensure warm crystalloids, use of a fluid warmer and covering the patient to prevent hypothermia.

Check Coagulopathy

- The point to emphasize is the importance of viscoelastic measurement of coagulopathy, which no doubt depicts the pathology as well as the components to be replaced to treat coagulopathy. Thrombelastography, ROTEM and Sonoclot are well-established methods to assess coagulopathy.
- Anticipate ongoing requirement for Pack B until bleeding is controlled. Request early; don't wait until the previous pack is finished. Give in sequential packs, keeping in view active haemorrhage control.
- Avoid crystalloids/colloids until acid–base balance and base deficit are corrected.
- Keep K+ less than 5.5.
- Keep ionized serum Ca++ > 1.0 mEq/L.
- Check blood glucose.

Table 9.2: Steps and Adjuncts to Code Crimson

T **Tranexamic acid**	15 mg/kg bolus (max 1g) followed by 2 mg/kg/hr over 8 hours
R **Resuscitation**	Rapid infusion of products Code Crimson Pack A Code Crimson Pack B
A **Avoid**	Avoid hypothermia Avoid vasoconstrictors
U **If unstable?**	Prepare for damage-control surgery
M **Metabolic**	Avoid acidosis Administer calcium
A **Assess**	Imaging Investigations, coagulation especially

Catch Up on Early Targets

- Control of bleeding
- Systolic blood pressure of 90 mmHg
- Heart rate < 120/min
- Haematocrit > 25%
- Lactate: decreasing trend as compared to the initial presentation
- Base deficit: decreasing deficit as compared to the initial presentation
- Blood gas analysis: no respiratory acidosis; metabolic acidosis not severe and not worsening
- Capillary refill time < 2 seconds
- Euthermia maintained
- Urine output > 0.5 ml/kg/min

Clinical resuscitation continues until caught up on deficit. Avoid excessive crystalloids. Consider noradrenaline infusion once blood loss is controlled and fully caught up.

Call Off the Code

Once bleeding is controlled and targets are achieved, step down Code Crimson, return unused products to blood bank to inform that code has been called off.

Complications and Postcode Management

Manage complications and keep the targets as

- No bleeding
- Systolic blood pressure 100 mmHg or within normal limits
- Heart rate < 100/min
- Haematocrit > 20%
- Lactate: normal
- Base deficit: normal
- Euthermia maintained
- Urine output > 0.5 ml/kg/min

Post-stabilization care of the patient should be in an intensive care unit or high dependency unit.

CONCLUSION AND ACKNOWLEDGEMENTS

A careful and systematic approach to the bleeding and unstable patient can help medical professionals to hold their nerves and manage the case efficiently. This material has drawn inspiration from Advanced Trauma Life Support, European Resuscitation Council and ATACC Royal College of Surgeons.

SUGGESTED READING

1. American College of Surgeons. *Advanced Trauma Life Support: Student Course Manual.* Chicago, IL: American College of Surgeons; 2018.
2. Mallinson, Tom. Anaesthesia Trauma and Critical Care (ATACC) course. *Journal of Paramedic Practice.* 2012;4:362–64.
3. Soar J, Perkins GD, Abbas G, et al. European Resuscitation Council Guidelines for Resuscitation 2010 Section 8. Cardiac arrest in special circumstances: electrolyte abnormalities, poisoning, drowning, accidental hypothermia, hyperthermia, asthma, anaphylaxis, cardiac surgery, trauma, pregnancy, electrocution. *Resuscitation.* 2010;81(10):1400–33.

10 Traumatic Cardiac Arrest

Bisman Jeet Kaur and Nidhi Bhatia

LEARNING OBJECTIVES

- Define traumatic cardiac arrest
- Knowledge of the difference between traumatic and medical cardiac arrest
- Learning the common causes of and management priorities in traumatic cardiac arrest
- Role of conventional cardiopulmonary resuscitation in traumatic cardiac arrest

DEFINITION

Traumatic cardiac arrest (TCA) is agonal or absent spontaneous respiration with absence of carotid pulsations having traumatic origin (in patients of trauma).

It is important to differentiate TCA from medical cardiac arrest (see Table 10.1).

Common Causes of TCA

- Haemorrhage (60%)
- Tension pneumothorax (33%)
- Cardiac tamponade (10%)
- Hypoxia/airway obstruction (7%)

Common Initial Rhythm Associated with TCA

- Pulseless electrical activity (PEA): 66%
- Asystole: 30%
- Ventricular fibrillation: 6%

It is important to differentiate patients with true mechanical cardiac standstill (classical PEA or asystole) from those with cardiac motion but impalpable pulses due to profound hypotension (pseudo-PEA).

MANAGEMENT PRIORITY IN TCA

Controlling haemorrhage, restoring the circulating blood volume, managing the airway and relieving hypoxia are a priority over conventional cardiopulmonary resuscitation (CPR) during the management of TCA. These priorities should be met quickly, followed by (or together with) initiation of conventional CPR. The reversible causes of TCA should be treated first (Table 10.2).

Hypovolaemia

The treatment of severe hypovolaemic shock is multifaceted and involves simultaneous employment of measures to control bleeding and resuscitation. The primary goal is to achieve early haemostasis.

Stop the bleeding. External haemorrhage should be treated with direct or indirect compression. Non-compressible haemorrhage should be addressed with application of a tourniquet, splinting of long bone and pelvic fracture, and packing of wounds with haemostatic dressing.

Intravenous or interosseous access. Intravenous or interosseous access should be established as soon as any trauma patient is received. Ideally at least two wide-bore 18G or 16G cannula should be secured while resuscitating a patient with traumatic cardiac arrest.

Interosseous access can be secured rapidly and safely in patients where peripheral access is difficult. The preferred site for insertion are the humeral head or medial aspect of the tibia on the non-affected limb for rapid administration of fluid.

Central venous access can be secured once the patient is stabilized, using the Seldinger technique in either the internal jugular vein, subclavian vein or femoral vein.

Fluid resuscitation. If hypovolaemia is the cause of TCA, an initial bolus of 20 ml/kg of crystalloid solution (preferably warm) should be given, followed by early administration of blood and blood products (fresh frozen plasma, platelets, cryoprecipitates). The blood bank should be alerted of the same, and the massive blood transfusion protocol should be activated. Placement of a resuscitative endovascular balloon occlusion of the aorta (REBOA) or clamping of the descending aorta can be considered for below diaphragm bleeding, but this requires expertise and a well-equipped operating room.

Hypoxia

Hypoxia in TCA can be due to airway trauma, airway obstruction, asphyxia, ventilatory failure or loss of consciousness. Adequate oxygenation and ventilation should be maintained by using basic or advanced methods of securing the airway. The basic head tilt and chin lift or jaw thrust (in patients with cervical spine injury) can be used to maintain patency of the airway. Definitive methods for securing the airway include endotracheal intubation. If airway trauma is present, an emergency tracheostomy

DOI: 10.1201/9781003291619-12

Table 10.1: Difference between TCA and Medical (Non-traumatic) Cardiac Arrest

- In medical cardiac arrest, there is an underlying primary cardiac disease.
- In TCA, clinicians are frequently confronted by a healthy heart that has arrested due to haemorrhage, hypoxia or obstructive shock, so management priorities are different.
- Patients with medical cardiac arrest are mostly euvolaemic, whereas patients with TCA are commonly hypovolaemic from blood loss.

Table 10.2: Reversible Causes of TCA

- Hypovolaemia: rapid infusion of blood and blood products; damage control resuscitation
- Hypoxia: oxygenate
- Tension pneumothorax: decompress chest
- Pericardial tamponade: decompress tamponade

or tube cricothyroidotomy should be considered for securing the airway.

Positive pressure ventilation can have detrimental effects in patients with hypovolaemia by decreasing the venous return, hence fluid resuscitation should be done continuously.

Tension Pneumothorax

Tension pneumothorax develops when a "one-way valve" air leak occurs from the lung or through the chest wall. Tension pneumothorax is a clinical diagnosis, and treatment should not be delayed for want of radiological confirmation. Bilateral decompression of the chest should be considered in patients of TCA with suspected/confirmed tension pneumothorax, along with simultaneous resuscitation measures. A bilateral finger/tube thoracostomy can be done in the fourth or fifth intercostal space in the mid-axillary line. Bilateral thoracostomies have shown better results in comparison to needle decompression.

Pericardial Tamponade

The commonest cause of pericardial tamponade is penetrating injury and requires immediate resuscitative thoracotomy via the clamshell technique or anterolateral approach. The important prerequisites for resuscitative thoracotomy are:

- Availability of an expert team in operating theatres that is well equipped to deal with the intraoperative findings
- Time elapse between TCA and thoracotomy of no more than 15 minutes

Resuscitative thoracotomy can:

- Release tension pneumothorax or cardiac tamponade
- Allow direct control of intrathoracic haemorrhage
- Allow cross-clamping the descending aorta (in so doing, stopping blood loss below the diaphragm and improving brain and cardiac perfusion)
- Permit open cardiac compression and defibrillation

Needle pericardiocentesis is not the ideal choice for decompressing the pericardium in trauma patients since the myocardial injury is not addressed and the clotted blood cannot be aspirated. However, in blunt trauma involving complex pathology, pericardiocentesis may be a reasonable intermediate step. If this is not followed by return of spontaneous circulation, an immediate thoracotomy should be done.

Favourable Prognostic Signs

- Short duration of TCA (< 10 minutes)
- Presence of cardiac contractility on point-of-care ultrasonography
- Presence of vital signs, organized electrical activity, and spontaneous movements at any time since first medical contact

ROLE OF CHEST COMPRESSIONS

The role of chest compressions in patients with traumatic cardiac arrest is highly debatable. External chest compressions deliver approximately one-third of the blood flow to the brain in non-TCA patients and rely on adequate venous return. However, the presence of hypovolaemia, tension pneumothorax and cardiac tamponade severely impedes venous return and significantly reduces the effectiveness of chest compressions. Furthermore, in the presence of significant thoracic trauma, chest compressions could theoretically exacerbate underlying parenchymal injuries. Given these concerns, consideration should be given to delaying compressions until preload and obstructive causes have been addressed. Hence chest compressions should be started after ensuring airway patency and instituting measures to restore circulating blood volume, giving fluids and blood products or decompression of the chest if required. If there is cardiac arrest during resuscitative thoracotomy, then internal cardiac compressions are preferred to external compressions.

ADRENALINE USE IN TCA

There is little evidence for or against the use of adrenaline in cardiac arrest due to trauma.

During hypovolaemic cardiac arrest, patient deterioration is associated with maximal catecholamine release and vasoconstriction. Thus, it is believed that giving patients vasopressors may worsen tissue perfusion. Further, epinephrine may adversely affect cerebral microvascular blood flow and may worsen cerebral ischaemia. Thus, combined with the fact that

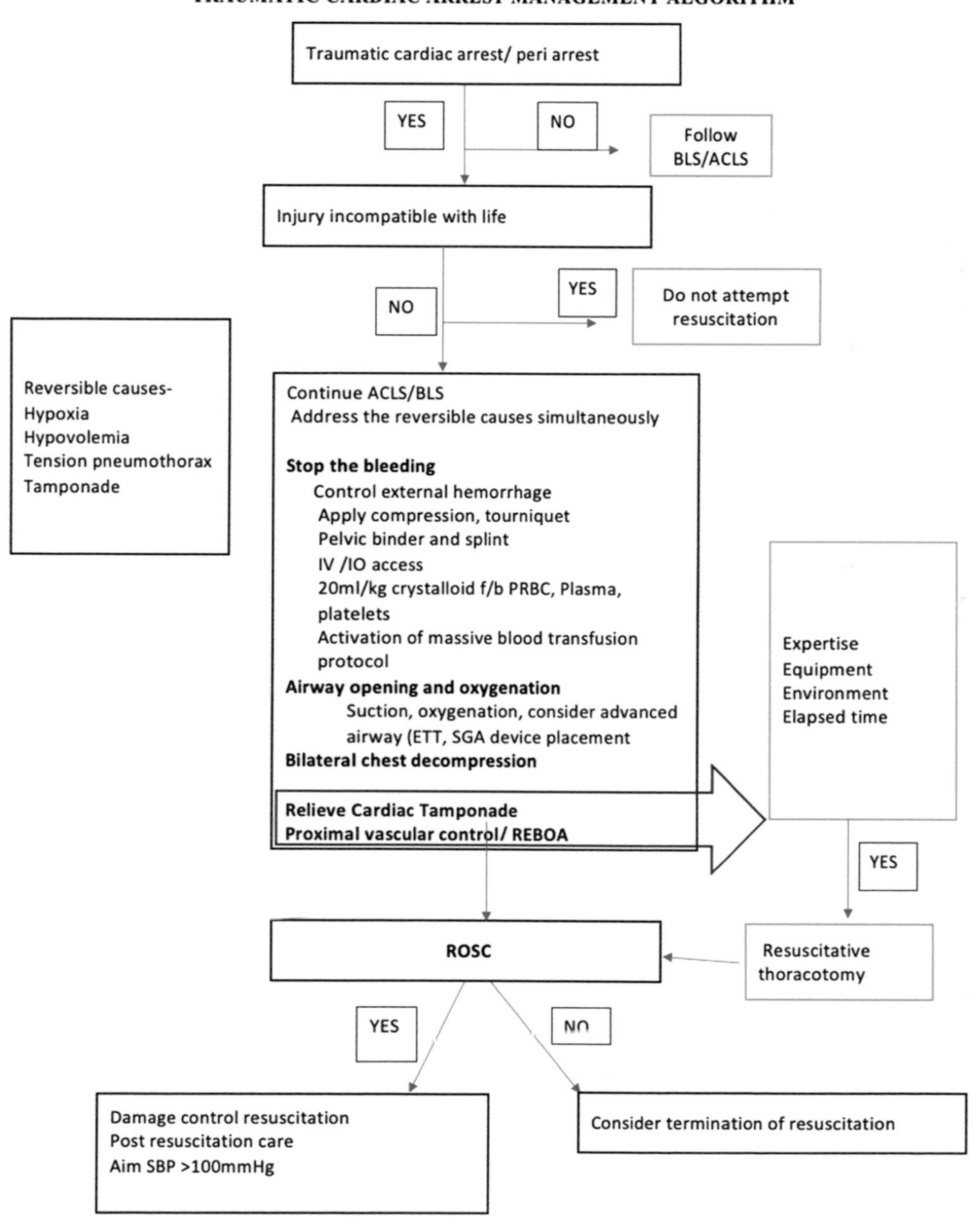

Figure 10.1 Traumatic cardiac arrest management algorithm

hypovolaemic TCA patients are already hypoperfused, severely acidaemic and maximally vasoconstricted, the role of epinephrine may be limited in this setting.

ROLE OF CONVENTIONAL CPR

Basic and Advanced Cardiac Life Support (BLS/ACLS) can occur simultaneously, provided they do not interfere with the interventions essential to manage the reversible causes of TCA. It is important to keep in mind that CPR will not be of much benefit until circulating volume is restored. Some patients may also present with medical causes of cardiac arrest. This should be considered when the mechanism of injury and the injury are not severe enough to directly attribute to cardiac arrest. In all patients with TCA, after addressing the aforementioned causes, assessment for the "4 H's and 4 T's" (hypoxia, hypovolaemia, hyper-/hypokalaemia, hypo-/hyperthermia and metabolic disorders; tension pneumothorax, tamponade, thrombosis and toxins) should be addressed and ruled out simultaneously.

WITHHOLDING RESUSCITATION EFFORTS

There are certain indications for withholding resuscitation in patients of TCA:

- Injuries that are incompatible with life, like decapitation or hemicorporectomy
- No signs of life in the preceding 15 minutes
- Signs of prolonged cardiac arrest (dependent lividity, rigor mortis)

INDICATIONS TO STOP RESUSCITATION

Cessation of resuscitative efforts must be considered in patients who are not responding to interventions, have no return of spontaneous circulation even after the reversible causes have been addressed and have no detectable cardiac activity on eFAST (extended focused assessment sonography for trauma).

The sequence of steps that should be followed while managing TCA are depicted in Figure 10.1.

CONCLUSION

- TCA is different from medical (non-traumatic) cardiac arrest.
- The most common causes of TCA are haemorrhage, tension pneumothorax, cardiac tamponade and hypoxia.
- Controlling haemorrhage, restoring blood volume, managing airway and relieving tension pneumothorax, and relieving cardiac tamponade are a priority over conventional CPR during the management of TCA.
- BLS/ACLS can occur simultaneously, provided it does not interfere with the interventions essential to manage the reversible causes of TCA.

SUGGESTED READING

1. Zwingmann J, Mehlhorn AT, Hammer T, et al. Survival and neurologic outcome after traumatic out-of-hospital cardiopulmonary arrest in a pediatric and adult population: a systematic review [Internet]. 2012 [cited 2021 May 27]. Available from: http://ccforum.com/content/16/4/R117.
2. Khalifa A, Avraham JB, Kramer KZ, et al. Surviving traumatic cardiac arrest: identification of factors associated with survival. *American Journal of Emergency Medicine*. 2021;43:83–7.
3. Huber-Wagner S, Lefering R, Qvick M, et al. Outcome in 757 severely injured patients with traumatic cardiorespiratory arrest. Working Group on Polytrauma of the German Trauma Society (DGU) 1. *Resuscitation*. 2007;75:276–85.
4. Kleber C, Giesecke MT, Lindner T, Haas NP, Buschmann CT. Requirement for a structured algorithm in cardiac arrest following major trauma: epidemiology, management errors, and preventability of traumatic deaths in Berlin. *Resuscitation*. 2014;85:405–10.
5. Millin M. Termination of resuscitation for adult traumatic cardiopulmonary arrest. *Prehospital Emergency Care* [Internet]. 2012 [cited 2021 May 29];16(4):571. Available from: https://www.tandfonline.com/action/journalInformation?journalCode=ipec20.
6. Mattox KL, Feliciano D. Role of external cardiac compression in truncal trauma. *Journal of Trauma: Injury, Infection and Critical Care* [Internet]. 1982 [cited 2021 Jun 1];22(11):934–6. Available from: https://pubmed.ncbi.nlm.nih.gov/7143499/.
7. Watts S, Smith JE, Gwyther R, Kirkman E. Closed chest compressions reduce survival in an animal model of haemorrhage-induced traumatic cardiac arrest. *Resuscitation* [Internet]. 2019 Jul 1 [cited 2021 Jun 1];140:37–42. Available from: https://pubmed.ncbi.nlm.nih.gov/31077754/.

8. Endo A, Kojima M, Hong ZJ, Otomo Y, Coimbra R. Open-chest versus closed-chest cardiopulmonary resuscitation in trauma patients with signs of life upon hospital arrival: a retrospective multicenter study. *Critical Care* [Internet]. 2020 Sep 1 [cited 2021 Jun 1];24(1):1–9. Available from: https://doi.org/10.1186/s13054-020-03259-w.

9. Lott C, Truhlář A, Alfonzo A, et al. European resuscitation council guidelines 2021: cardiac arrest in special circumstances. *Resuscitation*. 2021 Apr 1;161:152–219.

10. Aoki M, Abe T, Oshima K. Association of prehospital epinephrine administration with survival among patients with traumatic cardiac arrest caused by traffic collisions OPEN. Available from: www.nature.com/scientificreports.

11 Airway Management in Trauma Bay

Anudeep Jafra

LEARNING OBJECTIVES

- Identify clinical situations with airway compromise
- Recognize signs and symptoms of acute airway obstruction
- Recognize signs of inadequate ventilation
- Techniques to maintain and establish a patent airway
- Definitive airway management
- Drug-assisted intubation
- Rapid sequence intubation versus delayed sequence intubation
- Steps of oxygenation before attempting to secure a definitive airway

INTRODUCTION

Hypoxia and airway obstruction remain significant contributors to death following trauma. Approximately 7%–28% of trauma victims require definitive airway management. Literature suggests a high incidence of peri-intubation hypoxia and hypotension in emergency intubations in head injury victims.

The incidence of cervical spine injury is 2% in general trauma victims, whereas it is 6%–8% in patients with head and maxillofacial injuries. Immobilization of the cervical spine is recommended for any trauma victim unless proven.

PRIMARY SURVEY (ABCDE)

For any trauma victim wheeled in, a quick primary survey is required to recognize life-threatening scenarios (Table 11.1).

Airway Assessment of Trauma Victim

1. A responsive and talking patient reassures the airway patency. Failure to respond or talk suggests hypoxemia or brain injury.
2. Look for the mental status of patient: obtunded, agitated, cyanosed.
3. Watch out for signs of respiratory difficulty: breathing pattern, use of accessory muscles of respiration.
4. Observe the oral cavity: broken teeth, bone fragments, rolled over tongue, blood, secretions and vomitus.
5. Listen for abnormal breath sounds, stridor, gurgling, snoring or crackles.
6. Inspect and palpate the anterior aspect of the neck for any laceration, hematoma, crepitus, and swelling or deviated trachea.
7. Identify landmarks for cricothyroidotomy.

In the presence of a compromised airway, all patients should receive oxygen supplementation and C-Spine immobilization via a cervical spine collar.

Certain conditions/situations that can threaten the airway in trauma victims include:

- Vomitus – roll patient laterally while stabilizing cervical spine, suction from oral cavity
- Facial fractures – broken teeth, bone fragments, displaced tongue, foreign body, blood clots; remove using Magill forceps
- Midface fractures/maxillofacial injury – can lead to oro- and nasopharynx obstruction
- Mandibular fracture – especially bilateral will lead to loss of support to airway structures which leads to airway obstruction
- Neck trauma/penetrating injury to neck – haematoma, vascular injury, laryngotracheal injury, bleeding into tracheobronchial tree
- Laryngeal trauma – presentation is a classic triad, i.e. hoarseness of voice, subcutaneous emphysema and palpable fracture

Caveat: Noisy breathing suggests partial airway obstruction. Absence of breath sounds suggests complete airway obstruction.

Breathing and Ventilation

A number of conditions can compromise ventilation in trauma victims (Table 11.2). Of these, chest trauma accounts for 20%–25% of trauma-related deaths. Thus, a rapid assessment of oxygenation and ventilation is required. Ultrasonographic eFAST examination is a bedside assessment that may help in immediate diagnoses and management of impaired ventilation.

Objectives signs to determine inadequate ventilation include:

1. Look for asymmetrical rise and fall of chest wall

DOI: 10.1201/9781003291619-13

Table 11.1: Primary Survey in Advanced Trauma Resuscitation Guidelines

Airway assessment and protection, along with cervical spine stabilization
Breathing and ventilation assessment
Circulation assessment and control of haemorrhage
Disability assessment
Exposure

Table 11.2: Conditions Which Compromise Ventilation in Trauma Victims

Blunt trauma chest – pneumothorax, haemothorax, cardiac tamponade, flail chest
Head injury – intracranial injury with abnormal breathing pattern
C-Spine injury – above level of C3, diaphragm dysfunction and abdominal breathing

Table 11.3: Indications for Intubation in Trauma Victims

Need for airway protection (blood, vomitus, secretions)
Low GCS < 8
Severe maxillofacial injury
Neck trauma/laryngotracheal injury
Airway burns
Hypoxaemia (SpO_2 < 90 mmHg) despite oxygen supplementation
Cardiac arrest

2. Listen for breath sounds in bilateral lung fields and all zones
3. Feel for crepitus
4. Use of pulse oximetry and capnography

Table 11.3 enumerates the conditions that necessitate intubation in trauma victims.

AIRWAY ASSESSMENT OF TRAUMA VICTIMS

For all trauma victims requiring an airway intervention, a quick history and airway assessment is required. History can be obtained using a pneumonic SAMPLE (Table 11.4) and airway assessment can be done quickly using LEMON and BONES (Tables 11.5 and 11.6, respectively). Another modality, a bedside ultrasound scan of the neck, can be done for identification of cricothyroid membrane and tracheal rings for surgical access (Figure 11.1, Table 11.7).

MANOEUVRES TO OPEN THE AIRWAY

After an adequate and quick airway assessment, techniques are employed to open the airway. Two manoeuvres that can be used are the head tilt chin lift and jaw thrust technique (Table 11.8). However, airway adjuncts (oropharyngeal airway and nasopharyngeal airway) can play an important part in maintaining a patent airway (Table 11.9).

Table 11.4: A Quick History (SAMPLE) in Trauma Victims

S	Any signs and symptoms
A	History of any allergies
M	Any medications
P	Significant past medical history
L	Last meal when and what
E	Events prior to the injury

CERVICAL SPINE STABILIZATION

Unless proven otherwise, in all trauma victims keep a high suspicion of C-Spine injury. So, during any airway manoeuvre it is recommended to use manual in-line stabilization (MILS) for preventing aggravation and movement at C-Spine. Correct application of MILS requires immobilization of head and neck, while avoiding immobilization of the mandible. Problems that can be encountered during application of MILS are tabulated in Table 11.10. It is important to remember that videolaryngoscope improves the glottic view, and direct laryngoscopy with use of gum elastic bougie yields better results in the setting of MILS.

PREOXYGENATION

The goals of preoxygenation in the emergency department remain bringing oxygen saturation

Table 11.5: Airway Assessment Tool (LEMON)

L	Look for any faciomaxillary trauma, mandibular displacement, neck trauma, thyromental distance and receding chin
E	Evaluate using 3-3-2 rule: 3 fingers for mouth opening 3 fingers for submandibular space 2 fingers for distance between chin and thyroid notch
M	Mallampati grade ≥2, alert for difficult laryngoscopy and difficult intubation
O	Airway obstruction, fixed or dynamic or burns
N	Neck mobility, presence of halo frame or cervical collar

≥2 parameters: Alert for difficult mask ventilation.

Table 11.6: Airway Assessment Tool (BONES)

B	Presence of beard
O	Obese (BMI > 26 kg/m²)
N	No teeth (edentulous)
E	Elderly patient (age > 55 years)
S	Snoring

levels close to 100% and denitrogenation before attempting intubation.

Techniques of preoxygenation/paraoxygenation include:

1. Use of non-rebreather mask – provides 80%–90% FiO_2
2. Bag valve mask device – provides nearly 90% FiO_2
3. Use of nasal cannula or prongs to supply high flow oxygen 15 L/min – increases safe apnoea time

Patient position: A 20-degree head-up position during preoxygenation, and in case of cervical spine injury, a possibly reverse Trendelenburg position improves the oxygenation levels.

DEFINITIVE AIRWAY MANAGEMENT TECHNIQUES

A definitive airway can be achieved either by endotracheal intubation or through surgical access.

Endotracheal Intubation

The various techniques of securing the airway through endotracheal intubation include:

- Direct laryngoscopy and intubation
- Videolaryngoscope-guided intubation
- Flexible fibre-optic intubation
- Lightwand-guided intubation
- Intubating laryngeal mask airway–guided intubation
- Retrograde intubation
- Blind nasal intubation

The technique of choice for intubation remains direct laryngoscopy due to the vast experience of using the modality in all sorts of scenarios. Vision is usually not hampered during securing the airway, and a direct laryngoscope is robust enough

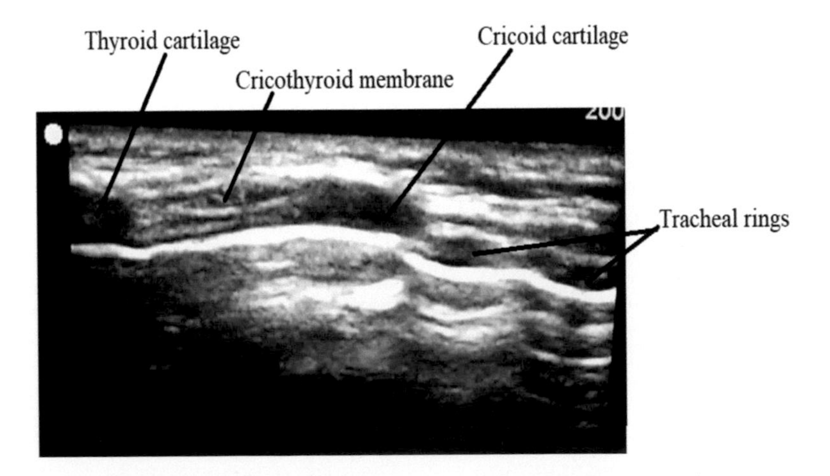

Figure 11.1 Neck scan to demonstrate cricothyroid membrane and tracheal rings

Table 11.7: Ultrasound Application in Trauma Critical Care (FAST ABC)

A	B	C
Airway Cervical USG	Breathing and Ventilation Lung scan	Circulation ECHO
⇩	⇩	⇩
Patency of airway	Lung fields Pneumothorax Presence of fluid Atelectasis Diaphragmatic movement Fractures	Cardiac tamponade
⇩	⇩	⇩
Subcutaneous emphysema Haematoma Tracheal injury/deviation USG stomach	Guide to management of intervention and ventilation	Pericardiocentesis
⇩		
Guide to definitive airway management		

Table 11.8: Manoeuvres to Open Airway

Head Tilt Chin Lift	Jaw Thrust
• Gentle placement of one hand on the head to stabilize it and tilt it a little. • With other hand, chin is brought forward to open airway and relieve obstruction. • Caution to be exercised in patients with suspected C-Spine injury.	With two hands, lower jaw is brought in front of upper jaw, to open and maintain the airway. Preferred technique in suspected C-Spine injury, as there is minimal movement at level of cervical spine.

Table 11.9: Use of Airway Adjuncts

Nasopharyngeal Airway (NPA)	Oropharyngeal Airway (OPA)
• Can be used in a conscious or semiconscious patient • Passed into posterior oropharynx • Size determination – tip of nose to tragus • Contraindicated with base of skull fractures	• Can be used in semiconscious or unconscious patient (results in gag reflex in conscious patient) • Size determination – angle of mouth to angle of mandible • Can suction through it, acts as a bite block

Table 11.10: Problems Encountered When Using MILS

- MILS worsens the glottic view obtained by direct laryngoscopy in 50% cases.
- MILS, along with cricoid pressure, increases CL grade to III in 20% cases.
- MILS application results in greater force application during laryngoscopy.

to handle the tissue and an agitated patient during laryngoscopy. A gentle direct laryngoscopy and intubation with manual in-line stabilization does not aggravate C-Spine injury.

Videolaryngoscopes have shown to have better success rates for securing an airway in trauma settings. They can be used as a teaching aid and act as feedback devices for the assistant applying the external laryngeal manipulation during intubation.

The incidence of unanticipated difficult intubation in the emergency department ranges from 3% to 5.3%, and that of failed intubation is 0.5%–1.2%. The existing difficult airway guidelines are not suitable for trauma victims, as there does not stand an option of awakening the patient. Hence, a backup in the form of surgical airway access should be sought.

Drug-Assisted Intubation

Drug-assisted intubation is required in the cases of awake patients with intact gag reflex and agitated patients. Commonly used drugs are enumerated in Table 11.11.

Table 11.11: Commonly Used Induction and Paralytic Agents in Trauma Victims

Induction Agent	Dosage
Thiopentone	3–5 mg/kg
Etomidate	0.3 mg/kg
Ketamine	1–2 mg/kg
Paralytic Agent	**Dosage**
Succinylcholine	1.5–2 mg/kg
Rocuronium	0.6–1.2 mg/kg

Rapid Sequence Intubation (RSI)

RSI is a preferred method for intubation in the emergency department and especially in agitated patients. It is a near-simultaneous administration of a sedative and hypnotic agent followed by a paralytic agent for intubation (Figure 11.2). However, use of RSI before adequate resuscitation may lead to more episodes of post-intubation instability in the form of hypercarbia, hypoxaemia and hypotension. Hence a preferred method in such scenarios is delayed sequence intubation (DSI). This technique, first described by Weingart et al., utilizes ketamine in a dissociative dose (Table 11.12).

DSI allays anxiety, allows airway manipulation and allows adequate preoxygenation while maintaining airway reflexes.

Cricoid Pressure (CP)

To date no studies have validated the role of CP in the emergency department. CP can itself lead to increased airway obstruction via increasing peak airway pressures and decreasing tidal volume.

Surgical Airway Access

Surgical airway access can be achieved through:

- Percutaneous tracheostomy
- Cricothyroidotomy
- Surgical tracheostomy

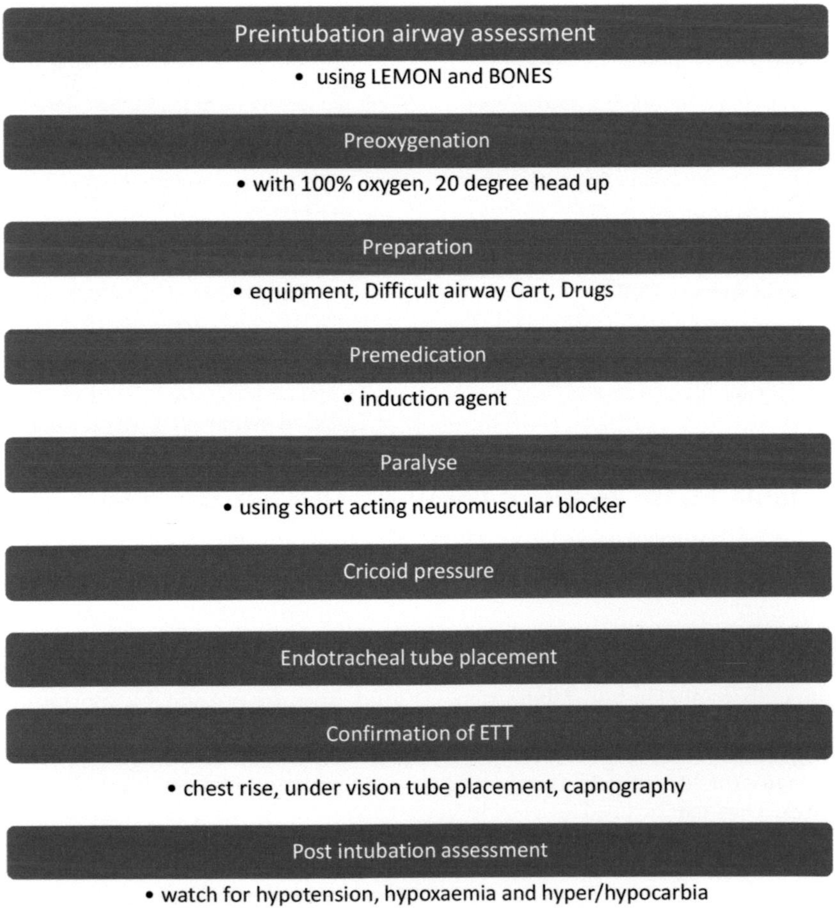

Preintubation airway assessment
- using LEMON and BONES

Preoxygenation
- with 100% oxygen, 20 degree head up

Preparation
- equipment, Difficult airway Cart, Drugs

Premedication
- induction agent

Paralyse
- using short acting neuromuscular blocker

Cricoid pressure

Endotracheal tube placement

Confirmation of ETT
- chest rise, under vision tube placement, capnography

Post intubation assessment
- watch for hypotension, hypoxaemia and hyper/hypocarbia

Figure 11.2 Steps of rapid sequence intubation

Table 11.12: Rapid Sequence Intubation versus Delayed Sequence Intubation

Rapid Sequence Intubation

3 minutes of preoxygenation

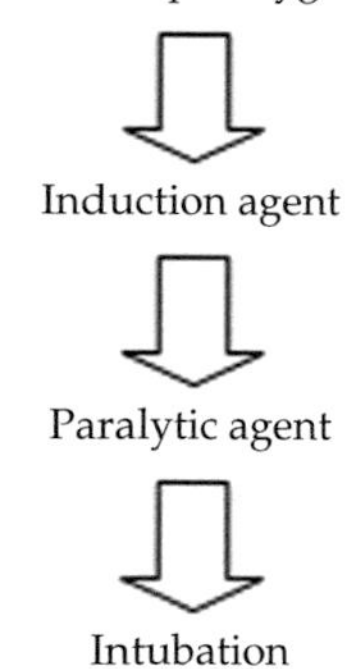

Induction agent

Paralytic agent

Intubation

Delayed Sequence Intubation

Dissociative dose of ketamine (0.5 mg/kg)

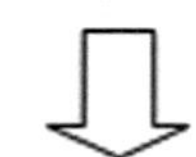

3 minutes of preoxygenation

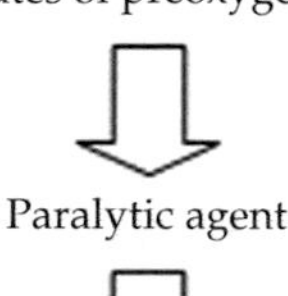

Paralytic agent

Intubation

Table 11.13: Indications for Surgical Airway Access

- Failed multiple attempts at intubation
- Cannot ventilate, cannot intubate
- Laryngotracheal injury
- Severe glottic oedema or haematoma
- Severe oropharyngeal bleeding

Table 11.13 depicts the indications for surgical airway access.

Surgical cricothyroidotomy is preferred to tracheostomy for most patients who need an immediate airway access, as it is easier to perform and minimal. But in scenarios where there is limited expertise and the patient requires airway access for a longer duration, a tracheostomy is preferred. The incidence of cricothyroidotomy in the emergency department ranges from 0.3% to 12.4%. The steps of cricothyroidotomy are depicted in Table 11.14.

AIRWAY MANAGEMENT SCHEME AND CHECKLIST

The management scheme that needs to be followed while managing a basic airway and an unanticipated difficult airway are depicted in Figures 11.3 and 11.4, respectively. It is important to keep at hand a checklist for equipment required for intubation in the trauma bay (Table 11.15, Figure 11.5).

MINIMUM MONITORING IN EMERGENCY DEPARTMENT

The minimum monitoring required for emergency department patients includes electrocardiography, non-invasive blood pressure, temperature monitoring and pulse oximetry, along with capnometry.

PROBLEMS ENCOUNTERED IN TRAUMA BAY DURING OR AFTER EMERGENCY AIRWAY MANAGEMENT

1. Failure to adequately assess the airway
2. Failure to recognize need for intervening and securing the airway
3. Failure to recognize need for ventilation and maintenance of oxygenation
4. Failure to establish a clear and patent airway
5. Failure to recognize the displacement of already placed airway device
6. Regurgitation or aspiration of gastric contents
7. Failure to recognize the need for alternative modality to secure airway in case of repeated failed attempts at intubation

These problems, leading to mismanagement, could be due to various reasons:

A. Environmental factors
   1. Unfavourable conditions – darkness, inadequate space, limited access to patient's airway
   2. Faulty patient positioning
   3. Assistants with different levels of training for managing airways
   4. Odd times

Table 11.14: Steps of Cricothyroidotomy

Try to keep patient conscious and on spontaneous ventilation
For sedation intravenous midazolam 0.1 mg/kg can be given

Avoid overextension of neck

Disinfect and prepare (local anaesthetic with epinephrine for analgesia and haemostasis)

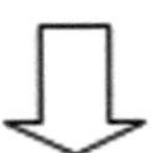

2 cm long vertical incision on skin below the laryngeal prominence

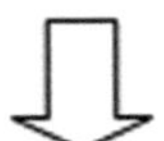

Identify cricothyroid membrane

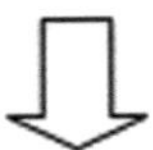

Give a transverse incision on cricothyroid membrane

Insert the tracheostomy or endotracheal tube and inflate

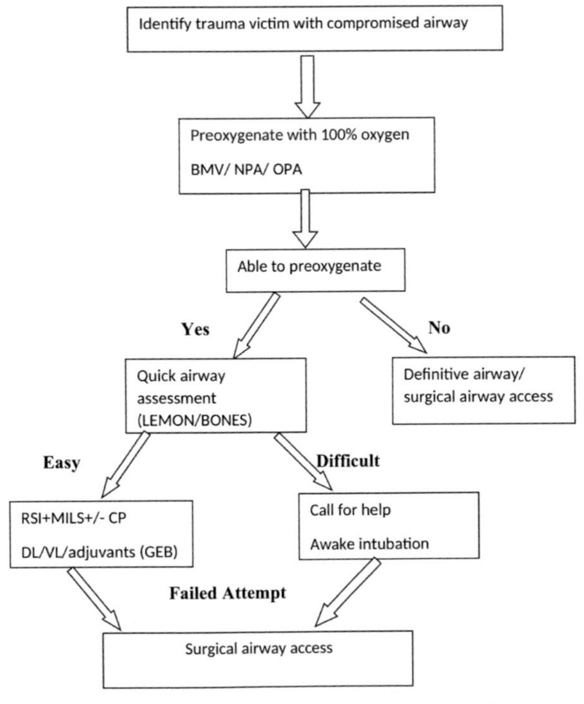

BMV: Bag Mask Ventilation; OPA: Oropharyngeal Airway; NPA: Nasopharyngeal Airway; RSI: Rapid Sequence Intubation; MILS: Manual In-Line Stabilisation; CP: Cricoid Pressure; DL: Direct Laryngoscopy; VL: Videolaryngoscopy; GEB: Gum Elastic Bougie

Figure 11.3 Airway management scheme

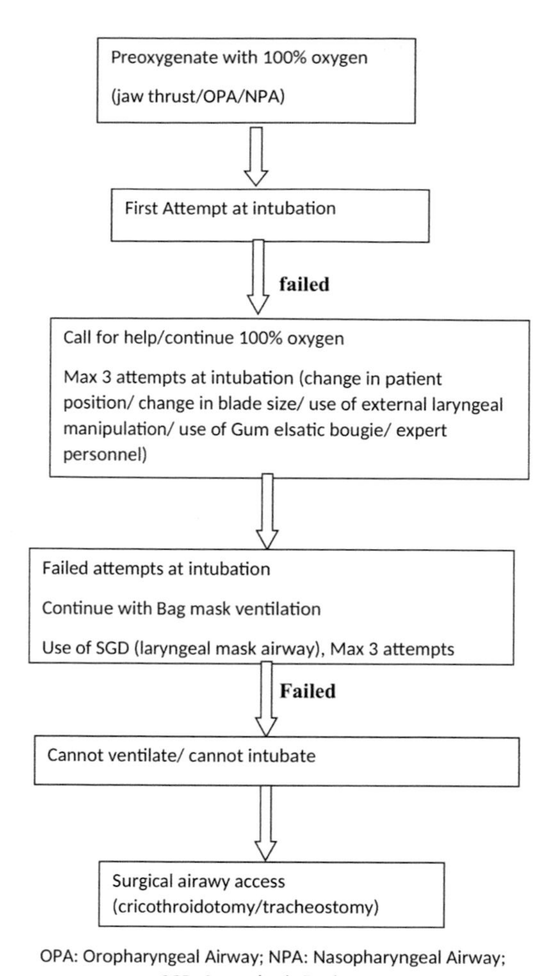

Figure 11.4 Airway management scheme for patients with an unanticipated difficult airway

Table 11.15: Checklist for Airway Management in Trauma Bay

Bag and Mask Device
Working suction
Magill forceps
Face mask
Nasopharyngeal/oropharyngeal airway
Different type of laryngoscope blade
Different size of endotracheal tubes
Laryngeal mask airway
Videolaryngoscope
Bougie
Fibre-optic bronchoscope

B. Patient factors
   1. Blood, secretions and vomitus obscuring the airway
   2. Uncooperative/agitated patient
   3. An immobilized C-Spine
   4. Faulty cricoid pressure
   5. Full stomach of the patient
   6. Volume status of patient

Post-Intubation Complications

Post-intubation complications are defined as events occurring within 30 minutes post-intubation. These include:

- Post-intubation hypotension: mean arterial pressure < 65 mmHg or systolic blood pressure < 90 mmHg; incidence ranges from 23% to 46%
- Hypoxaemia (oxygen saturation < 90%)
- Transient tachycardia, hypertension and arrythmia

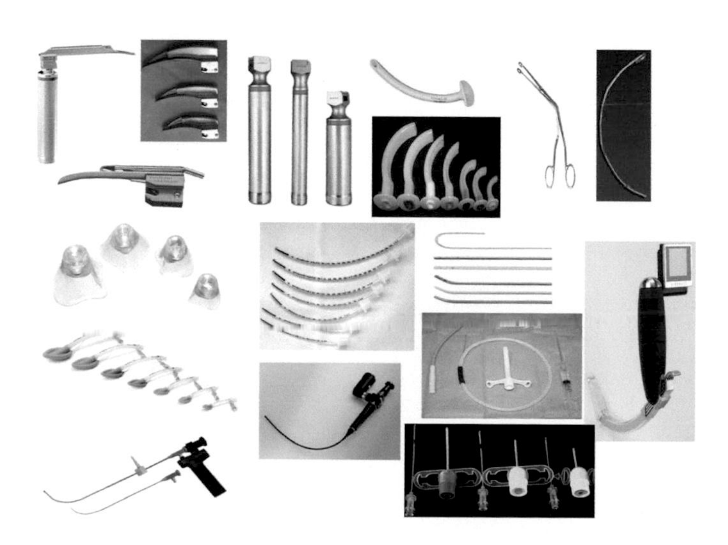

Figure 11.5 Difficult airway cart in trauma bay

- Cardiac arrest
- Vomiting/regurgitation and aspiration of abdominal contents

CONCLUSION

An effective trauma care requires multidisciplinary teamwork. Ensure adequate oxygenation and ventilation. Securing the airway effectively, safely and at the right time will play a significant role in trauma care.

SUGGESTED READING

1. Ollerton JE. *Adult Trauma Clinical Practice Guidelines: Emergency Airway Management in the Trauma Patients.* NSW: NSW Institute of Trauma and Injury Management, North Ryde; 2007.

2. American College of Surgeons. Committee on Trauma. *Advanced Trauma Life Support: Student Course Manual.* Tenth edition. Chicago, IL: American College of Surgeons; 2018.

3. Manoach S, Paladino L. Manual in line stabilization for acute airway management of suspected cervical spine injury: historical review and current questions. *Ann Emerg Med.* 2007;50:236–45.

4. Reed MJ, Rennie LM, Dunn MJ, et al. Is the 'LEMON' method an easily applied emergency airway assessment tool? *Eur J Emerg Med.* 2004;11:154–7.

5. Neri L, Storti E, Lichtenstein D. Toward an ultrasound curriculum for critical care medicine. *Crit Care Med.* 2007;35(Supplement):290–304.

6. Mayglothling J, Duane TM, Gibbs M, et al. Emergency intubation immediately following traumatic injury: an eastern association for the surgery of trauma practice management guideline. *J Trauma Acute Care Surg.* 2012;73(Supplement 4):S333–40.

7. Conroy MJ, Weingart GS, Carlson JN. Impact of checklists on peri intubation care in ED trauma patients. *Am J Emerg Med.* 2014;32:541–4.

8. Weingart SD , Trueger NS, Wong N, et al. Delayed sequence intubation: a prospective observational study. *Ann Emerg Med.* 2015;65:349–55.

9. Weingart SD, Levitan RM. Preoxygenation and prevention of desaturation during emergency airway management. *Ann Emerg Med.* 2012;59:165–75.

10. Vender JS, Szokol JW. Oxygen delivery systems, inhalation therapy, and respiratory therapy. In: Hagberg CA, ed. *Benumof's Airway Management: Principles and Practice.* Second ed. Philadelphia, PA: Mosby; 2007:321–45.

12 Front of Neck Access

Haneesh Thakur and Kajal Jain

LEARNING OBJECTIVES

- Anatomical knowledge for achieving front of neck access (FONA)
- Indications and contraindications of FONA
- Various techniques of achieving FONA
- Equipment required, preparation and steps of the procedure

INTRODUCTION

Airway access through the anterior part of the neck is defined as front of neck access (FONA). Depending upon the access location, it can be technically a tracheostomy or cricothyroidotomy when proceeded through the trachea or cricothyroid membrane, respectively. Technically, a tracheostomy is also front of neck airway access, but it is an elective procedure and not an emergency.

eFONA, or emergency front of neck access, however, is an emergency method of securing the airway through the cricothyroid membrane to facilitate alveolar oxygenation. It is also addressed by the following terms:

- Cric
- Cricothyroidotomy

It is an emergency life-saving procedure aimed at reversing hypoxia, thus preventing neurological, cardiac or life-endangering complications. All healthcare providers who work in emergency and operation theatre settings should be geared with adequate hands-on training and skill for performing front of neck procedures.

INDICATIONS

The main indication for achieving front of neck access is "can't intubate, can't oxygenate". As per the Royal College of Anaesthetists and Difficult Airway Society audit, the incidence of serious airway events is 1 in 22,000 general anaesthesia cases. This method of rescue airway is highlighted in various algorithms, for example:

- UK Difficult Airway Society
- American Society of Anaesthesiologists (ASA)
- Vortex approach (Australia)

CONTRAINDICATIONS

- Inability to identify surface landmarks (thyroid cartilage, cricoid, cricothyroid membrane) due to, e.g., obesity, cervical trauma
- When there are options to easily secure airway through less invasive techniques
- In case of trauma to the area of interest, e.g. laryngeal trauma or laryngotracheal trauma
- Relatively contraindicated in children below 10 years of age because of increased incidence of complications; however, there are reports of lifesaving cricothyroidotomy through surgical technique successfully performed in children
- Airway obstruction distal to subglottis, e.g. tracheal stenosis or transection
- Laryngeal cancer; other than for an extreme airway emergency, avoid a cricothyroidotomy so as not to seed the soft tissue of the neck with cancer cells
- Coagulopathy (other than an emergency)

SURFACE LANDMARKS FOR FONA

The anatomical landmarks for the procedure are thyroid cartilage with laryngeal prominence of the thyroid cartilage/the thyroid notch (Adam's apple). Below the thyroid prominence, the cricoid cartilage ring is easily palpable. Between both cartilages, lies the cricothyroid membrane (CTM), which is the landmark for emergency access. It can be identified by palpation, though there is huge variability in the palpatory method and requires frequent practice. The cricothyroid membrane can also be identified ultrasonographically (Figure 12.1). However, ultrasonographic guidance cannot be advised in an emergency setting.

TECHNIQUE

eFONA can be achieved by various techniques:

- Needle technique
- Surgical technique
- Knife–finger–bougie technique

EQUIPMENT REQUIRED

- 4 × 4 gauze pieces
- Chlorhexidine solution

DOI: 10.1201/9781003291619-14

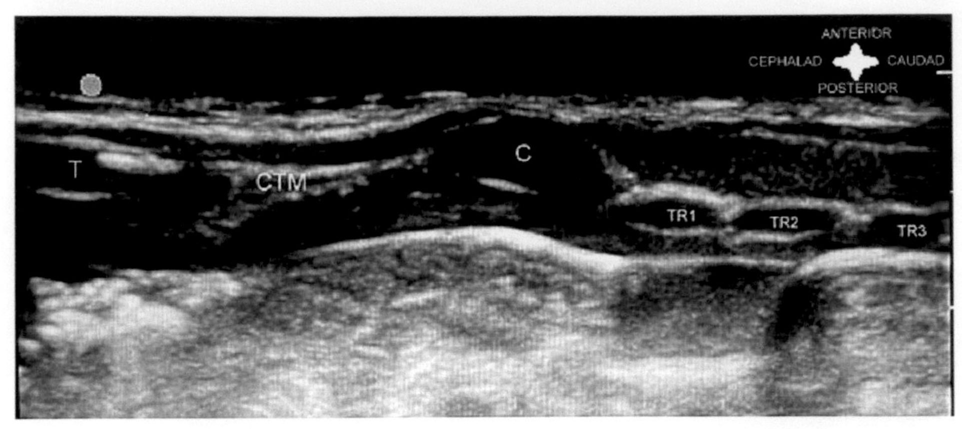

T: Thyroid Cartilage; CTM: Cricothyroid Membrane; C: Cricoid Cartilage; TR: Tracheal Ring

Figure 12.1 Ultrasonographic image depicting the cricothyroid membrane as appreciated with point-of-care ultrasound (POCUS)

- Yankauer suction
- Gum elastic bougie
- 5 cc, 10 cc syringes
- Angiocath/cricothyroid cannula
- #10 blade with a handle
- Cuffed 6.0 size tracheostomy tube or endotracheal tube
- Securement device

Steps

- **Needle technique**
  1. Palpate the neck structures in the midline and identify the thyroid cartilage, cricoid cartilage and cricothyroid membrane in between the two cartilages.
  2. Using a small calibre angiocath and saline-containing syringe, the cricothyroid membrane is punctured at a 45 degree angle in the caudad direction, the airway is confirmed (using aspiration) and the angiocath is inserted percutaneously.
  3. High-pressure oxygen is insufflated into the trachea. The expiration is passive. This technique is known as jet ventilation.
- **Surgical technique**

  The surgical technique differs from other techniques in that in this technique tissue dissection is done.
  1. The patient is positioned with the neck extended. Position yourself as per your surgical ease, either on the right or left shoulder of the patient.
  2. Palpate the structures in the midline. Identify the thyroid and cricoid cartilage, and the cricothyroid membrane in between the two cartilages.
  3. Give a generous vertical incision over the skin on the palpated structures. Fix the larynx in between your fingers of the non-dominant hand.
  4. Tissue dissection should be done till a cricothyroid membrane is identified. The dissection can be done by finger, the handle of the scalpel or Trousseau dilator.
  5. A horizontal incision is made in the midline of the cricothyroid membrane. The lateral part of CTM is thickened and provides resistance to movement of the scalpel. It has a role to protect the vascular structures.
  6. With a tracheal hook inserted horizontally, lift the thyroid cartilage from the caudal end of the cartilage to increase the space between the thyroid and cricoid cartilage.
  7. Insert the cricothyroid cannula with a preloaded dilator in a scooping fashion through the CTM.
  8. Remove the dilator and connect the cannula (which has a 15 mm universal connector) with the ventilating circuit or Ambu.
- **Knife–finger–bougie technique**

  This is one of the most preferred approaches.
  1. Stand by the side of the patient.
  2. With the non-dominant hand, grasp the entire cricothyroid complex and taut the overlying skin. This is known as a laryngeal handshake.
  3. With a #10 scalpel, make a vertical midline incision. The incision should extend

from the middle of the thyroid cartilage to the top of the cricoid cartilage.
4. Perform the laryngeal handshake firmly.
5. With your non-dominant index finger feel the cricothyroid membrane between the thyroid cartilage and the cricoid cartilage.
6. After identifying the cricothyroid membrane using a #10 scalpel, make a horizontal incision past the membrane.
7. Shift the scalpel to a non-dominant hand, and hold it like a shoehorn to make room for the bougie.
8. With the dominant hand, insert a preloaded bougie through the incision into the airway.
9. Rail-road the preloaded endotracheal tube over the bougie. Use an endotracheal tube or tracheostomy tube with an inner diameter no larger than 6.0 mm.
10. Feed the tube over the bougie into the airway. The size of CTM may differ and offer variable resistance to the tube. Depending upon the resistance, variable pressure may be applied.
11. Inflate the cuff as soon as the tube is in the trachea.
12. Confirm the tube placement using an auscultatory method or capnography, and later on with a chest X-ray.

Double Set-Up in the Emergency

A double set-up includes an approach in the anticipated difficult airway in which one person attempts intubation and another person goes ahead with preparations for performing FONA with sterile donning (gown gloves, mask, etc.), identifies and prepares the part, infiltrates the skin with a local anaesthetic and keeps the surgical equipment cart ready. In case of an emergent need, FONA is performed, thus saving time for preparation.

ADVANTAGES OF EMERGENCY CRICOTHYROIDOTOMY

- Provides a definitive airway for ventilating the patient
- Can be performed quickly and has few complications associated with the procedure

DISADVANTAGES OF EMERGENCY CRICOTHYROIDOTOMY

- Has a learning curve
- Humidification of air is bypassed
- Respiratory resistance (with smaller size tube/needle)
- Improper placement of airway may happen
- Can be catastrophic if complicated

COMPLICATIONS

Immediate

1. Injury to the thyroid gland
2. Bleeding
3. False tract
4. Vocal cord injury
5. Subcutaneous emphysema
6. Pneumothorax
7. Pneumomediastinum

Late

1. Dislodgement or blockage of the tube
2. Subglottic stenosis
3. Vocal cord paralysis or paresis
4. Granulation at cuff site
5. Infected stoma
6. Plugging of tube
7. Persistent stoma
8. Difficulty ventilating

CONCLUSION

- eFONA is an emergency procedure that can be life-saving for the patient in case of an unanticipated difficult airway.
- eFONA requires quick presence of mind and expertise in an emergency.
- Understanding and learning this procedure is a pressing need for every healthcare provider.

SUGGESTED READING

1. Onrubia X, Frova G, Sorbello M. Front of neck access to the airway: a narrative review. *Trends Anaesth Crit Care*. 2018;22;45.
2. Greenland KB, Bradley WPL, Chapman GA, et al. Emergency front-of-neck access: scalpel or cannula–and the parable of Buridan's ass†. *BJA: Br J Anaesth*. 2017;118:811–14.
3. Rai Y, You-Ten E, Zasso F, et al. The role of ultrasound in front-of-neck access for cricothyroid membrane identification: a systematic review. *J Crit Care*. 2020;60:161–68.

4. Humble AGR, Phu T, Ryan K. Emergency front of neck access after a can't intubate can't oxygenate scenario in a patient with achondroplasia. *Can Anesth*. 2020;67:779–80.
5. Henderson MA. Front-of-neck access: a practical viewpoint, from experience. *BJA: Br J Anaesth*. 2011;118:468.

13 Shock in Trauma Patients

Jeetinder Kaur Makkar and Mandeep Tundak

LEARNING OBJECTIVES

- Understand the pathophysiology of shock
- Response of body systems to shock
- Management and resuscitation priorities in a trauma patient in shock
- Pathogenesis of trauma-induced coagulopathy

INTRODUCTION

Shock is defined as a failure of the circulatory system to provide adequate organ perfusion to meet the oxygen demand of cellular metabolism. Based on its root cause, shock can be classified into one of four subtypes: hypovolaemic, cardiogenic, obstructive or distributive. Haemorrhage is the most common cause of shock in trauma and accounts for up to 40% of deaths following trauma. Hypovolaemic shock brought on by blood loss is called haemorrhagic shock.

PATHOPHYSIOLOGY

Problem

Imbalance between systemic oxygen delivery and consumption.

Sequalae

1. Haemodynamic instability
2. Coagulopathy
3. Decreased oxygen delivery
4. Decreased tissue perfusion
5. Cellular hypoxia

The initial response is microcirculatory, followed by a microcirculatory response.

Macrocirculatory Response

Changes: release of catecholamines to preserve blood flow to vital organs, i.e. heart, kidney and brain, via vasoconstriction in other regional beds

Mediators: renin, angiotensin, vasopressin, antidiuretic hormone, growth hormone, glucagon, cortisol, epinephrine and norepinephrine

Microcirculatory Response

Ischaemic cells take up interstitial fluid

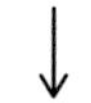

Cellular oedema and depleted intravascular fluid

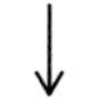

Choking adjacent capillaries

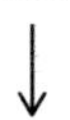

No-reflow phenomenon (prevents reversal of ischaemia even in the presence of adequate macroperfusion)

Ischaemic cells produce lactate, free radicals and inflammatory factors (prostacyclin, thromboxane, prostaglandins, leukotrienes, endothelin, complement, interleukins and tumour necrosis factor), which accumulate in the circulation if perfusion is diminished and directly damage the cells. This bulk of toxic load washes back to the central circulation later. This inflammatory response, once started, becomes a disease process independent of its origin and is responsible for multiple-organ failure and accounts for high mortality rates.

Role for Endothelial Injury in Pathophysiology

Endothelium is one of the "largest" organs in the body with a surface area of up to 5000 m^2. It is anticoagulated by a number of natural anticoagulant systems, including the negatively charged luminal surface layer and the glycocalyx, which is rich in heparinoids and interacts with antithrombin. During shock, the high catecholamine levels directly injure the endothelium, as evidenced by an increase in *syndecan-1 levels*, a marker of endothelial glycocalyx degradation. This leads to glycocalyx shedding, breakdown of tight junctions with capillary leakage, and a pro-coagulant microvasculature, which reduces oxygen delivery due to the increased tissue and microvascular thrombosis.

DOI: 10.1201/9781003291619-15

RESPONSE OF SPECIFIC SYSTEMS

Central Nervous System

1. *Prime trigger* of neuroendocrine response.
2. Maintains perfusion to vital organs.
3. Reflexes and cortical electrical activity are both depressed.
4. Response to shock is reversible with mild hypoperfusion but becomes permanent with prolonged ischaemia.
5. *Failure to recover preinjury neurologic function is a marker for a poor prognosis.*

Kidneys and Adrenal Glands

1. *Prime responders* to neuroendocrine changes.
2. Produce renin, angiotensin, aldosterone, cortisol, erythropoietin and catecholamines.
3. Maintain glomerular filtration by vasoconstriction and concentration of blood flow in the medulla and deep cortical area.

Heart

1. Preserved from ischaemia during shock.
2. Lactate, free radicals and other humoral factors released act as negative inotropes.
3. A fixed stroke volume inhibits the body's ability to increase blood flow in response to hypovolaemia and anaemia, leaving tachycardia as the only option with potentially disastrous consequences on the oxygen supply–demand balance.
4. Therefore, shock in older patients may be rapidly progressive and doesn't respond predictably to fluid.

Lungs

1. Immune complex and cellular factors accumulate in pulmonary capillaries.
2. This leads to neutrophil and platelet aggregation, increased capillary permeability, destruction of lung architecture and, finally, acute respiratory distress syndrome.
3. They act as the sentinel organ for the development of multiple-organ dysfunction.

Gut

1. Earliest organ affected.
2. Intense vasoconstriction occurs early, leading to a no-reflow phenomenon.
3. Breakdown of gut barrier function causes increased translocation of bacteria to liver and lung.

Liver

1. Suffers reperfusion injury during recovery.
2. Failure of synthetic function after shock is almost always lethal.

Skeletal Muscles

1. They are not metabolically active during shock and thus tolerate ischaemia better.
2. They act as an important source in generation of lactic acid and free radicals.
3. Sustained ischaemia of muscle cells leads to an increase in intracellular sodium and free water, thus causing intravascular depletion.

TRAUMA-INDUCED COAGULOPATHY (TIC)

TIC is the multifactorial, global failure of the coagulation system to sustain adequate haemostasis following haemorrhage. It can manifest as a spectrum of phenotypes from hypocoagulation to hypercoagulation due to interaction of several factors including (but not limited to) tissue injury, presence of shock and time from injury. Understanding of the pathogenesis is based on the concept of the cell-based model of coagulation. This model emphasizes the role of platelets as a platform for clotting factor assembly. Interaction with the endothelium results in thrombin generation and incorporation of fibrin to form a haemostatic plug. There are several hypotheses on the driving mechanisms of tissue injury and shock:

(1) Both activate the endothelium, platelets and the immune system.

(2) There is the generation of an array of mediators that reduce fibrinogen, impair platelet function and compromise thrombin generation.

(3) Ultimately, the above lead to inadequate clot formation for haemostasis.

(4) Increased fibrinolysis via plasmin generation further compromises haemostatic capacity.

These defects are aggravated by the ongoing blood loss, haemodilution, metabolic acidosis and hypothermia. The mechanism can result in both hypocoagulation and hypercoagulation. The conventional tests include a platelet count, Clauss assay to measure fibrinogen level, prothrombin time (PT) and activated partial thromboplastin time (aPTT). Major limiting factors with these assays are the time to obtaining results from multiple tests and the inability to identify hyperfibrinolysis. The alternative currently is viscoelastic haemostatic assays (VHAs), which provide several measurements in a single readout in half the time (newer ones in 5 min). Use of VHAs to guide resuscitation are associated with reduced mortality. Though the ITACTIC study found no difference in clinical outcomes between resuscitations guided by VHAs and those guided by conventional coagulation tests, this can be attributed to use of similar thresholds in both groups.

GENERAL APPROACH TO RESUSCITATION

See Figure 13.1.

Clinical Features on Primary Assessment

1) **Level of consciousness**

Patients might be confused or demonstrate rowdy, unruly behaviour. Differential diagnosis includes traumatic brain injury, hypoxia or severe pain due to long bone trauma.

2) **Peripheral vasoconstriction**

- Cold and clammy skin
- Prolonged capillary refill time
- Decreased urine output in advanced stages

3) **Vital signs**

Tachycardia has traditionally been regarded as an early sign of haemorrhage because the heart rate may rise slightly above normal with as little as 15% blood loss. However, the heart rate may be affected by a number of factors, including pain, anxiety and spinal injuries, and is not a predictor in early shock. Systolic blood pressure might remain normal in early stages of shock. Table 13.1 shows the stages of haemorrhagic shock. The pulse becomes rapid and thready in severe shock. Peripheral pulses might not be palpable. The femoral artery or the common carotid artery can be palpated in these patients.

Clinical Diagnosis and Investigations

"One on the floor and four more" – The focus is not only on the obvious extremity injury but

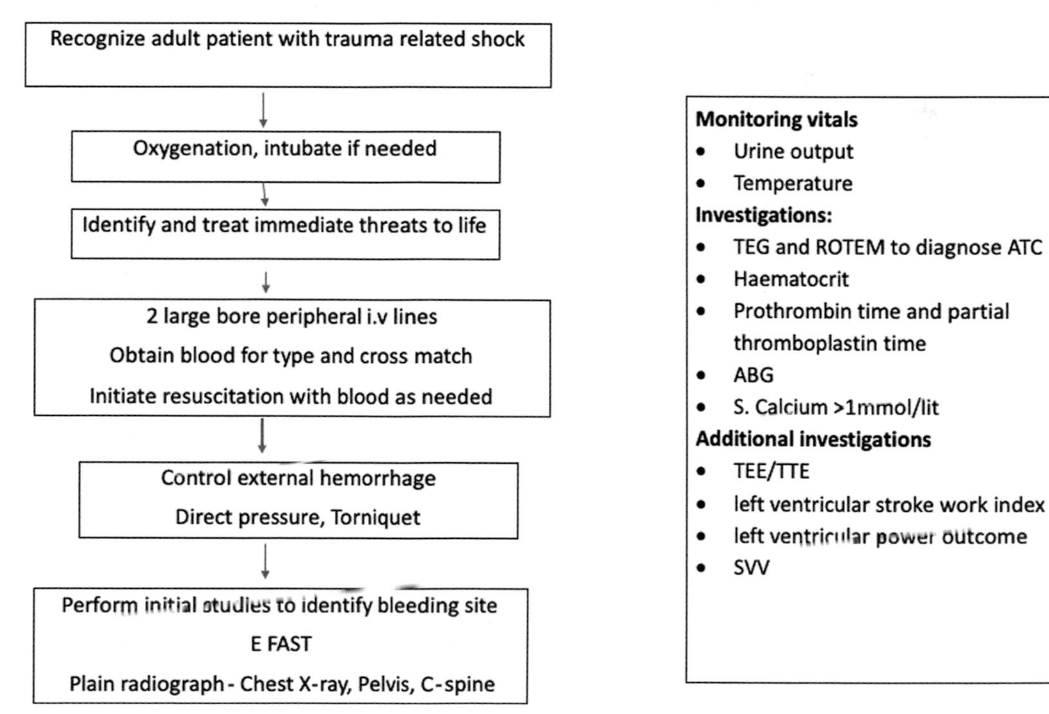

Figure 13.1 General approach to resuscitation of a trauma patient in shock

Table 13.1: Stages of Shock

Parameter	Stage 1 (Stage of Compensation)	Stage 2 (Stage of Decompensation)	Stage 3 (Stage of Deterioration)	Stage 4 (Stage of Impending Mortality)
Blood loss	< 750 ml	450–1500 ml	1500–2000 ml	> 2000 ml
Heart rate (beats/min)	< 100	100–200	121–140	> 140
Blood pressure	Normal	Reduced	Reduced	Reduced
Pulse pressure	Normal or increased	Reduced	Greatly reduced	Significantly reduced
Respiratory rate (per min)	14–20	21–29	30–35	More than 35
Urine output	Normal	Oliguria	Oliguria	Anuria
Neurological status	Normal	Agitated	Confused	Lethargic
Base deficit	<2	2.1–6	6–10	> 10
Type of intravenous fluid	Crystalloid	Crystalloid	Crystalloid Blood-type specific	Crystalloid Blood O negative Massive transfusion protocol

also on concealed, silent, life-threatening bleeding that can occur in the body cavities, such as the pleural space, retroperitoneal space and intra-abdominal space. So, patients without a need for immediate bleeding control and an unidentified source of bleeding should undergo immediate further investigation of the chest, abdominal cavity and pelvic ring, which can be a major source of acute blood loss following traumatic injury. Besides clinical examination, imaging studies, including ultrasonography and computed tomography, blood gas analysis and coagulation profiles, together with functional assays, are recommended diagnostic modalities during the primary survey.

Arterial blood gas estimation – Normal pH is 7.4. Acidosis can be diagnosed if the base excess is less than –6 mmol/L. Higher mortality and morbidity were observed if the base deficit exceeded –6 mmol/L. Serum lactate > 4 mmol/L is an additional indicator of acidosis.

eFAST (extended focused abdominal sonography for trauma) – Examination in the emergency room to diagnose haemothorax, cardiac tamponade and free fluid in the abdomen.

General Interventions

- Compression – Use local compression, if possible, to limit life-threatening bleeding.
- Oxygen – Administer 100% O_2 (15 L/min), as there is wide discrepancy between demand and supply of oxygen. It is better to administer O_2 using a non-rebreather mask.
- Wide-bore intravenous cannula – Since the rate of administration of intravenous fluids is directly proportional to the diameter of the veins, it is preferrable to insert a wide-bore (16G) intravenous cannula. Blood samples are drawn for haemogram, blood gases including base deficit, blood group and crossmatching. If peripheral veins are difficult to cannulate due to vasoconstriction, then the intraosseous cannula or central vein such as the femoral vein or jugular vein might need cannulation.
- Crystalloids – Crystalloids need to be used judiciously until blood products become available. Excessive use of intravenous crystalloid fluids is detrimental due to risk of worsening coagulopathy, hypothermia and acidosis. Warmed crystalloid isotonic solutions such as 0.9% normal saline or Ringer's lactate are given rapidly. Intravenous fluids of 1 to 1.5 L are administered, and response to the fluid challenge is noted. It is preferable not to exceed 2 L of crystalloid solution. Liberal and injudicious use of 0.9% normal saline and Ringer's lactate can lead to hyperchloremic metabolic and respiratory acidosis, respectively.

Colloids such as hydroxyethyl starch (Voluven), polygeline (Haemaccel), gelatine polysuccinate (Gelofusine) are not currently recommended. Starch-based colloids can precipitate coagulopathy, anaphylaxis type reaction and renal failure.

- Blood and blood products – Blood is the best replacement for haemorrhagic blood loss. Replacement of only packed red blood cells is likely to affect blood coagulation. Hence, a massive transfusion protocol has been developed to give packed red blood cells, fresh frozen plasma and platelets in the ratio of 1:1:1. Administration of platelets early during the course of treatment in haemorrhagic shock reduces mortality in critically injured patients.

Each institute needs to have a protocol for massive transfusion. Most accepted indications for activation of massive transfusion are the presence of haemodynamic instability despite transfusion of four units of packed red blood cells, replacement of > 1 blood volume in 24 h or replacement of > 50% of blood volume in 4 h.

- Intravenous tranexamic acid – Tranexamic acid works by preventing disruption of the fibrin clots that are formed as the body's response to prevent blood loss. Tranexamic acid works best when given within 3 h from the time of trauma. It is given intravenously as a 1 gm loading dose over 10 min followed by 1 gm maintenance dose over 8 h as an intravenous infusion.
- Vasopressors – Routine use of vasopressors in the trauma setting in order to avoid further tissue hypoperfusion and hypoxia due to vasoconstriction as part of the physiological response to haemorrhagic shock is not advocated. If more than 1.5 L of intravenous fluids are given and patient continues to be haemodynamically unstable and blood products are awaited, then vasopressors can be given to buy time till blood products become available.
- Prevention of hypothermia – It is important to prevent hypothermia from setting in due to higher risk of associated mortality. Blankets, warming blankets (Bair Huggers), use of room warmers and administration of warmed crystalloid solutions can be helpful in prevention and management of hypothermia.
- Serum lactate and/or base deficit measurements are recommended as sensitive tests to estimate and monitor the extent of bleeding and shock.
- Early and repeated monitoring of haemostasis, using either a combined traditional laboratory determination [prothrombin time (PT), platelet counts and Clauss fibrinogen level] and/or point-of-care (POC) PT/international normalized ratio (INR) and/or a viscoelastic method (VEM) should be done.
- Permissive hypotension is recommended, with a target systolic blood pressure of 80–100 mmHg (mean arterial pressure 50–60 mmHg) until major bleeding has been stopped in the initial phase following trauma without brain injury.
- Ionized calcium levels should be monitored and maintained within the normal range during massive transfusion.

GOALS OF RESUSCITATION

- Maintain systolic blood pressure (SBP) of 80–100 mm Hg with mean arterial pressure (MAP) between 50 to 60 mmHg
- Maintain haematocrit of 25%–0%
- Maintain prothrombin time and partial thromboplastin time in normal ranges
- Maintain platelet count at greater than 50,000 per high-power field
- Maintain normal serum ionized calcium
- Maintain core temperature higher than 35°C
- Maintain saturation
- Prevent increase in serum lactate
- Prevent acidosis from worsening
- Achieve adequate anaesthesia and analgesia

PATTERN OF PATIENT RESPONSE

The patient's response to initial volume is a key factor to determine further resuscitation.

Rapid response – The patient quickly responds to initial fluid bolus and become hemodynamically stable. The clinician can slow the fluid to maintenance rate. Less than 15% blood volume is usually lost.

Transient response – The patient responds to initial fluid bolus; however, they show deterioration of perfusion indices once the clinician slows the fluid to maintenance rate. About 15%–40% blood volume is lost, and transfusion of blood and blood products is indicated.

Minimal or no response – No response to crystalloids and blood indicates an immediate need for definitive intervention (operation or angiography) to control haemorrhage. Massive transfusion protocol should be initiated.

End point of resuscitation – Serum lactate (can be measured from arterial blood gas evaluation) is an indicator of adequacy of resuscitation. The normal serum lactate level is ≤ 2.0 mmol/L.

SUGGESTED READING

1. Barbee RW, Reynolds PS, Ward KR. Assessing shock resuscitation strategies by oxygen debt repayment. *Shock.* 2010;33(2):113–22. PMID: 20081495.

2. De Backer D. Detailing the cardiovascular profile in shock patients. *Crit Care.* 2017;21(Suppl 3):311. PMID: 29297372.

3. Goonzalez E, Moore EE, Moore HB, et al. Goal-directed hemostatic resuscitation of trauma-induced coagulopathy: a pragmatic randomized clinical trial comparing a viscoelastic assay to conventional coagulation assays. *Ann Surg.* 2016;263:1051–9. PMID: 26720428.

4. Baksaas-Aasen K, Gall LS, Stensballe J, et al. Viscoelastic haemostatic assay augmented protocols for major trauma haemorrhage (ITACTIC): a randomized, controlled trial. *Intens Care Med.* 2020;4:49–59. PMID: 33048195.

5. Spahn DR, Bouillon B, Cerny V, et al. The European guideline on management of major bleeding and coagulopathy following trauma: fifth edition. *Crit Care.* 2019;23:98. PMID: 30917843.

14 Vascular Access in Bleeding Patients

Amarjyoti Hazarika

LEARNING OBJECTIVES

- To be aware of the importance of fluid resuscitation, employing a good, working vascular access
- To know the common areas/sites of vascular access needed for resuscitation and how to perform it
- To know other sites and methods of vascular access when common areas of access are not easy or impossible
- To manage/take care of the vascular access achieved and be aware of its complications

WHY VASCULAR ACCESS IS REQUIRED

- Fast resuscitation with IV fluids
- Immediate start of blood and blood products
- Immediate start of hemodynamic supportive treatment, i.e. inotropes, vasopressors

PERIPHERAL VENOUS CANNULATION

When to Achieve Peripheral Vascular Access

Most trauma patients already have one or two peripheral IV cannulas that are inserted from the referring centres. It is important to check that the cannulas are of adequate calibre and are functioning in full flow. For example, in a patient with polytrauma where haemodynamic parameters are not stable, a cannula of 22G or even 20G in situ may not be appropriate for fluid resuscitation and starting haemodynamic supporting treatment.

If vascular access is not already in place, we need to secure it once the person enters the triage area/resuscitation bay. This access will be concurrent with the primary survey, which is initiated on patient arrival.

Where to Achieve Peripheral Vascular Access

In most injured patients, two large-bore (preferably 16G) peripheral IV lines in the upper limb are sufficient for initial resuscitation and volume replacement. The vascular access should preferably be in the cubital fossa veins. In a stable patient, one can look into the dorsum of the hand/forearm for access. In situations where hand access is not there, one can try veins in the legs around the ankle region. Other sites for achieving vascular access include the femoral vein and external jugular vein. In a young child/infant, the scalp vein can be used. Figure 14.1 shows different sites for achieving vascular access. It is important to remember that:

1. An intravenous cannula should never be placed in an extremity with burns/crush injuries or fractures.
2. In pelvic fracture, to ensure that the administered fluid reaches the central circulation, place IV lines below and above the diaphragm.

How to Achieve Peripheral Vascular Access

Prerequisites

- Intravenous cannula of all sizes and dimensions, preferably size 16G and 18G
- A tourniquet or any device that can be used to make the veins prominent
- Cannula dressing, sticking/adhesive material for fixing the cannula
- Clean procedure tray, sterile gloves, sterile dressing pack (to provide a sterile field)
- Gauze swab, alcohol swab (2% chlorhexidine gluconate in 70% isopropyl)

Step 1: Choose a vein that is large, visible, straight, clear and accessible, where a 16G or 18G cannula can be inserted, preferably veins in and around the cubital fossa.

Step 2: Make the veins prominent by applying a tourniquet either by using an actual device or just using hands (manual limb compression). The tourniquet should be applied approximately four to five finger widths above the planned cannulation site. (The tourniquet should be left on for no longer than 2 minutes.)

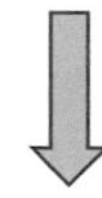

Step 3: After securing the cannula and confirming free flow of IV fluid, one needs to fix it with adhesive/stickers firmly, ensuring no dislodgement or obstruction in the flow of fluid.

DOI: 10.1201/9781003291619-16

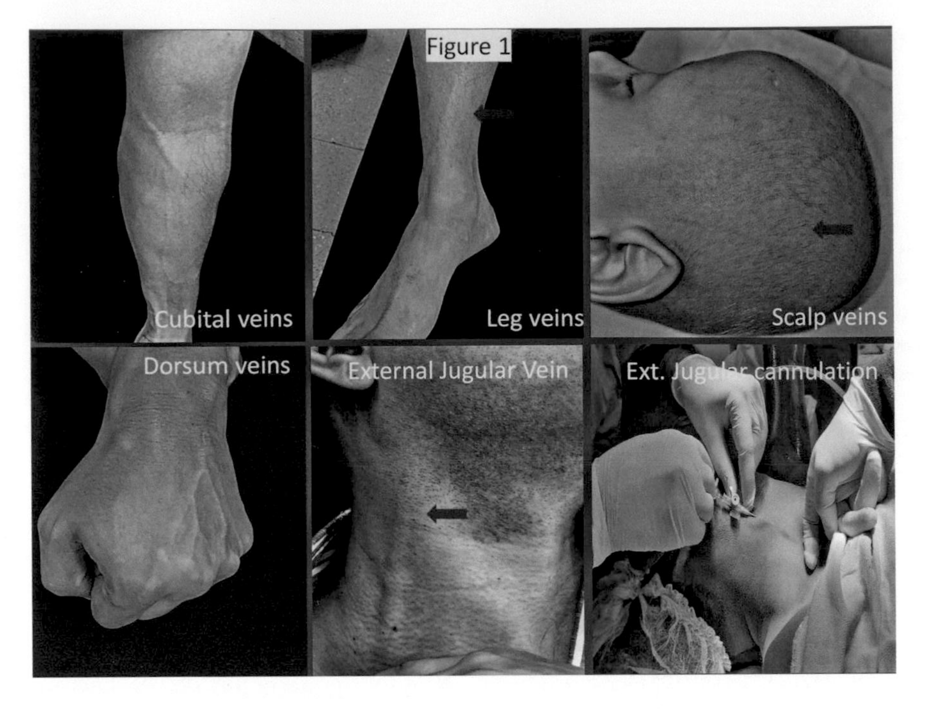

Figure 14.1 Different sites for achieving vascular access

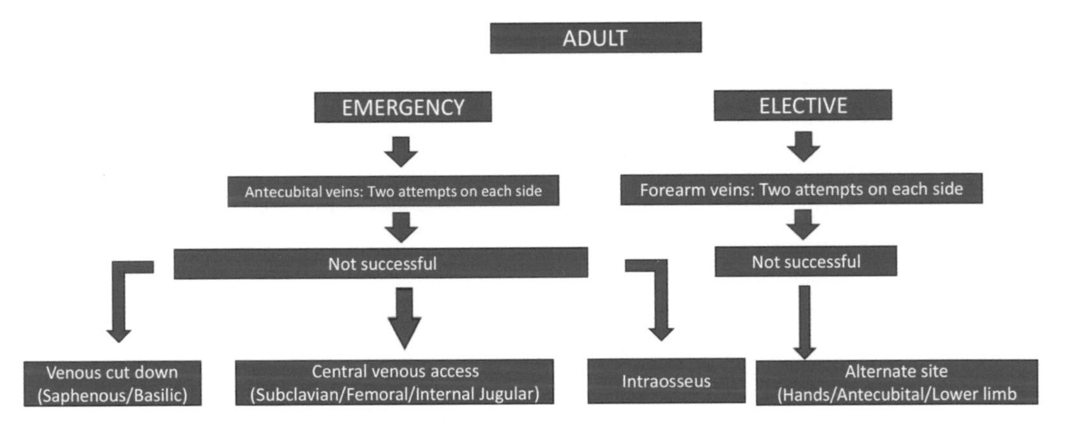

Figure 14.2 Sequential algorithmic approach for achieving successful venous access

Key Points to Keep in Mind

1. Although 16G or 18G is preferable, one should not be too preoccupied with size, rather go ahead with whatever cannula size is available so that treatment is not delayed.
2. Avoid cannulating veins that are around joints, as they tend to get kinked with movement.
3. Kindly confirm free flow as it helps in quick and judicious resuscitation.

Figure 14.2 describes methods to improve peripheral venous access in a sequential algorithmic approach.

Complications

- Phlebitis
- Extravasation of IV fluids
- Bruising
- Haematoma formation

Recommendations for achieving vascular access are summarized in Figure 14.3.

CENTRAL VENOUS CANNULATION (CVC)

Why Do We Need It?

Early peripheral IV access in the critically hypovolaemic patient may be difficult with

Vascular Access Recommendations

- Upper extremity is the preferred site in adults. In case lower extremity site used for catheter insertion, it should be replaced to an upper extremity as soon as possible
- In paediatric patients, catheter insertion site can be any upper or lower extremities or the scalp (esp. in neonates or young infants)
- While selecting a catheter, one should do it on the basis of its intended purpose, duration of use and individual operators experience
- Catheter insertion site must be evaluated daily by palpation through the dressing to discern tenderness
- Peripheral venous catheters should be removed if the patients develop signs of phlebitis (warmth, tenderness, erythema, or palpable venous cord), infection, or a malfunctioning catheter.

Figure 14.3 Recommendations for achieving vascular access

collapsed circulation. In these cases, early central access should be achieved. Besides, it allows the delivery of potent vasoactive drugs. However, a central venous cannula is small in diameter, associated with high resistance to flow. It thus proved ineffective in the volume resuscitation required in major trauma patients.

Which Vein(s) to Canulate?

For central vein cannulation, commonly, the internal jugular vein is preferred. Other veins include the subclavian and femoral veins that can be cannulated based on requirement and expertise.

The internal jugular vein is often the site of choice due to the following advantages:

- Superficial location
- Proper surface marking
- Easy ultrasonic visualization
- Straight course to the superior vena cava (on the right)

Steps and Techniques

The patient is positioned supine with the head rotated 30 to 40 degrees away from the side of the puncture. Most commonly the right side is the first choice, as the route follows a more linear course. A roll may be placed anywhere under the chest to facilitate extension of the neck. Use of the Trendelenburg position increases engorgement of the neck veins and facilitates cannulation, more so in hypovolaemic patients.

The techniques can broadly be divided into anterior, central and posterior approaches, depending on their relationship to the sternocleidomastoid (SCM). However, for easy and quick cannulation, a central approach is commonly employed. The central approach has a site of puncture at the intersection of the clavicular and sternal heads of the SCM; this should be at the level of the cricoid cartilage. The needle is directed towards the ipsilateral nipple at an angle of 45 degrees to the skin. Entry is made to the vein where it lies lateral to the pulsation of the carotid artery (Figure 14.4).

Complications

- Pneumothorax, the most common complication
- Vascular injuries
- Arterial puncture is more common with the internal jugular vein (the carotid artery is at risk)
- Line malposition, air embolism, cardiac dysrhythmias, chylothorax, and peripheral plexus or nerve damage

Notes

1. Weigh the risks and benefits of CVC.
2. CVC should only be done by those fully trained in the technique.
3. The best predictor of complications during CVC insertion is the number of insertion attempts.
4. If available, use ultrasound to place catheters.
5. Promptly remove catheters that are no longer essential.

Figures 14.5 and 14.6 highlight CVC care and danger signs, respectively.

Role of Ultrasound

Ultrasound-guided cannulation is associated with a significantly lower failure rate both overall and on the first attempt. However, the technique requires a good learning curve and may not be suitable in an emergency where time is a factor. But it is to be used when available, especially whenever a difficult central venous access is suspected. Its merits and demerits are summarized in Figure 14.7.

PERIPHERAL VENOUS CUTDOWN

Peripheral venous cutdown is an emergency procedure where the vein is surgically exposed and then a cannula is inserted into the vein.

When to Do Peripheral Venous Cutdown

The peripheral venous cutdown is done to get vascular access in trauma and hypovolaemic

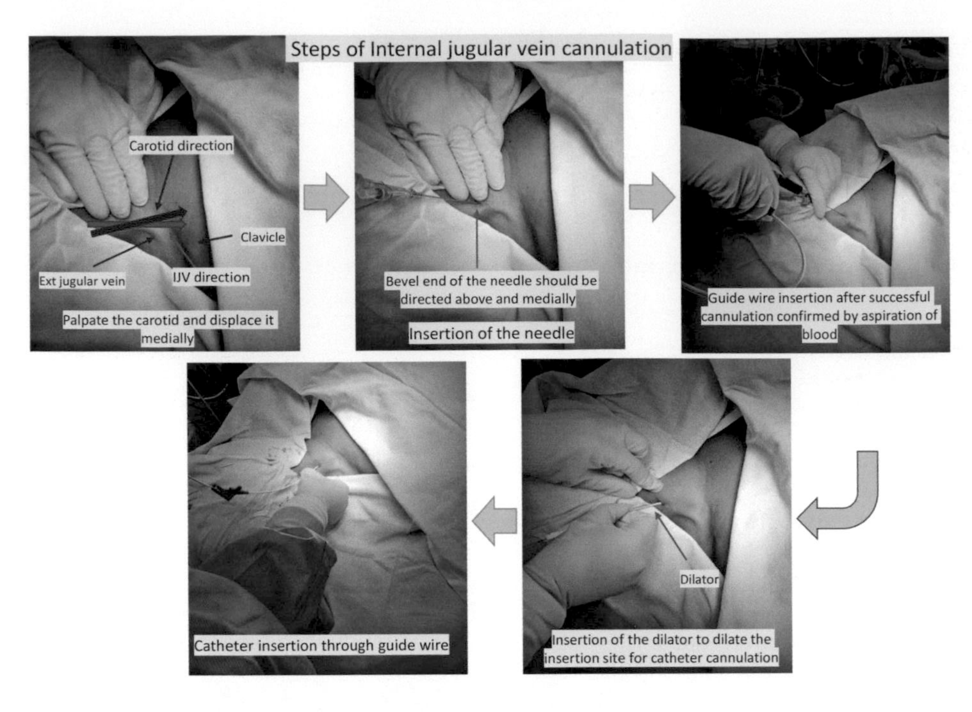

Figure 14.4 Steps of internal jugular vein cannulation

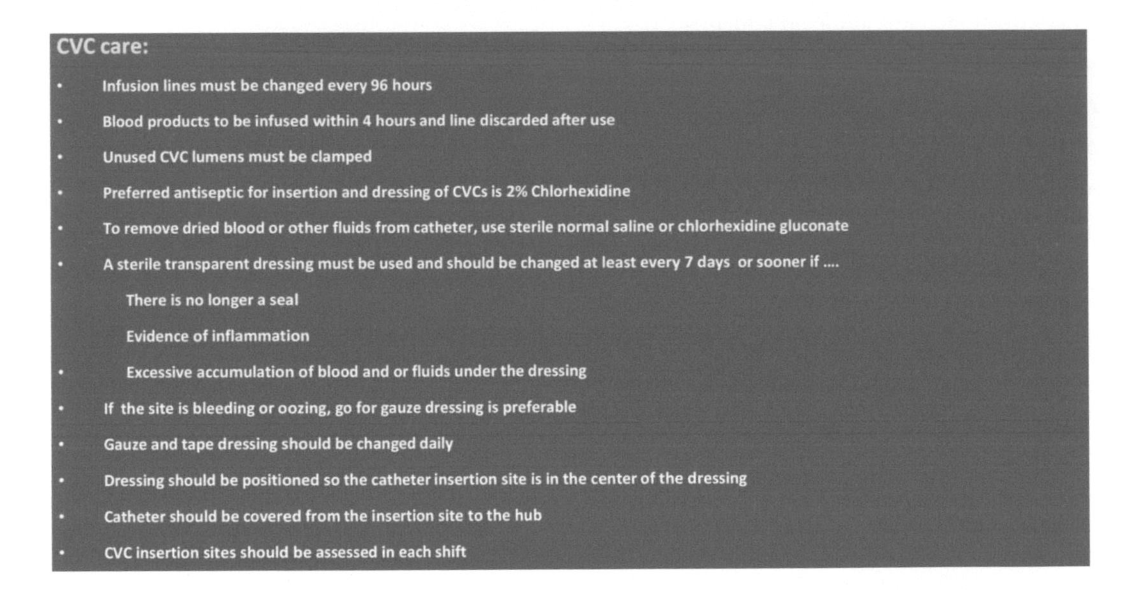

Figure 14.5 Care following central venous cannulation

shock patients where peripheral cannulation is difficult or impossible and access to techniques for central venous catheterization are not there. Although resuscitation via venous cutdown techniques takes a long time when compared to percutaneous vein cannulation, a cutdown remains a viable option where percutaneous access proves impossible.

Where to Do Peripheral Venous Cutdown

Most commonly, the greater saphenous vein at the level of the medial malleolus in the ankle is the best preferred site. Another possible site includes the basilic vein in the cubital fossa. This site helps in patients with pelvic injuries or if the leg veins have been spoilt in previous vein surgery or bypass operations.

Danger signs of CVC:

- Redness, swelling, or fluids draining around the catheter site
- Swelling, tenderness, or redness in arm or neck ipsilateral to the site of catheter insertion
- Inability or resistance to flush the catheter
- Displacement/lengthening of the catheter
- Tightness in chest or shortness of breath

Figure 14.6 Danger signs following central venous cannulation

How to Do Peripheral Venous Cutdown

A proper surgical kit with drape, antiseptic, blades, suture and equipment for skin retraction and stabilization should be ready. The technique of performing a peripheral venous cutdown is enumerated in Figure 14.8.

Complications

- Infection, most common
- Bleeding, due to dislodgement

INTRAOSSEOUS ACCESS

Intraosseous (IO) vascular access is a valuable tool in the initial resuscitation of trauma patients in whom intravenous access is difficult/not possible. Commercial kits are available on the market to achieve access quickly and safely. It is essential that one is familiar with this access.

Merits	Demerits
• Good to visualize vascular structures • Needle placement is precise • Protection against unwanted puncture of other vascular structures • Confirmation of the guidewire position • Lower complication and attempt rates	• Technical equipment dependent • May be loss of skill in anatomical technique • Rise in false sense of surety • Increase cost

Figure 14.7 Advantages and disadvantages of ultrasound-guided central venous cannulation

Technique to perform venous cutdown

- Prepare the area anterior to the medial malleolus in aseptic manner. Infiltrate local anaesthetic in awake patient.
- An incision of two finger breadths proximal to the medial malleolus along the length of the flat tibial edge.
- Isolate the vein, and prepare for the venotomy.
- Two absorbable sutures pilled under the exposed vein with a clamp.
- Vein ligated as far distally as possible with a distal suture without cutting the ends of the suture.
- Put a knot in the proximal suture without tying it.
- Give a transverse cut in the vein, not too small Dilate the cut with the tip of a small clamp.
- Insert cannula catheter of 8 Fr without stylet and put a tie in the proximal to fix it.
- Patency and flow confirmed by connecting it to an infusion system and then close the wound with suture.

Figure 14.8 Technique of performing peripheral venous cutdown

Where to Place Intraosseous Access

- Proximal tibia: anteromedial surface, 2–3 cm below the tibial tuberosity
- Distal tibia: proximal to the medial malleolus
- Less common sites: distal femur, humeral head, sternum, iliac crest

How to Achieve Intraosseous Access

Step 1: Prepare the skin over the identified site.

Step 2: Insert the needle through the skin in a screwing motion. There is a feeling of give away as the marrow cavity is entered (feeling of loss of resistance).

Step 3: The trocar is removed and needle position is confirmed by aspirating bone marrow. Use a 5 ml syringe; marrow cannot always be aspirated, but it should flush easily.

Step 4: Secure the needle and start the fluids.

Contraindications: Ipsilateral fracture and vascular injury.

Complications

- Failure to enter the bone marrow, with extravasation or subperiosteal infusion
- Through and through penetration of the bone
- Osteomyelitis (rare in short-term use)
- Local infection, skin necrosis, pain, compartment syndrome
- Fat and bone microemboli

SUGGESTED READING

1. Wahlberg E, Olofsson O, Goldstone J. Chapter 11: Vascular access in trauma. In: *Emergency Vascular Surgery: A Practical Guide*. Verlag Berlin Heidberg: Springer; 2007:137–40. Available from: http://eknygos.lsmuni.lt/springer/628/137-140.pdf.

2. Mbamalu D, Banerjee A. Methods of obtaining peripheral venous access in difficult situations. *Postgrad Medical Journal*. 1999;75:459–62. doi:10.1136/pgmj.75.886.459.

3. O'Grady NP, Alexander M, Burna LA, et al. Summary of recommendations: guidelines for the prevention of intravascular catheter-related infections. *Clinical Infectious Diseases*. 2011;52:1087–99. doi:10.1093/cid/cir138.

4. Internet. Health.qld.gov.au. 2021 [cited 21 August 2021]. Available from: https://www.health.qld.gov.au/__data/assets/pdf_file/0028./444493/icare-pcvc-guideline.pdf

5. Vinci RJ. Venous cutdown catheterization. In: Henraiting FM, King C, eds. *Textbook of Pediatric Emergency Procedures*. Philadelphia, PA: Williams & Wilkins; 1997:284.

6. Klofas E. A quicker saphenous vein cutdown and a better way to teach it. *Journal of Trauma*. 1997;43:985–7. doi:10.1097/00005373-199712000-00025.

7. Melbourne, T. 2021. Clinical practice guidelines: intraosseous access. [online] Rch.org.au. Available from: https://www.rch.org.au/clinicalguide/guideline_index/Intraosseous_access/ [Accessed 20 August 2021].

8. Sá RA, Melo CL, Dantas RB, Delfim LV. Vascular access through the intraosseous route in pediatric emergencies. Acesso vascular por via intraóssea em emergências pediátricas. *Revista Brasileira de Terapia Intensiva*. 2012;24:407–14. doi:10.1590/s0103-507x2012000400019.

15 Central Venous Access in Trauma Bay

Anjuman Chander, Ashish Aditya, Tanvir Samra and Harshit Singla

LEARNING OBJECTIVES

- Indications and contraindications of central venous catheterization in trauma victims
- Site selection, preparation, procedure and checklist
- Use of ultrasonography in central venous catheterization

INTRODUCTION

Establishment of adequate vascular access is challenging, but of utmost importance for the management of patients with traumatic injuries. As recent as the 20th century, peripheral intravenous (PIV) access complemented by venous cutdown was the standard of care for vascular access in the trauma bay. These intravascular access techniques were revolutionized by the development of central venous catheterization (CVC), which was first attempted in 1929 by Dr Werner Forssmann and has now gained popularity in emergent and elective situations. Intraosseous (IO) access is another underutilized technique for vascular access of adult patients. But IO access has recently gained popularity in light of the American Heart Association (AHA) guidelines that call for prompt administration of resuscitation agents and minimal interruption of chest compressions for patients in cardiac arrest.

The American College of Surgeons' Advanced Trauma Life Support (ATLS) course mandates the insertion of two large-bore intravenous (IV) lines or the equivalent for patients with trauma. An audit in 2016, however, demonstrated that only 36.4% of patients with major trauma were receiving at least two ≥ 18-gauge IV lines during their resuscitative phase of care. Various non-modifiable factors like collapsed veins secondary to hypovolaemia, obesity, and small intravenous access already in place in the antecubital area or other areas limit the potential success rate.

Though not widespread, some reports suggest the usefulness of CVC as an alternative route for medications and resuscitative fluid, as well as IV contrast for diagnostic procedures in specific circumstances in emergency areas like trauma triage centres. Placement of CVC in the trauma bay is more challenging than placement in controlled or elective settings. Improper positioning, cervical immobilization, altered anatomical landmarks, the emergent nature of the procedure, concurrent medical or surgical procedures, and overcrowding around the patient contribute to difficulty in placing CVC in this clinical setting.

INDICATIONS FOR CENTRAL VENOUS CATHETERIZATION

The foremost indication of central venous catheterization in the trauma bay is for hemodynamic resuscitation of the patient following a failed attempt of peripheral venous catheter insertion. Administration of warm isotonic crystalloids and blood products to maintain haemodynamic stability is the main goal during the primary survey. The indications are as elaborated next:

1. Intravenous access (fluid, blood, drugs, nutrition)
   a. Difficult peripheral venous access (collapsed veins secondary to hypovolaemia, obesity)
   b. Administration of irritant drugs known to cause phlebitis (hypertonic saline, calcium and potassium supplements)
   c. Vasopressors or inotropes
2. Haemodynamic monitoring
   a. Central venous pressure monitoring
   b. Central venous oxyhaemoglobin saturation monitoring
3. Access for interventions
   a. Temporary transvenous pacing

Before the insertion of central venous catheters in the trauma bay, it is important to make a note of any factor which precludes the insertion/use of the same.

CONTRAINDICATIONS OF CVC FOR PATIENTS IN TRAUMA BAY

1. Patient refusal (absolute contraindication)
2. Coagulopathy (do risk–benefit analysis)
3. Venous thrombosis (another vein should be chosen)
4. Contralateral haemothorax/pneumothorax (ipsilateral side to the pneumothorax should be cannulated to avoid bilateral pneumothorax)

SITE SELECTION

There are three main sites that have been explored for central venous catheterization. They are the internal jugular vein (IJV), subclavian vein (SCV) and femoral vein (FV). Each of

DOI: 10.1201/9781003291619-17

Table 15.1: Advantages/Disadvantages of Three Main Sites of Central Venous Cannulation

	Advantages	Disadvantages
Internal jugular vein (IJV)	• Good external anatomical landmarks • Good sonographic image and easy access • Carotid artery easily identified and compressible • Less risk of pneumothorax • Less chance of malposition	• More inconvenient for patient • Higher infection and thrombosis risk than SCV
Subclavian vein (SCV)	• Least risk of infection • Relatively more convenient for patients than IJV or FV	• Inability to compress bleeding vessel • Risk of pneumothorax • Higher chance of catheter insertion failure and malposition
Femoral vein (FV)	• No risk of pneumothorax • Vessels are directly compressible	• High risk of thrombosis and infection • More inconvenient for patient • Cannot be used for central venous pressure measurements

these sites has its own advantages and disadvantages (Table 15.1).

Previous studies have shown less thrombotic and infectious complications in SCV cannulation as compared to IJV or FV cannulation. But still femoral CVC has been adopted into routine use in many resuscitation protocols in various trauma centres. Femoral site cannulation is technically easier as compared to the subclavicular or jugular site. The biggest advantage is the relative safety in a resuscitation situation where other operators can still access the patient to perform concurrent interventions while femoral cannulation is being performed. During the primary survey it is a team of clinicians who perform a fast, intense, full-body exam in the trauma bay, and any intervention chosen should not hinder the assessment and resuscitation of the patient. The supraclavicular approach to the SCV also shares the same advantage, as cannulation does not require any special patient positioning and can be performed simultaneously with chest compressions. A large diameter, absence of valves and ability to remain patent in hypovolemic patients is an added advantage.

A retrospective review at an urban, level I trauma centre compared infraclavicular subclavian versus femoral CVC complications during initial trauma resuscitations and concluded that both subclavian and femoral CVCs caused significant complications. Contrary to non-trauma situations, subclavian catheter-related pneumothoraxes occurred more commonly and femoral catheter-related blood stream infections (CRBSI) less commonly. This supports the use of femoral CVC during initial trauma resuscitations. But it is to be noted that femoral CVC was used for initial resuscitation and later removed within 48 hours. There is a lack of evidence on the use of the supraclavicular approach of subclavian vein cannulation for resuscitation in the trauma bay. Inline cervical spine immobilization is generally done in the trauma bay, and IJV cannulations are not encouraged as they need patient positioning and some amount of neck mobilization.

USE OF ULTRASONOGRAPHY IN CENTRAL VENOUS CATHETERIZATION

Earlier CVCs were done using a landmark technique based on anatomical structures and palpation of nearby arteries. Currently, ultrasound-guided cannulation is being widely practised, as it increases the first-attempt success rate and decreases the total number of attempts, time until successful catheterization and overall complications.

A linear array, high frequency (8–13 Hz) probe is best for visualizing superficial structures like veins for cannulation, as penetration is inversely proportional to frequency. On the ultrasound screen, blood vessels are anechoic structures and muscles are hypoechoic in comparison to fascia, whereas bone appears to be hyperechoic. Arteries are pulsatile structures and difficult to compress, whereas veins are compressible, non-pulsatile and their diameter usually varies with respiration, patient's position and volume status. Ultrasound-guided cannulations can be performed either in transverse or longitudinal plane, and the chosen vein can be visualized as a round to tubular structure depending on the orientation of the probe to the vein. The in-plane approach is the one in which the probe is placed parallel to the anatomical course of the vein and the needle is entered from the side, whereas, in the out-of-plane approach, the orientation of probe is perpendicular to the vein.

PREPARATION AND PROCEDURAL TECHNIQUE OF CENTRAL VENOUS CATHETERIZATION

Central venous cannulation is to be performed in a designated sterile area/zone, equipped with a resuscitation cart/essential monitoring device and USG machine with high frequency probe. Written informed consent should be obtained from the patient or from the attendants (Table 15.2). The American Society of Anesthesiologists (ASA) Advisory emphasizes the need of a checklist for the same.

CONCLUSION

In emergency conditions like massive haemorrhage commonly encountered in trauma bay, a wide-bore catheter is required to rapidly replace the lost blood volume with intravenous fluids or blood products. The flow rate through a catheter is determined using the Hagen–Poiseuille equation: $Q = \pi Pr^4/8\eta l$. As flow rate is directly proportional to radius and inversely with the length of the catheter, thus for trauma resuscitation, a short catheter with a large diameter should be used along with an introducer sheath. Insertion of two large-bore IV cannulas is a priority, but in circumstances in which peripheral venous access cannot be established, central venous cannulation is considered. The most important point is that CVC insertion in the trauma bay should not delay the primary survey and expedient management in a bleeding patient, and should only be performed by a trained trauma team member.

Table 15.2: Preparation and Technique for Central Venous Catheterization

Consent

Equipment

- Syringes
- 2% lidocaine
- Central line set
  - Central venous catheter
  - Tissue dilator
  - Introducer needle
  - Guidewire
  - Scalpel
- Suture with needle
- Sterile transparent dressing
- Sterile cleaning solution (2% chlorhexidine)
- Sterile heparinized solution (2 units unfractionated heparin per millilitre of saline)
- Sterile drape sheet
- Sterile gown, cap, mask, gloves and face mask
- Ultrasound machine with linear high frequency probe and sterile ultrasound gel

Monitoring Devices

Continuous ECG monitoring, pulse oximeter, non-invasive blood pressure

Positioning of the Patient

For IJV/SCV

- Reverse Trendelenburg with head turned to opposite side and extension with a sandbag in between scapulae is not encouraged as cervical mobilization is discouraged

For Femoral Vein

- Supine with exposed inguinal area
- Chosen side leg should be bent at knee with lateral aspect touching the bed

(Patient with pelvic fractures/leg injuries may be difficult to position)

Donning

Put on sterile gown, gloves, cap, mask

Painting and Draping

- Clean the desired area with 2% chlorhexidine skin preparing solution or 5% betadine solution
- Full body patient drape, only insertion site should be exposed
- Clean ultrasound probe with alcohol-containing solution and cover with sterile transparent sheet

Identification of Vein and Cannulation

- Identify vein either using ultrasound scanning or landmark technique
- Skin infiltration with 2% lidocaine at the expected site of cannulation
- Continuous aspiration and advancement of introducer needle with attached syringe
- Once venous blood is aspirated or needle tip in vein is confirmed using USG/manometry/continuous ECG, stop advancement of needle
- Carefully thread guidewire using introducer needle hub and remove introducer needle holding guidewire in place
- Confirm guidewire in selected central vein using ultrasound or continuous ECG
- Insert tissue dilator over the guidewire in a twisting motion
- If required, then use scalpel to make a nick at insertion site
- Remove dilator and thread CVC over the guidewire
- Remove guidewire carefully holding CVC in place; check all ports for backward and forward flow
- Fix with sutures and apply transparent sterile dressing

IJV, internal jugular vein; SCV, subclavian vein; CVC, central venous catheter.

SUGGESTED READING

1. Kalso E. A short history of central venous catheterization. *Acta Anaesthesiol Scand Suppl.* 1985;81:7–10. PMID: 3909712.

2. Beheshti MV. A concise history of central venous access. *Tech Vasc Interv Radiol.* 2011;14:184–5. doi: 10.1053/j.tvir.2011.05.002.

3. Engels PT, Erdogan M, Widder SL, et al. Use of intraosseous devices in trauma: a survey of trauma practitioners in Canada, Australia and New Zealand. *Can J Surg.* 2016;59:374–82. doi: 10.1503/cjs.011215.

4. Engels PT, Passos E, Beckett AN, Doyle JD, Tien HC. IV access in bleeding trauma patients: a performance review. *Injury.* 2014;45:77–82. PMID: 23352673.

5. American College of Surgeons. Committee on Trauma. *Advanced Trauma Life Support: Student Course Manual.* Tenth edition. Chicago, IL: American College of Surgeons; 2018.

6. Verhoeff K, Saybel R, Mathura P, et al. Ensuring adequate vascular access in patients with major trauma: a quality improvement initiative. *BMJ Open Qual.* 2018;7:e000090. doi: 10.1136/bmjoq-2017-000090.

7. Westfall MD, Price KR, Lambert M, et al. Intravenous access in the critically ill trauma patient: a multicentered, prospective, randomized trial of saphenous cutdown and percutaneous femoral access. *Ann Emerg Med.* 1994;23:541–5. PMID: 8135430.

8. Scalea TM, Sinert R, Duncan AO, et al. Percutaneous central venous access for resuscitation in trauma. *Acad Emerg Med.* 1994;1:525–31. doi: 10.1111/j.1553-2712.1994.tb02547.x.

9. Parienti JJ, du Cheyron D, Timsit JF, et al. Meta-analysis of subclavian insertion and nontunneled central venous catheter-associated infection risk reduction in critically ill adults. *Crit Care Med.* 2012;40:1627e1634. doi: 10.1097/CCM.0b013e31823e99cb.

10. Hamada SR, Fromentin M, Ronot M, et al. Femoral arterial and central venous catheters in the trauma resuscitation room. *Injury.* 2018;49:927–32. doi: 10.1016/j.injury.2018.03.026.

11. Patrick SP, Tijunelis MA, Johnson S, Herbert ME. Supraclavicular subclavian vein catheterization: the forgotten central line. *West J Emerg Med.* 2009;10:110–4. PMID: 19561831.

12. Saini V, Samra T. Ultrasound guided supraclavicular subclavian cannulation: a novel technique using "hockey stick" probe. *J Emerg Trauma Shock.* 2015;8:72–3. doi: 10.4103/0974-2700.150408.

13. Choron RL, Wang A, Orden KV, Capano-Wehrle L, Seamon MJ. Emergency central venous catheterization during trauma resuscitation: a safety analysis by site. *Am Surg.* 2015;81:527–31. doi: 10.1177/000313481508100538.

14. Brass P, Hellmich M, Kolodziej L, Schick G, Smith AF. Ultrasound guidance versus anatomical landmarks for internal jugular vein catheterization. *Cochrane Database Syst Rev.* 2015;1:CD006962. doi: 10.1002/14651858.CD006962.pub2.

16 A Guide to Use of Crystalloids

Jeetinder Kaur Makkar and Mandeep Tundak

LEARNING OBJECTIVES

- Early use of blood, if available, remains the optimal resuscitation fluid for hypovolemic patients
- Where blood is not available or delayed, balanced salt solution/Ringer's lactate is the preferred alternative for initial resuscitation of hypovolaemic trauma patients. Caution should be exercised in trauma patients with liver disease and head injury
- 0.9% normal saline is an acceptable alternative. Large volumes, however, may result in metabolic acidosis
- Vigilance is needed to provide only fluid that is necessary to maintain perfusion. Excessive administration has negative consequences

INTRODUCTION

Major cause of potentially preventable death in injured patients is uncontrolled haemorrhage. Fluid resuscitation in trauma includes optimal type and volume. It helps in restoring lost blood volume, regaining tissue perfusion and reducing mortality. Fluid administration is useful only when it increases stroke volume (SV) and cardiac output.

A patient will be fluid responsive if fluid bolus increases the stressed blood volume with a resultant increase in mean circulating filling pressure, thereby increasing the gradient of venous return if ventricles are functioning on an ascending limb of the Frank–Starling curve. Fluid responsiveness can be defined by various parameters:

- Passive leg raise (PLR) test – Passively raising the lower limbs mobilizes almost 300 ml of fluid from the lower limb to intravascular space. A more than 10% increase in pulse pressure or stroke volume indicates patient is fluid responsive.
- An increase in SV by at least 10% after 500 ml of crystalloid infusion indicates fluid responsiveness.
- Pulse pressure variation or SV variation more than 12% upon arterial pressure contour analysis indicates fluid responsiveness.

FLUID RESUSCITATION STRATEGIES

These strategies are based on volume, rate and time of fluid resuscitation.

- Immediate aggressive fluid resuscitation – This aims at restoring circulating volume and maintaining organ perfusion. Large volume resuscitation leads to dislodgement of soft clots, dilutional coagulopathy, increased mortality, increased extremity and abdominal compartment pressure, electrolyte disturbances and hypothermia.
- Delayed resuscitation – Fluid is administered after bleeding has been controlled. This technique showed better results compared to immediate resuscitation in patients with penetrating injuries to the torso. Ideal in the scenario where transfer time is very short (< 10–15 min). Delayed fluid resuscitation intends to maintain minimally adequate organ perfusion (SBP > 70 or MAP 50–65) until the bleeding is controlled.
- Permissive hypotension – Fluid is administered to increase systolic blood pressure (SBP) without reaching normotension. If patient transfer time is more than 15 min, then low volume resuscitation should be used. Goal-directed resuscitation [SBP/mean arterial pressure (MAP) is targeted based on patient physiology] or controlled resuscitation (predetermined fixed rates are infused such that normotension is not achieved) is associated with decreased blood loss, intra-abdominal bleeding, risk of intra-abdominal hypertension, acidaemia, haemodilution, thrombocytopenia, coagulopathy, tissue injuries, sepsis, volume of crystalloid needed and blood product utilization. It improves organ perfusion and survival. If the duration of permissive hypotension (SBP < 65) is more than 8 hours, it may lead to increased metabolic stress, tissue hypoxia and mortality.
- Haemostatic resuscitation – It involves early use of blood and blood products. It entails use of plasma, platelets and red blood cells in an optimal ratio of 1:1:1, as well as use of antifibrinolytic agents.

Restrictive volume replacement has been recommended by international guidelines to achieve target blood pressure until the bleeding has been controlled. Commonly used targets of blood pressure before controlling bleeding include:

- Penetrating trauma: SBP 60–70 mmHg
- Blunt trauma: SBP 80–90 mmHg

DOI: 10.1201/9781003291619-18

- Traumatic brain injury: SBP 100–110, MAP > 80 mmHg

CHOICE OF FLUID FOR RESUSCITATION

Blood is the best resuscitation fluid, as it provides simultaneous volume expansion and oxygen carrying capacity. The concerns associated with its use include issues of compatibility, cost and storage requirements.

The use of crystalloids or colloids for resuscitation is still a debatable issue. Crystalloids expand plasma volume to a lesser degree than colloids, as they hydrate both plasma and interstitial space. Hypotonic fluids (e.g. D5) do not stay intravascular, so isotonic and hypertonic crystalloids are used. Ringer's lactate (RL) or normal saline (NS) are the primary resuscitation fluids.

Table 16.1 shows the composition of commonly used crystalloids.

Plasmalytes. Plasmalytes are balanced solutions which closely resemble human plasma in their content of electrolyte, osmolality and pH. They have additional buffer capacity, as they contain acetate and gluconate. These are converted to bicarbonate, CO_2 and water quickly and efficiently, thus consuming less oxygen. Lack of calcium allows for their use in combination with most drugs and blood.

Ringer's lactate. RL is the preferred alternative for blood as the initial resuscitation fluid in the hypovolemic trauma patient. It replaces some of interstitial fluid and electrolyte in trauma patients. It is slightly hypotonic, so can increase brain cell mass in neurotrauma patients. RL and blood should be infused through separate lines because of the risk of clotting. Lactate is cleared by the liver, so it should be used with caution in patients with severe liver injuries.

Saline. A 0.9% solution of saline is isotonic, but it has supraphysiological concentration of chloride. It is widely used because of cheaper availability. It is devoid of calcium, so blood can be transfused along with it. Because of the isotonic nature, it is used as the first fluid in neurotrauma patients. Serious complications occur if more than two litres of isotonic saline is used. Complications include hyperchloremic metabolic acidosis and abdominal pain. Hypertonic saline (HTS) (3% or 7.5%) can be used in hypotensive neurotrauma patients where massive crystalloid administration can lead to more harm than benefit. Compared to isotonic crystalloid, use of permissive hypotension with HTS in patients undergoing damage control surgery resulted in reduced 30-day mortality; increased urine output; and reduced risk of acute respiratory distress syndrome, sepsis and organ failure. HTS is beneficial in patients with brain oedema, traumatic brain injury (TBI), or massive haemorrhage requiring damage control surgery. HTS is associated with increased renal failure, need for renal replacement therapy and mortality.

Problems associated with all crystalloids includes fluid overload, oedema with weight gain, lung oedema and compartment syndrome.

Colloids. Preparations include albumin, dextran, hydroxyethyl starch (HES) and gelatins. Comparison of saline versus 4% albumin have shown clinical equivalent efficacy in a saline versus albumin fluid evaluation (SAFE) study. This has been attributed to use of less saline with albumin. However, TBI patients had high mortality when resuscitated with albumin. Colloids can be used when patients do not tolerate large volume of crystalloids and overload is a concern.

Table 16.1: Constituents and Properties of Commonly Used Crystalloids

	Plasma	Plasmalyte-A	RL	0.45% Saline with Soda Bicarb	0.9% Saline	3% HTS
Na^+ (mEq/L)	135–145	140	130	141	154	513
K^+ (mEq/L)	3.5–5.0	5	4			
Ca^{2+} (mEq/L)	2.2–2.6		2.7			
Mg^{2+} (mEq/L)	0.8–1.0	3.0				
Cl^- (mEq/L)	94–111	98	109	72	154	513
Lactate (mEq/L)	1–2		28			
Acetate (mEq/L)		27				
Gluconate (mEq/L)		23				
Bicarbonate (mEq/L)	24–32			70		
pH	7.35–7.45	7.4	6.5		5.0	5.0
Osmolarity (mOsm/L)	275–295	294	273	283	308	1027
SID		27	28			

RL, Ringer's lactate; HTS, hypertonic saline; SID, strong ion difference.

Newer gelatins have low molecular weight and are easily excreted by kidneys. They have a lower risk of dilutional coagulopathy. Further studies are needed to prove their benefit over crystalloids.

European guidelines recommend:

- Fluid therapy using isotonic crystalloid solution to be initiated in hypotensive bleeding trauma patients (Grade 1A)
- Balanced electrolyte solution to be used and saline solution to be avoided (Grade 1B)
- Hypotonic solution, e.g. RL, be avoided in severe head injury patients (Grade 1B)
- The use of colloids to be restricted due to adverse effect on haemostasis (Grade 1C)

PRACTICAL APPROACH TO A MAJOR TRAUMA PATIENT IN TRIAGE

See Figure 16.1.

1. Initial fluid resuscitation in haemorrhagic shock – One litre or 20 ml/kg isotonic crystalloid, preferably Ringer's lactate, bolus as rapidly as possible using short, large-gauge peripheral intravenous access. Target: SBP = 90 mmHg or blood products available. Send blood sample for crossmatch and blood typing simultaneously.
2. Check for patient responsiveness using vital signs (blood pressure, pulse pressure, pulse rate), decreasing lactate and normalization of base deficit.
    a. Rapid response – Patient responds quickly to initial fluid bolus and become hemodynamically stable, without sign of inadequate tissue perfusion and oxygenation. Change to maintenance rate after resuscitation. Type and crossmatch blood should be available.
    b. Transient response – Patient responds to initial fluid bolus but shows deterioration of perfusion when maintenance fluid given, indicating ongoing loss or inadequate resuscitation. Blood and blood product transfusion is indicated. May need operative or angiographic control of haemorrhage.
    c. Minimal/non-responsive – Patient fails to respond to fluids. Needs immediate definitive intervention to control bleeding. Massive transfusion protocol needs to be initiated.
3. Observe for evidence of adequate tissue perfusion and oxygenation.
4. Achieve definite control of haemorrhage.

POST-RESUSCITATION FLUID MANAGEMENT

This is the period after haemostasis has been achieved and coagulopathy corrected, microcirculatory flow improved (improving lactate and blood gas parameters) and haemodynamic parameters are stabilized (SBP > 100; MAP > 65 mmHg). In this phase, crystalloids are required both for drug administration

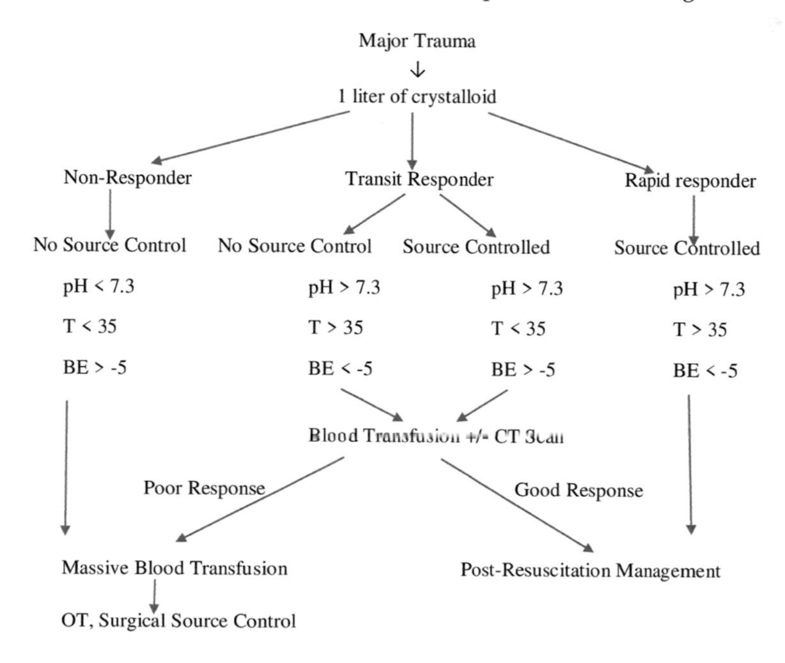

Figure 16.1 Flow diagram of initial fluid resuscitation in trauma patients

and fluid supplementation. Maintenance fluid should be less than 2 ml/kg/h. Balanced fluid is better than normal saline.

SUGGESTED READING

1. Cherkas D. Traumatic hemorrhagic shock: advances in fluid management. *Emerg Med Pract.* 2011;13:1–19. PMID: 22164397.
2. Marik PE. Fluid responsiveness and the six guiding principles of fluid resuscitation. *Crit Care Med.* 2016;44:1920–2. PMID: 26571187.
3. Monnet X, Teboul JL. Passive leg raising: five rules, not a drop of fluid! *Crit Care.* 2015;19:18. PMID: 25658678.
4. Paravar M, Hosseinpour M, Mohammadzadeh M, Mirzadeh AS. Prehospital care and in-hospital mortality of trauma patients in Iran. *Prehosp Disaster Med.* 2014;29:473–7. PMID: 25196346.
5. Santry HP, Alam HB. Fluid resuscitation: past, present, and the future. *Shock.* 2010;33:229–41. PMID: 20160609.
6. Rossaint R, Bouillon B, Cerny V, et al. The European guideline on management of major bleeding and coagulopathy following trauma: fourth edition. *Crit Care.* 2016;20:100. PMID: 27072503.
7. Wise R, Faurie M, Malbrain MLNG, Hodgson E. Strategies for intravenous fluid resuscitation in trauma patients. *World J Surg.* 2017;41:1170–83. PMID: 28058475.
8. Finfer S, Bellomo R, Boyce N, French J, Myburgh J, Norton R; SAFE Study Investigators. A comparison of albumin and saline for fluid resuscitation in the intensive care unit. *N Engl J Med.* 2004;350:2247–56. PMID: 15163774.
9. Duchesne JC, Simms E, Guidry C, et al. Damage control immunoregulation: is there a role for low-volume hypertonic saline resuscitation in patients managed with damage control surgery? *Am Surg.* 2012;78:962–8. PMID: 22964205.

17 Blood Transfusion Strategies in Trauma Patients

Lakhvinder Singh

LEARNING OBJECTIVES

- Various blood components and their role in trauma
- Pathophysiology of trauma-induced coagulopathy
- Concept of damage control resuscitation
- Transfusion therapy in massively bleeding patients

INTRODUCTION

Transfusion plays a vital role in the management of massively bleeding trauma patients. These patients generally present with bleeding and coagulopathy in the emergency department. Patients presenting with coagulopathy carry a higher risk of mortality. Early initiation of blood component therapy has the potential to improve the clinical outcome and prevent mortality in these patients. Inappropriate blood transfusions can cause haemodilution, which can worsen acidosis, hypothermia and coagulopathy (the lethal triad of massive blood loss) in bleeding patients. Ratio-based balanced blood component therapy as a part of damage control resuscitation is the most accepted strategy for blood transfusion in trauma patients with massive bleeding. Tables 17.1 and 17.2 describe various blood components and products, respectively, and their role in trauma resuscitation.

Figure 17.1 shows the importance of maintaining haematocrit in a bleeding patient. Higher haematocrit (as shown in Figure 17.1b) causes margination of platelet towards the endothelium and enhanced P-selectin on the platelet surface, which causes endothelial platelet interaction and better haemostatic control.

COAGULOPATHY IN TRAUMA

Trauma-Induced Coagulopathy (TIC)

TIC is early onset coagulopathy which is induced by trauma itself. It is complicated by the iatrogenic coagulopathy which occurs due to dilutional and metabolic effects (hypocalcaemia) of hemodynamic resuscitation with crystalloids and blood products. As shown in Figure 17.1, trauma and resultant tissue hypoperfusion lead to synergistic activation of platelets and endothelium with initiation of coagulation at the site of injury. This leads to depletion of coagulation factors and fibrinogen leading to further bleeding. Endothelial dysfunction in trauma, which is also known as endotheliopathy of trauma (EOT), leads to activation of protein C, which leads to fibrinolysis due to activation of tissue plasminogen activator (t-PA). During the initial phase of trauma, thrombin generation is not sufficient to cause thrombosis. A decrease in coagulation factors, acidosis and hypothermia with depletion of endogenous anticoagulant mediator leads to excessive thrombin generation. Hence, trauma can also induce a hypercoagulable state due to excessive release of thrombin leading to systemic thrombotic events. The clinical picture in TIC simulates hyperfibrinolytic disseminated intravascular coagulation (DIC). Early identification of the mechanism of coagulopathy is essential for effective management of trauma patients (Figure 17.2).

Coagulopathy in Patients with Traumatic Brain Injury (TBI)

Trauma-induced coagulopathy develops rapidly in patients with brain injury. Cerebral tissue releases phospholipids and brain-derived microvesicles, which are procoagulant leading to depletion of coagulation factors and platelet dysfunction. Also, release of von Willebrand factor from the cerebral tissue plays an important role in trauma-induced coagulopathy. In patients with TBI, there is a rapid transition to the hypercoagulable state and the patient may require anticoagulation therapy. Blood component therapy should be planned meticulously to balance hypocoagulation and hypercoagulation in these patients.

MANAGEMENT STRATEGIES FOR POST-TRAUMATIC HAEMORRHAGE

Damage Control Resuscitation

Damage control resuscitation is the management strategy being used by most trauma teams for the management of acutely bleeding patients. It aims at preventing the development of coagulopathy by reducing the blood loss and breaking the vicious circle of the lethal triad of acidosis, hypothermia and coagulopathy. It includes:

1. Rapid diagnosis:
   a. Rapid diagnosis and identification of the source of bleeding.

DOI: 10.1201/9781003291619-19

Table 17.1: Various Blood Components and Their Role in Trauma

Blood Component	Volume	Storage Temperature	Role in Bleeding Patients
Packed red blood cells	220–280 ml	2°C–6°C	• Improves oxygen delivery and prevent tissue hypoxia • Maintains blood flow haemodynamics • Controls bleeding by margination of platelets, as shown in Figure 17.1
Fresh frozen plasma	150–220 ml	< –30°C	• Replacement of coagulation factors and prevention of dilutional coagulopathy
Platelet components	RDP 50–60 ml SDAP 200–220 ml	20°C–24°C	• Corrects dilutional thrombocytopenia due to bleeding and transfusion of other blood components • Improves haemostasis in patients with trauma-induced platelet dysfunction
Cryoprecipitate	15–20 ml	< –30°C	• Provides fibrinogen, which supports the formation of a stable clot and maintains effective haemostasis

RDP, random donor platelet; SDAP, single-donor apheresis platelets.

Table 17.2: Blood Products and Their Role in Trauma

Blood Product	Role in Trauma
Prothrombin complex concentrate	After reconstitution, it provides factor II, IX and X, and helps in clot formation.
Fibrinogen concentrate	It provides fibrinogen and factor XIII, and has a similar role as cryoprecipitates.
Recombinant activated factor VIIa	It bypasses the coagulation pathways and helps in formation of stable clot, but its usage is limited due to its alleged association with post-trauma thrombosis and better damage control resuscitation strategies.

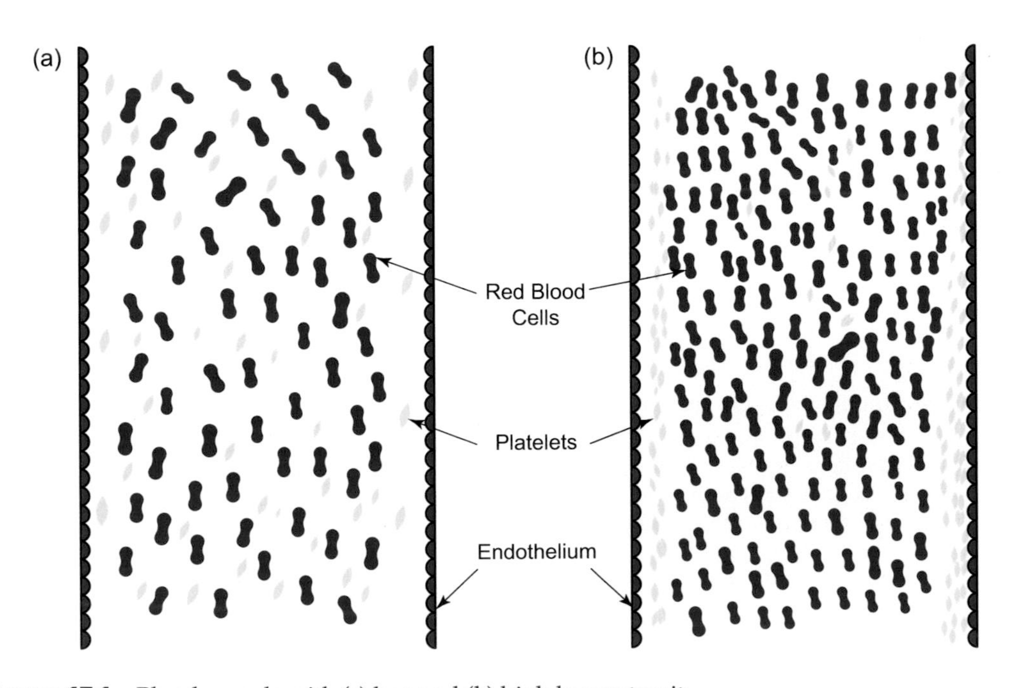

Figure 17.1 Blood vessels with (a) low and (b) high haematocrit

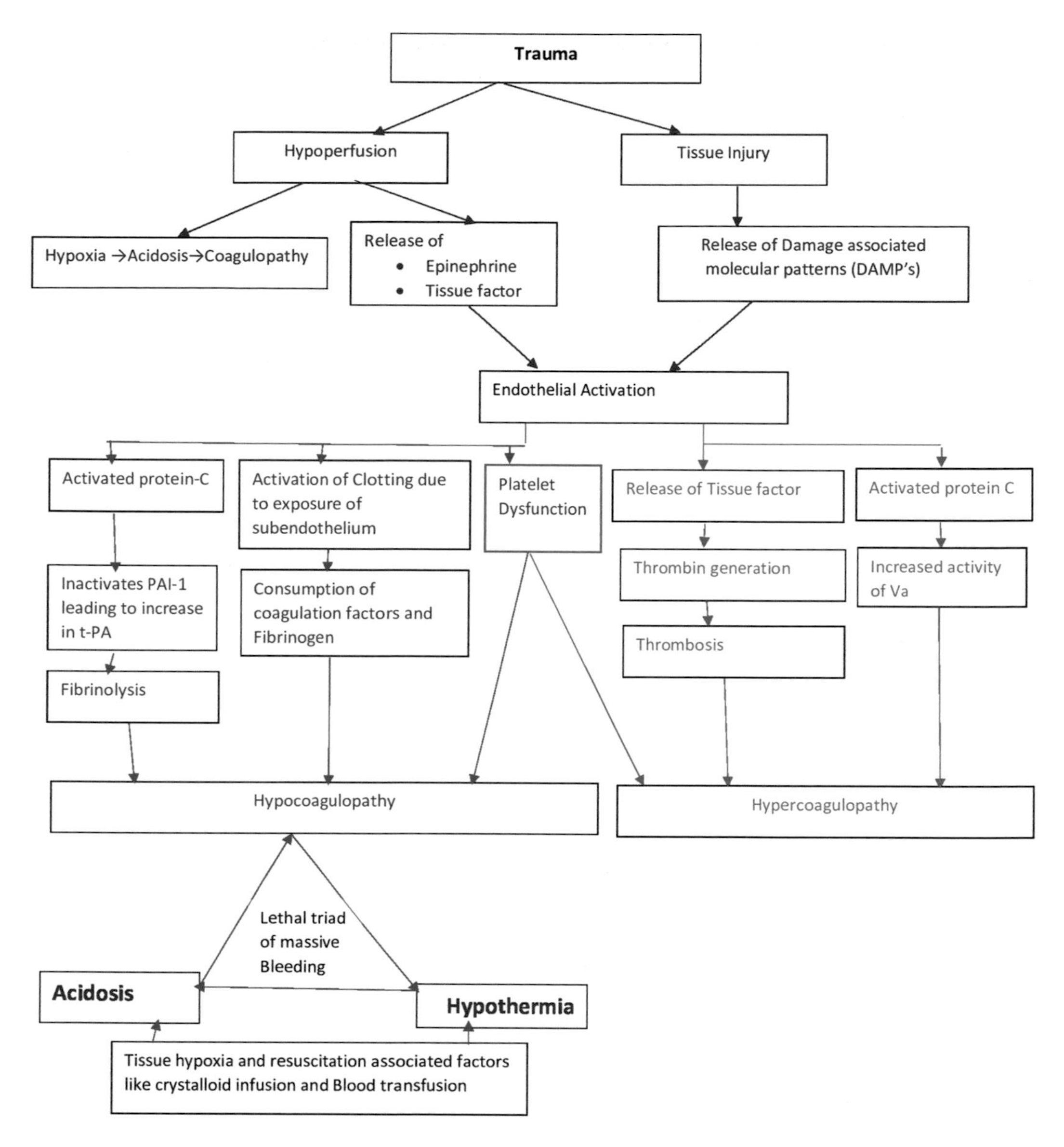

Figure 17.2 Pathophysiology of trauma-induced coagulopathy and lethal triad of massive bleeding

b. Identification of triggers for initiating the massive transfusion.
   i. ABC score of two or more: An ABC score has four variables (HR> 120, systolic BP < 90, +FAST and penetrating torso injury, each assigned one point). Other injury severity scores can also be used to assess the level of injury and requirement of blood transfusion.
   ii. Active bleeding requiring surgical repair.
   iii. Persistent haemodynamic instability.

2. Damage control surgery: Massive blood loss is prevented by controlling the bleeding using surgical and radiological techniques. It gives time for adequate resuscitation of the patient and prevention of complications of massive bleeding and transfusion before the patient is taken up for a definitive surgical procedure.
3. Limit crystalloids: Infusion of crystalloids in acutely bleeding patients is aimed at restoring the intravascular volume. However, it has been found that excessive crystalloid infusion may cause hydrostatic pressure on primary haemostatic plugs leading to further bleeding and dilution of coagulation factors. It can aggravate hypothermia and acidosis with worsening of coagulopathy.

On the other hand, prolonged hypoperfusion due to decreased intravascular volume can deteriorate organ function. Hence, crystalloid administration should be used with caution. Early initiation of blood component therapy maintains intravascular volume and prevents the development of deleterious effects of crystalloid infusion.

4. Anti-fibrinolytics: Administer anti-fibrinolytics like tranexamic acid within three hours of injury to prevent bleeding. They prevent bleeding by reversing the effect of increased t-PA after trauma.
5. Permissive hypotension: Systolic blood pressure between 90 and 100 mm Hg prevents blood loss due to hydrostatic pressure and maintains organ perfusion. For patients with traumatic brain and spinal cord injuries, permissive hypotension should not be practised and systolic blood pressure above 100 mg Hg should be maintained.
6. Early initiation of blood component therapy.

Blood Component Therapy

1. Blood component therapy during the active bleeding phase:
   a. Initiate blood transfusion in the ratio of fresh frozen plasma (FFP) to platelets to packed red blood cells (PRBC) of 1:1:1.
   b. Administer calcium chloride to prevent hypocalcaemia due to citrate present in various blood components. Acidosis due to lactate accumulation can also cause hypocalcaemia. Hypocalcaemia, in turn, can worsen coagulopathy, as it is required for fibrin polymerization and platelet function. Calcium also helps to maintain vascular contractility and tone.
   c. Ratio of blood components can be altered depending on the patient's comorbid condition and results of point-of-care tests like viscoelastic assays.

   Important points to remember while transfusing blood components in emergency:

   - Requisition form and blood sampling: A blood sample should be taken after positive patient identification. The requisition form and sample labelling should be completed by a single person and performed as one continuous, uninterrupted event.
   - Before starting the transfusion, identify the patient and match details with the blood unit to prevent incidents like issuing and transfusing of the wrong blood. These types of errors are common with unknown patients.
   - Emergency issues: Red blood cells require routine anti-human globulin (AHG) crossmatch before transfusion. But if transfusion is life-saving, then it can be transfused with emergency crossmatch (blood grouping and saline phase crossmatch only) after obtaining the consent in view of the life-saving nature of transfusion. In critically injured patients, O group PRBC (universal donor PRBC) can be issued with consent. For plasma transfusion, AB group can be transfused to patient with non-AB blood group.
   - Plasma and platelet products are issued blood-group-wise and do not require any crossmatch.
   - Cryoprecipitates can be transfused across the ABO blood group barrier.
   - Warming of blood components:
     - Warming of blood components may be required in a patient receiving massive transfusion to avoid hypothermia.
     - Warming of blood components should be done only with blood warmers with temperature display and temperature-sensitive alarms approved by the US Food and Drug Administration.
     - High temperature exposure to red blood cells can cause haemolysis and severe reaction in the patient.
     - Do not warm blood components in contaminated bowls or directly under hot water.

2. Viscoelastic assays: These are point-of-care tests available to monitor the coagulation status in a patient. These tests can be used to guide appropriate transfusion therapy in a patient requiring blood transfusion by localizing the defect in the coagulation. There are various types of viscoelastic assays available like thromboelastography, rotational thromboelastometry and sonoclot. These assays are better than the conventional coagulation tests, as whole blood is used for testing and the effect of platelets is also studied. It can also differentiate between the hypofibrinolytic and hyperfibrinolytic state trauma-induced coagulopathy. Table 17.3 shows an

Table 17.3: Interpretation of Sonoclot and Blood Component Therapy

Parameter	Interpretation	Normal Value	Main Corrective Component
Activated clotting time (ACT)	It is the time until initial clot formation. During this phase, all coagulation factors trigger thrombin generation.	100–155 seconds	Fresh frozen plasma
Clot rate	It is the rate of fibrin gel formation. A lower clot rate means a decrease in fibrinogen level.	11–35	Cryoprecipitate
Platelet function	Platelet contraction stabilizes the clot and causes a secondary peak in the sonoclot signature graph. Platelet function is calculated using an algorithm.	1.5 (platelet function is graded from 0 minimum to 5 maximum)	Platelet components

Table 17.4: Transfusion Triggers for Blood Component Therapy in a Patient with Controlled Bleeding

Transfusion Trigger For	Transfusion Trigger
Red cell transfusion	Haemoglobin < 8 gm/dl
Platelet transfusion (one adult dose and then reassess)	Platelet count < 50,000/μl
Fresh frozen plasma (15–20 ml/kg body weight)	INR > 1.5
Cryoprecipitate (one unit/kg body weight)	Fibrinogen < 150 mg/dl

interpretation of sonoclot assay and its role in guiding blood component therapy.

3. Reassessment of the patient: Reassessment of the patient should be done every 30–60 min.
   a. Bleeding ongoing with laboratory tests not available: Continue with ratio-based transfusion therapy.
   b. Bleeding ongoing with laboratory test available:
      i. Use laboratory tests to guide transfusion therapy (Table 17.4).
      ii. Monitor for hyperkalaemia and hypercalcaemia. Give calcium if ionized calcium is less than 1 mmol/l.

SUGGESTED READING

1. Vernon T, Morgan M, Morrison C. Bad blood: a coagulopathy associated with trauma and massive transfusion review. *Acute Med Surg.* 2019;6:215–22. DOI: 10.1002/ams2.402.
2. David JS, Voiglio EJ, Cesareo E, et al. Prehospital parameters can help to predict coagulopathy and massive transfusion in trauma patients. *Vox Sanguinis.* 2017;112:557–66. DOI: 10.1111/vox.12545.
3. Fullenbach C, Zacharowski K, Meybohm P. Improving outcome of trauma patients by implementing patient blood management. *Curr Opin Anesthesiol.* 2017;30:243–9. DOI: 10.1097/ACO.0000000000000427.
4. Wagner SH, Kanz KG. Massive transfusion in trauma patients. *ISBT Sci Ser.* 2007;2:98–103. DOI: 10.1111/j.1751-2824.2007.00121.x.
5. Moore EE, Moore HB, Kornblith LZ, et al. Trauma induced coagulopathy. *Nat Rev Dis Primers.* 2021;29:7(1):30. DOI: 10.1038/s41572-021-00264-3.

18 Interpreting Arterial Blood Gases in Trauma Patients

Narender Kaloria

LEARNING OBJECTIVES

- To list normal arterial blood gas values
- To diagnose acid-base disorders
- Sample collection and transport
- Stepwise approach to interpretation of arterial blood gas

INTRODUCTION

Trauma patients pose a significate challenge to attending clinicians due to the multi-organ involvement and rapid change in clinical condition. However, the management of these patients starts with assessment of airway, breathing and circulation with their management in the same order. In serious patients, further management requires trauma intensive care. Arterial blood gas (ABG) analysis is a useful tool for management for these patients in an acute trauma setting as well as intensive care. Accurate interpretation of ABG provides additional information regarding respiration, circulation and metabolic changes. ABG requires arterial blood and analysis of the oxygenation by partial pressure of oxygen (PaO_2) and ventilation by partial pressure of carbon dioxide ($PaCO_2$). pH and $PaCO_2$ are measured directly from the blood, but bicarbonate (HCO_3^-) and base excess derive from the Hesselbach equation.

COMMON TERMINOLOGY AND NORMAL ABG VALUES

- pH: acid-base balance of the blood (7.35–7.45)
- PaO_2: partial pressure of oxygen in arterial blood (75–100 mmHg)
- $PaCO_2$: partial pressure of carbon dioxide in arterial blood (35–45 mmHg)
- HCO_3^-: concentration of bicarbonate in arterial blood (22–26 meq/L)
- Base excess/deficit (–4 to +2)
- SaO_2: arterial oxygen saturation (95%–100%)

ACID-BASE DISORDERS WHICH CAN BE DIAGNOSED WITH ABG

Metabolic Acidosis

In metabolic acidosis, pH is decreased either due to a decreased level of bicarbonate (HCO_3^-) or accumulation of acid in the blood. It can be seen with various clinical conditions. It is broadly divided in two categories as per status of the anion gap (AG), which is calculated by the subtraction of unmeasured anions with cations.

$AG = Na^+ - (Cl + HCO_3^-)$; normal AG: 12 ± 2 meq/L

High Anion Gap Metabolic Acidosis (HAGMA)

High anion gap metabolic acidosis (HAGMA) occurs due to consumption of HCO_3^- in response to increased H^+ from endogenous acids. HAGMA is commonly seen in trauma patients who are hemodynamically unstable.

Examples of HAGMA are uraemia, ketoacidosis (diabetic, alcoholic or starvation), lactic acidosis, tissue hypoxia, alcohol intoxication and salicylate intoxication.

Non- or Normal Anion Gap Metabolic Acidosis (NAGMA)

The basic pathophysiology in this is loss of HCO_3^- or increase in Cl^- concentration. A few examples of non-anion gap (NAGMA) metabolic acidosis include:

- Gastrointestinal loss of HCO_3^- (diarrhoea, ileostomy, proximal colostomy, ureteral diversion)
- Renal loss of HCO_3^- [renal tubular disease, proximal renal tubular acidosis (RTA), distal RTA, carbonic anhydrase inhibitor (acetazolamide), chronic renal disease, aldosterone inhibitors]
- Sodium chloride infusion
- Total parenteral nutrition (TPN)

To differentiate high AG or non-AG or metabolic acidosis or metabolic acidosis mixed with metabolic alkalosis, the delta-delta ratio should be calculated.

$$Delta - delta\ ratio\ (DD) = | \Delta AG / \Delta HCO_3$$

- Delta-delta ratio < 1 = Non-AG metabolic acidosis
- Delta-delta ratio 1–2 = High AG metabolic acidosis
- Delta-delta ratio > 2 = High AG metabolic acidosis with concurrent metabolic alkalosis

DOI: 10.1201/9781003291619-20

Once diagnosis of metabolic acidosis is established, look for respiratory compensation for it. There will be a decrease in the CO_2 level as per the value of HCO_3^-. Whenever compensation is complete, then the pH will be in normal range; and if incomplete, then the pH will not be fully corrected. The following formula can be used to calculate the expected level of CO_2 for respiratory compensation with metabolic acidosis:

$$Expected\ CO_2(mmHg) = (1.5 \times HCO_3) + 8 \pm 2$$

Metabolic Alkalosis

In metabolic alkalosis, pH is increased due to the increased level of HCO_3^-, either due to loss of hydrogen ions (H^+) or gain of HCO_3^-. The following clinical conditions may result in metabolic alkalosis:

- Hypovolaemia with Cl^- depletion
  - GI loss of H^+ (vomiting, gastric suction, diarrhoea with chloride-rich fluid, villous adenoma)
  - Renal loss of H^+ (use of diuretics, hypercapnia following mechanical ventilation)
- Hypervolaemia with Cl^- expansion
  - Renal loss of H^+: volume overload (heart failure, cirrhosis, nephrotic syndrome), bicarbonate administration, hyperaldosteronism, hypercortisolism, excess ACTH, exogenous steroids, severe hypokalaemia, renal artery stenosis

Here, too, the compensation is respiratory but in opposite direction as compared to metabolic acidosis. The expected $PaCO_2$ value will be as per the level of HCO_3^-:

$$Expected\ PaCO_2 = (0.7 \times HCO_3) + 20 \pm 5$$

Acute Respiratory Acidosis

A sudden rise in $PaCO_2$ is primarily responsible for the decrease in pH in case of acute respiratory acidosis. There is not sufficient time for compensation in an acute setting. Hence, partial compensation may be present and pH mostly reflects the level of $PaCO_2$. However, pH decreases by 0.008 with every 1 mmHg rise in $PaCO_2$. Further, there is a decrease of 1 mEq/l HCO_3^- for every 10 mmHg rise in $PaCO_2$.

Common conditions leading to acute respiratory acidosis include airway obstruction secondary to airway trauma or secretions, acute onset severe lung pathology, pneumothorax secondary to chest trauma, acute narcotics or sedative intoxication, head injury and residual neuromuscular weakness.

Chronic Respiratory Acidosis

Whenever chronic CO_2 retention occurs (> 24 hour), renal compensation of HCO_3^- starts, resulting in minimal change in pH with rise of $PaCO_2$ values. This results in chronic respiratory acidosis. Common causes include chronic obstructive pulmonary disease (COPD), morbid obesity, moderate to severe kyphoscoliosis, and neuromuscular disease.

Acute Respiratory Alkalosis

In acute respiratory alkalosis, a decrease in $PaCO_2$ is responsible for the increase in pH. There is insufficient time for compensation due to acute onset. Hence, pH increases by 0.008 with every 1 mmHg decrease of $PaCO_2$, and HCO_3^- decreases by 2 mEq/l for every 10 mmHg decrease of $PaCO_2$. Common causes include central nervous system stimulation (pain, anxiety, head injury), pneumonia, pregnancy, fever and thyrotoxicosis.

Chronic Respiratory Alkalosis

Here, also, pH increases due to a fall in $PaCO_2$, but the compensation is better as compared to acute respiratory alkalosis. The expected increase in pH is 0.0017 with a 1 mmHg decrease of $PaCO_2$, and HCO_3^- decreases by 5 mEq/l with a 10 mmHg decrease of $PaCO_2$.

Acid-Base Abnormality Coexisting with Each Other

Respiratory acidosis with metabolic acidosis: In this condition, a decrease in pH results from both a decrease in HCO_3^- and an increase in $PaCO_2$. Common examples are following cardiac arrest, intoxications multi-organ failure.

Respiratory alkalosis with metabolic alkalosis: Here, pH increases due to an increase of HCO_3^- and a decrease of $PaCO_2$. A few examples are cirrhosis with diuretics, pregnancy with vomiting and overventilation of COPD.

SAMPLE COLLECTION AND TRANSPORT

A sample for ABG analysis can be taken from any artery, but the radial artery is commonly used, preferably of the non-dominant hand, either via puncturing the artery or drawing blood from an indwelling catheter. A modified Allen's test must be performed before puncturing for sampling from the radial artery to ensure the patency of collateral blood flow. After making a tight fist, occlude both the radial and ulnar arteries and then open the fist. After ensuring blanching of the palm, release the ulnar artery and see the return of blood flow to the palm. If the return of blood flow occurs in 5–10 s, then it denotes the presence of sufficient collateral blood flow, denoting that the radial artery can be safely punctured for sampling. So, by performing the modified Allen's test, we can avoid catastrophic complications like ischaemia and necrosis to the palm and fingers. After taking the sample, the artery should be compressed to avoid extravasation of blood and its subsequent complications.

The ABG sample should be collected in a heparinized syringe of small size (1–2 ml), which can be prepared by taking heparin in the hub of the syringe and flushing it back. Only 0.05 ml of heparin is required for anticoagulation of 1 ml blood. Heparin should be in very low quantity and concentration (1:1000). The sample should be air-bubble free and should be transported within 30 min for processing and reporting. For best results, the

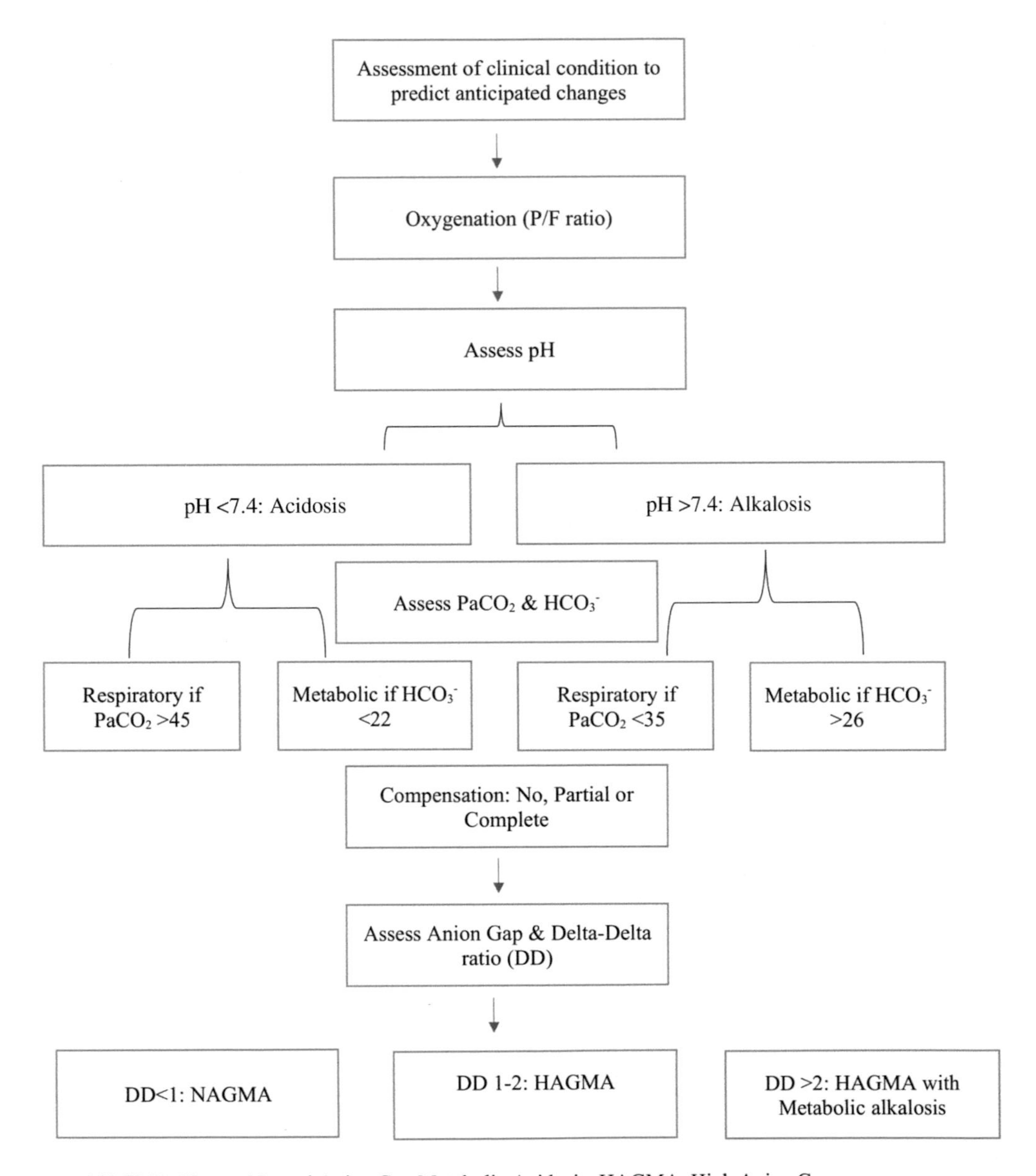

Figure 18.1 Algorithm for interpreting arterial blood gases

sample should be transported with ice pack coverings.

ABG INTERPRETATION STEPS

The ABG interpretation is very important in management for critically ill patients, especially in cases of polytrauma patients, where major fluid shifts occur and management is highly dependent upon ABG values. The interpretation should be in a systematic manner to identify the primary abnormality and to also look for its compensation. After interpretation, it should be correlated with the clinical condition and then management should be started as per findings. The ABG interpretation should be done in the following steps:

Step 1: ABG analysis starts with the clinical condition for which ABG is advised, and expected changes should be kept in mind. The severity of the clinical condition can be estimated with changes in ABG parameters.

Common clinical conditions and the expected ABG results are:

a. Hypotension/shock: lactic acidosis
b. Vomiting: metabolic alkalosis
c. Diarrhoea: metabolic acidosis
d. Bronchial asthma: respiratory alkalosis/acidosis
e. Diabetes mellitus: ketoacidosis
f. Renal disorder: metabolic acidosis
g. Septicaemia: lactic acidosis

Step 2: Assessment of oxygenation status by looking at PaO_2 and SaO_2 values. Always feed FiO_2 values to the ABG machine to get the accurate PaO_2:FiO_2 (P/F) ratio, which can tell the actual state of the body's oxygenation. A P/F ratio < 300 is considered to be abnormal, and if the value is less than 100, then it indicates severe hypoxia. All the corrective steps should be followed to correct hypoxia by checking the airway and breathing.

Step 3: Look for the values of pH. The cut-off value of pH for ABG interpretation is 7.4, so anything below 7.4 is considered acidosis and more than 7.4 as alkalosis.

Step 4: Check the $PaCO_2$ and HCO_3^- values to categorize the condition as respiratory or metabolic, respectively.

Step 5: Look for compensation, i.e. no compensation, partial compensation or complete compensation. The compensation should be checked according to disease process (either acute or chronic compensation as previously described in acid-base disorders). However, the following things need to be remembered for compensation:

a. If there is no compensation, then pH changes with only one parameter, either PaCO2 or HCO_3^-. In cases of partial compensation, both $PaCO_2$ and HCO_3^- change, but fail to normalise pH. However, if compensation is complete, then pH normalizes with a change in both $PaCO_2$ and HCO_3^-.
b. Acute compensation usually occurs within 6–24 hours and chronic may take 1–4 days.
c. The compensating parameter (either $PaCO_2$ or HCO_3^-) moves in the same direction as the primary abnormal parameter in the case of a simple acid-base disorder, but it moves in the opposite direction in case of a mixed acid-base abnormality. For example, HCO_3^- decreases in metabolic acidosis and $PaCO_2$ will decrease to compensate for pH (same direction). On the other hand, in mixed metabolic and respiratory acidosis, HCO_3^- decreases and $PaCO_2$ increases (opposite direction).

Step 6: Calculation of anion gap [$AG = Na^+ - (Cl^- + HCO_3^-)$] will help to differentiate the pathology of normal AG with high AG.

Step 7: Assess the delta gap ($\Delta AG/\Delta\ HCO_3^-$). This also helps to diagnose the state of metabolic acidosis (normal or high AG) or metabolic acidosis with alkalosis. The algorithm for interpreting ABG is depicted in Figure 18.1.

SUGGESTED READING

1. Gattinoni L, Pesenti A, Matthay M. Understanding blood gas analysis. *Intens Care Med*. 2018;44:91–3. doi: 10.1007/s00134-017-4824-y.

2. Cowley NJ, Owen A, Bion JF. Interpreting arterial blood gas results. *BMJ*. 2013;346:f16. doi: 10.1136/bmj.f16.

3. Larkin BG, Zimmanck RJ. Interpreting arterial blood gases successfully. *AORN J*. 2015;102(4):343–54; quiz 355–7. doi: 10.1016/j.aorn.2015.08.002. PMID: 26411819.

4. Zisquit J, Velasquez J, Nedeff N. *StatPearls* [Internet]. Treasure Island (FL): StatPearls Publishing; Jul 10, 2020. Allen Test.

5. Sood P, Paul G, Puri S. Interpretation of arterial blood gas. *Indian J Crit Care Med*. 2010;14(2):57–64. doi: 10.4103/0972-5229.68215. PMID: 20859488.

6. ARDS Definition Task Force, Ranieri VM, Rubenfeld GD, Thompson BT, Ferguson ND, Caldwell E, et al. Acute respiratory distress syndrome: the Berlin definition. *JAMA*. 2012;307:2526–33. doi: 10.1001/jama.2012.5669. PMID: 22797452.

19 Point-of-Care Ultrasound

Applications in Triage

Haneesh Thakur and Kajal Jain

LEARNING OBJECTIVES

- USG probes
- FAST and eFAST examinations
- POCUS in emergency resuscitation

INTRODUCTION

Point-of-care ultrasound (POCUS) is a valuable bedside instrument as it provides an edge over primitive methods by providing real-time ultrasonographic assessment identifying underlying life-threatening pathologies and rapidly sorting them out. A key goal is to become well-practised with a better understanding of the basics of POCUS, its role and its approach in trauma emergency care.

POCUS works on the principle of the piezoelectric effect (Figure 19.1). Probe or transducer components are assembled to produce and acquire images at the patient end. These can be classified on the basis of depth and resolution (depending upon the assembly and beam shapes) as mentioned in Table 19.1.

FAST AND EFAST EXAMINATION

FAST stands for focused assessment with sonography in trauma and consists of four views: the right upper quadrant view, the left upper quadrant view, the pelvic view and subcostal view.

eFAST exam expands as extended focused assessment with sonography in trauma and consists of the examination of lungs in addition to the aforementioned spaces. Figure 19.2 represents sites to examine in eFAST.

Indications

- Trauma patient with hemodynamic instability
- Blunt or penetrating neck, torso or pelvic trauma
- New acute haemodynamic or respiratory worsening in a previously stable trauma patient
- A patient with dangerous trauma mechanism in an unconscious or disoriented state

Preparation

- Patient position – supine or in the Trendelenburg position
- Position the machine by the right side of the patient
- Machine should be preset to eFAST exam or abdominal exam

Protocol for eFAST Sequence

Follow the protocol so that one doesn't forget to examine any particular region.

1. Right upper quadrant view (RUQ)
2. Left upper quadrant view (LUQ)
3. Pelvic view
4. Cardiac view (subxiphoid or parasternal long axis)
5. Lungs (right and left)

The purpose of the examination is to rapidly identify the result of injuries to the organ i.e. haemorrhage, rather than an assessment of organ injury (which is difficult to identify).

Questions to Be Kept in Mind before You Proceed

- What abnormality am I looking for?
- Is there free fluid in the right upper part of the abdomen or right thorax?
- Does my patient have free fluid in the left upper part abdomen or left lower thorax?
- Does my patient have free fluid in the pelvis?
- Am I suspecting pneumothorax?

Step 1: Right Upper Quadrant View (RUQ)

The RUQ probe position and hand positioning are illustrated in Figure 19.3a.

Probe: Curvilinear.

Probe marker: Towards the patient's head.

Position: Probe is placed vertically at the tenth intercostal space in midaxillary line.

Expected view: A coronal view of the liver and right kidney interface (Figure 19.4a).

Examines the right paracolic gutter, Morison's pouch, the hepato-diaphragmatic area and perirenal space.

DOI: 10.1201/9781003291619-21

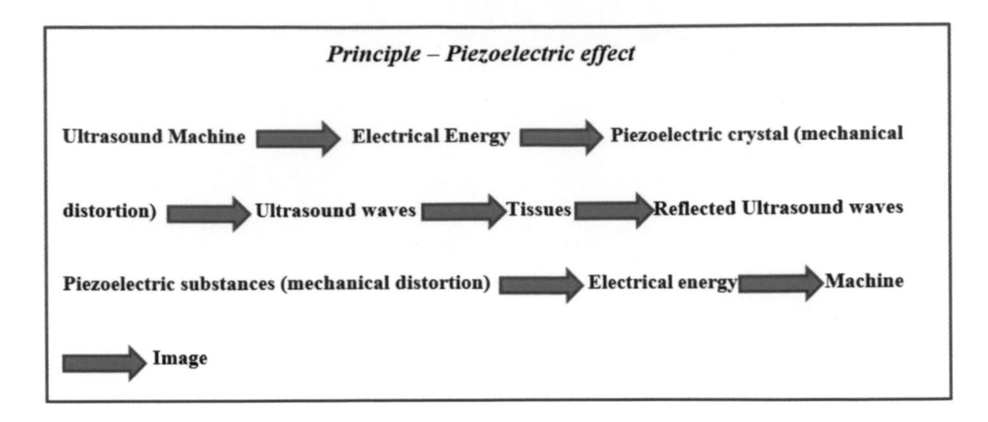

Figure 19.1 Flow chart depicting the principle of working of POCUS, the piezoelectric effect

Table 19.1: Types of Probes and Functions Pertaining to Trauma

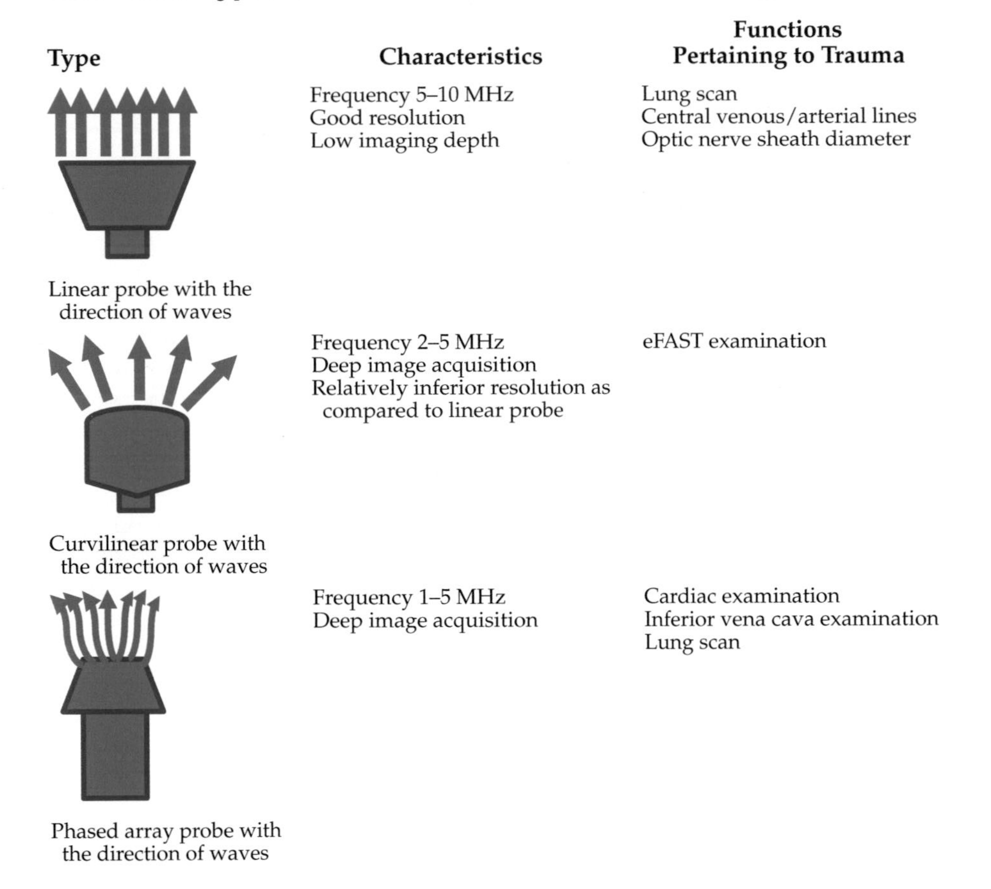

Type	Characteristics	Functions Pertaining to Trauma
Linear probe with the direction of waves	Frequency 5–10 MHz Good resolution Low imaging depth	Lung scan Central venous/arterial lines Optic nerve sheath diameter
Curvilinear probe with the direction of waves	Frequency 2–5 MHz Deep image acquisition Relatively inferior resolution as compared to linear probe	eFAST examination
Phased array probe with the direction of waves	Frequency 1–5 MHz Deep image acquisition	Cardiac examination Inferior vena cava examination Lung scan

Step 2: Left Upper Quadrant View (LUQ)

LUQ probe position is illustrated in Figure 19.3b.

Probe: Curvilinear.

Pointer: Towards the patient's head.

Position: At posterior axillary line level, around the eighth intercostal space; as the spleen is fairly posterior, one should have "knuckles to the bed".

Expected view: A coronal view of spleen and left kidney interface (Figure 19.4b).

Examines: Splenorenal recess, the subphrenic space, the left paracolic gutter, as well as the left lower hemithorax.

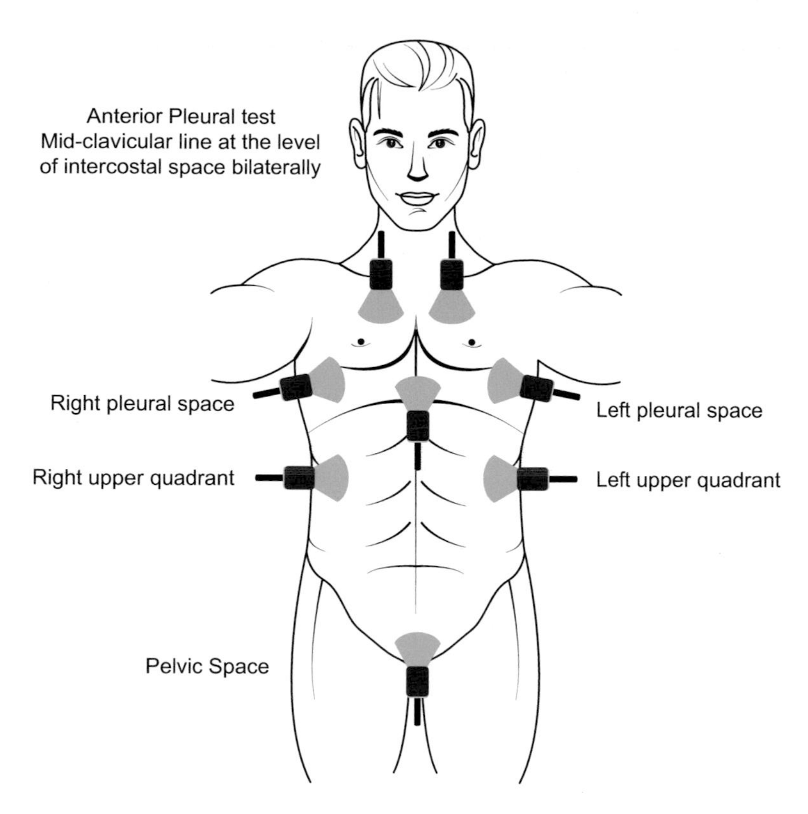

Figure 19.2 Diagrammatic representation of the sites to perform eFAST

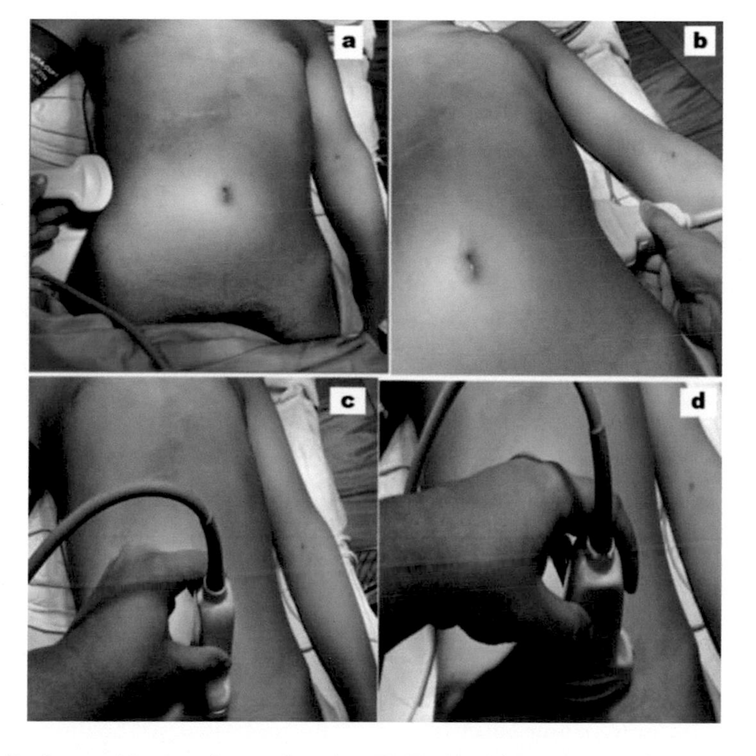

Figure 19.3 Probe positioning for performing FAST: (a) right upper quadrant; (b) left upper quadrant; (c) pelvis, longitudinal placement of probe; (d) pelvis, transverse placement of probe

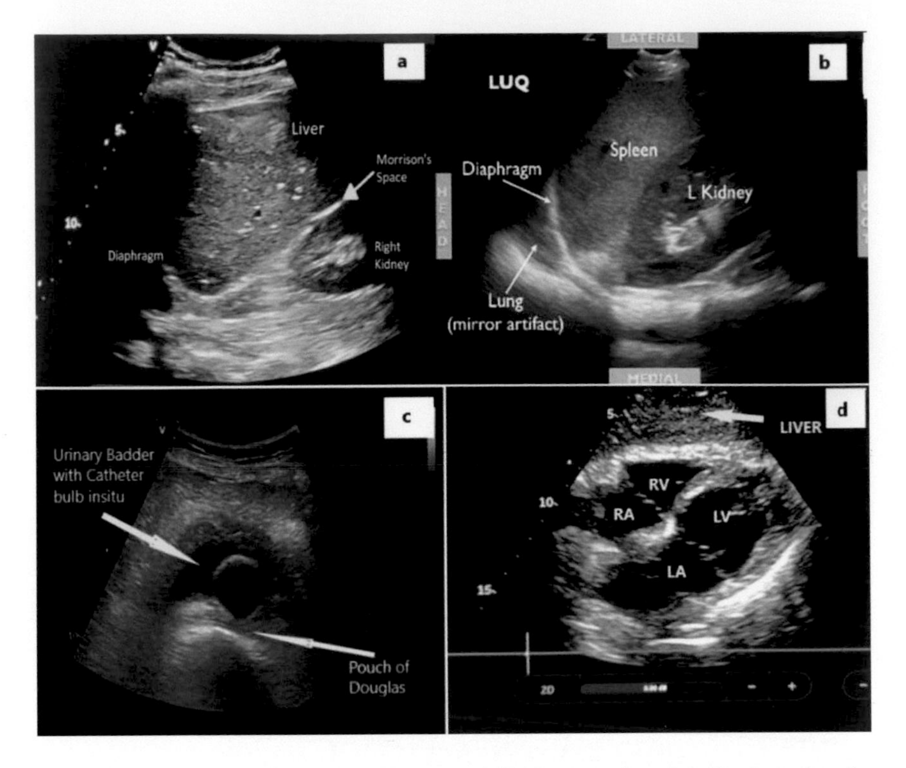

Figure 19.4 Normal FAST sonography: (a) normal RUQ view showing the interface between liver and kidney; (b) normal LUQ view showing the interface between spleen and kidney; (c) normal transverse view of the pelvis; (d) normal subcostal view showing the heart

Step 3: Pelvic View

The patient should be scanned in a full bladder status. The probe-holding method for performing an eFAST of pelvic view has been illustrated in Figure 19.3c, d.

Probe: Curvilinear.

Pointer: Towards the patient's head in vertical transducer placement and towards the right side in horizontal transducer placement.

Position: Along midline suprapubic region.

1. Vertical
2. Horizontal

Expected view: In males, the rectovesical pouch is the space where the fluid accumulates. The first step is to identify the bladder (containing urine confined by the wall), prostate/seminal vesicle and rectovesical pouch in the longitudinal view. Rotate the transducer perpendicularly, have a transverse view, identify the bladder and any perivesical collection if any.

In females, the first step is to identify the bladder, uterus, and recto-uterine pouch (also called the *pouch of Douglas*) (Figure 19.4c). Free fluid can accumulate in the pouch of Douglas.

Step 4: Cardiac Scan (Cardiac Subxiphoid View)

Pointer: Towards the patient's right shoulder. Figure 19.4d illustrates the cardiac view as seen during the eFAST examination.

Probe: Phased array (ideal) or curvilinear; depth of the ultrasound imaging to be set around 15–20 cm.

The probe should be kept as horizontal as possible over the subcostal area aiming towards the left shoulder of the patient over the subcostal area to get a good view of the heart. The examination can be followed by a parasternal long-axis view examination to get additional information if possible. Otherwise, the examiner should proceed to lung scanning.

Examines: Pericardial space, cardiac chambers, cardiac contractility.

CARDIAC PARASTERNAL LONG AXIS

Probe: Curvilinear or phased array probe. Hold the probe in a pen-holding fashion.

Pointer: Towards the patient's left hip.

Identify the cardiac structures outward to inward or vice versa (pericardium, left atrium, mitral valve, left ventricle, aortic valve, right ventricle and descending aorta). Look for fluid in the pericardial space.

Step 5: Lung Scan

Probe: Linear.

Pointer: Towards the patient's head.

Position: At the midclavicular line in the second intercostal space of the right and left lungs, respectively. This point provides the most sensitive place for looking at pneumothorax in a patient in the supine position. Always compare both sides.

Expected view: Sagittal view showing skin, subcutaneous tissue with underlying pleura showing sliding. Lung sliding is the appearance of movement of parietal pleura and visceral pleura against one another. It also looks like "ants marching on a line". The presence of lung sliding effectively rules out pneumothorax.

Other signs to look for:

Batwing sign: Image formed by two ribs shadow with pleura in between appearing as wings of a bat ensuring correct probe position.

Seashore sign: Using M-mode in ultrasound, lung sliding can be further evaluated (*M-mode for motion*). The ultrasound cursor should be placed over the lung field. The M-mode pattern appears like a seashore suggesting normal finding: sky = skin/subcutaneous tissue, ocean = muscle, beach = lung sliding motion (Figure 19.5a).

Barcode sign: M-mode appearance when the pleural lines are apart (as in pneumothorax). It appears as a barcode (Figure 19.5b).

"Lung point sign": Pneumothorax may also be suspected when there is a "lung point sign", which appears as the point where lung sliding and the absence of lung sliding transition is there. This appearance is due to the transition between a normal and a collapsed lung in a developing pneumothorax. Moreover, the location of the lung point at the intercostal space also helps to have an idea about the size of the pneumothorax.

Interpreting eFAST Findings

Advantages

- FAST sensitivities range from 85% to 96%, whereas specificities exceed 98%.
- A faster learning curve.
- Non-invasiveness.
- Repeated reproducibility allowing for serial monitoring of patients.
- Patient can be examined while another examination is being proceeded.
- It is less time-consuming, being at the bedside.
- No radiation exposure and can be safely used in pregnant people as well as children.

Limitations

- The resultant haemorrhage due to organ injury is assessed, but the injured abdominal organ is not localized.
- As air is an enemy of ultrasound, the views may be inadequate/limited in subcutaneous emphysema.
- A hollow viscus injury with free air in the abdomen may limit the view.

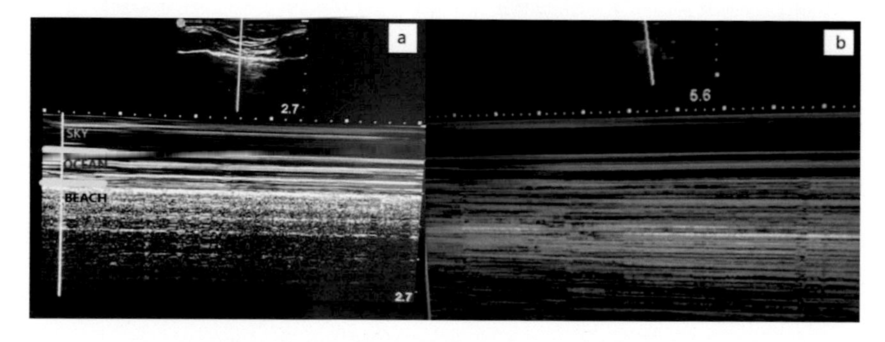

Figure 19.5 M-mode ultrasonography of the lung: (a) normal lung scan showing "seashore sign"; (b) abnormal lung scan showing "barcode sign"

- At least 200–250 ml of blood is required to be present before the eFAST scan becomes positive.
- Does not localize the bleeding to a specific organ. A CT scan is needed to localize the origin of abdominal bleeding in a trauma patient.

The three common locations for free fluid to accumulate in the RUQ of the eFAST scan are:

- Hepatorenal space or "Morison's pouch" (Figure 19.6a)
- Caudal tip of the liver
- Supra hepatic space

Figure 19.6 (a–d) depicts FAST positive images.

Haemothorax via eFAST

After evaluating the RUQ or LUQ, move the probe superiorly to one or two rib spaces to evaluate the thorax for fluid accumulation.

Mirror sign: A normal lung will have a mirror image artefact due to the reflection of ultrasound waves by the aerated lung and you will be unable to see the spine.

Spine sign: When there is free fluid (or blood) above the diaphragm (haemothorax), the ultrasound waves are not reflected and patient's spine can be visualized. This is known as a "spine sign".

Figure 19.7 illustrates the steps to proceed with FAST examination.

EMERGENCY RESUSCITATION

Advantages in Trauma

- POCUS has provided a dynamic way of diagnosing and managing shock rather than the use of traditional relay on the interpretation of blood pressure, heart rate and systemic vascular resistance to diagnose the type of shock encountered in trauma.
- Response to administered fluid and drugs (inotropes and pressors) can be seen in real time.

The purpose is to identify volume status of the patient using ultrasound.

- Look for the status in subcostal view. If the walls of the left ventricles (LV) are approximating or "kissing" (gap between walls $\leq$ 2.5 cm), then hypovolaemia is likely. If the gap between the LV walls is approximately $>$ 6 cm, then hypervolaemia/poor systolic function is likely.

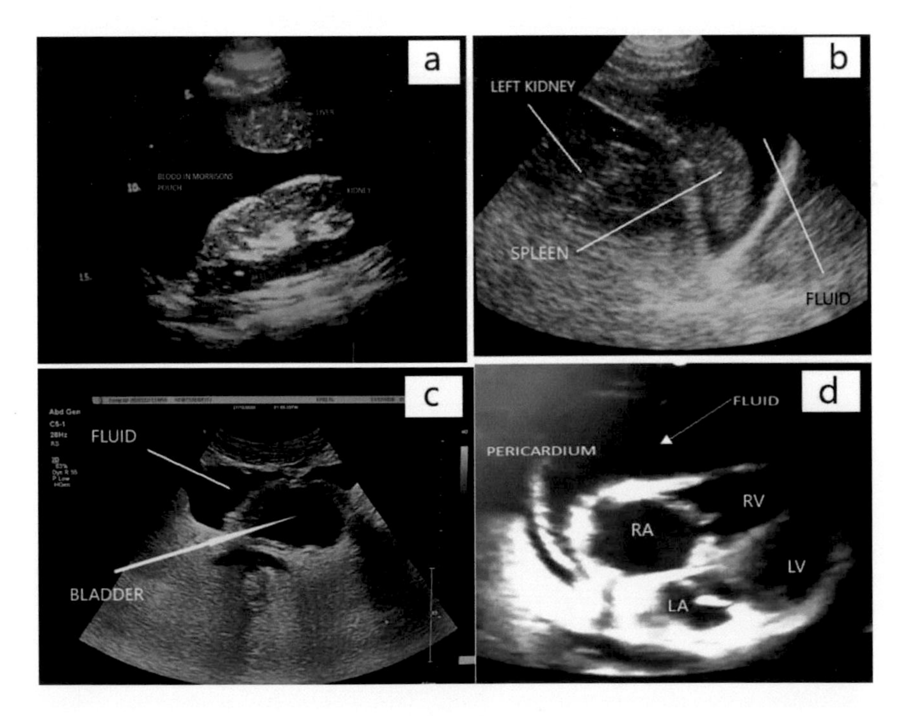

Figure 19.6 Abnormal FAST sonography: (a) fluid collection in Morison's pouch in RUQ view; (b) fluid collection around the spleen; (c) collection of fluid in pelvic space; (d) presence of fluid in pericardial space

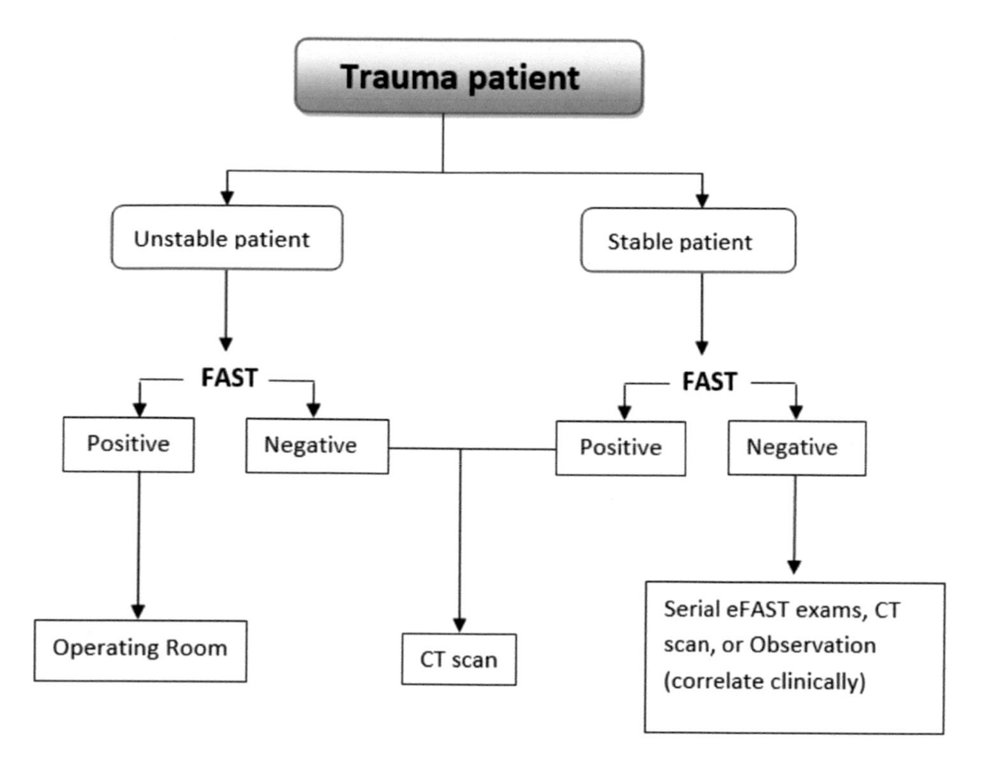

Figure 19.7 Flow chart depicting steps to proceed for FAST examination

- One can also look for the inferior vena cava (IVC) diameter.
- Correlation of IVC diameter with central venous pressure (CVP):
  - IVC diameter < 1.5 cm with 100% collapsibility: Approximate CVP is 0–5 mmHg.
  - IVC diameter 1.5–2.5 with > 50% collapsibility: CVP approximates 5–10 mmHg.
  - IVC diameter 1.5–2.5 with < 50% collapsibility: CVP is 10–15 mmHg.
  - IVC diameter > 2.5 with no collapsibility: CVP approximates > 20 mmHg.

EMERGENCY AIRWAY MANAGEMENT

Probe: Linear probe.

Position of the marker: Towards the head.

Position of the probe: Longitudinal and midline below the thyroid prominence.

Pointer: Towards patient's head.

Approach:

- The objective emergency is to identify the cricothyroid membrane.
- Position of the transducer: Longitudinal with pointer towards the head slightly lateral to the midline of the trachea. The probe should be held with the non-dominant hand to identify airway structures (thyroid, cricoid and tracheal cartilages). In between the thyroid and cricoid cartilages, identify the cricothyroid membrane.
- Once the cricothyroid membrane is identified, a single horizontal incision is made medial to the probe with the scalpel through the membrane and surgical front of neck access is achieved.

PROCEDURAL FOCUS: A Great Help

Probe: Linear probe.

Marker position: Medially.

Procedure:

- Identify the anatomy of the insertion site and localization of the artery or vein.
- Confirm and place a catheter in the artery or vein (e.g. central line/dialysis catheter/ arterial line).

CONCLUSION

Point-of-care ultrasound has provided an extra vision to the medical personnel and its utility cannot be denied. It has emerged from the confined radiology suite to almost every phase of a healthcare facility. Especially in trauma, where urgent decision-making is of utmost importance, this extra vision has been a boon and greatly aids better patient evaluation and management.

SUGGESTED READING

1. Gleeson T, Blehar D. Point-of-care ultrasound in trauma. *Semin Ultrasound CT MR*. 2018;39:374–83. doi: 10.1053/j.sult.2018.03.007.

2. Morrow D, Cupp J, Schrift D, Nathanson R, Soni NJ. Point-of-care ultrasound in established settings. *South Med J*. 2018;111:373–81. doi: 10.14423/SMJ.0000000000000838. PMID: 29978220.

3. Montorfano MA, Pla F, Vera L, Cardillo O, Nigra SG, Montorfano LM. Point-of-care ultrasound and Doppler ultrasound evaluation of vascular injuries in penetrating and blunt trauma. *Crit Ultrasound J*. 2017;9:5. doi: 10.1186/s13089-017-0060-5.

4. Rippey JC, Royse AG. Ultrasound in trauma. *Best Pract Res Clin Anaesthesiol*. 2009;23:343–62. doi: 10.1016/j.bpa.2009.02.011. PMID: 19862893.

5. American College of Surgeons. *Advanced Trauma Life Support: Student Course Manual*. Chicago, IL: American College of Surgeons; 2018.

20 Desaturating Patient with Long Bone Fractures

Diagnosis and Management

Devendra Kumar Chouhan and Narendra Chouhan

LEARNING OBJECTIVES

- What is desaturation
- Causes of desaturation in cases with long bone fractures
- How to diagnose the cause of desaturation
- Management of desaturating patient with long bone fractures

DEFINITION

A blood oxygen saturation value less than 92% is considered hypoxia (or desaturation). Hypoxia is a medical emergency and should be promptly treated. Identifying the cause of hypoxia, oxygen supplementation and problem-specific intervention are key to preventing secondary injury to the vital organs.

AETIOLOGY AND DIFFERENTIAL DIAGNOSIS

A long bone fracture with associated polytrauma in adult patients indirectly indicates a high velocity of trauma. Management consists of a quick primary survey (ABCDE), coupled with intervention and an outcome assessment. There could be multiple causes for hypoxia in cases with long bone fractures that can be readily diagnosed following the Advanced Trauma Life Support guidelines (Table 20.1).

Secondary Lung Injury

Respiratory decompensation can happen in reaction to the humoral response to traumatic incidence without any direct blow to the airway, chest wall or lungs in cases with long bone fractures. The common causes of lung injury in such cases are fat embolism syndrome (FES) and acute respiratory distress syndrome (ARDS).

FAT EMBOLISM SYNDROME (FES)

Fractures of long bones lead to the release of fat globules into the circulation, which can embolize to vital organs (e.g. lungs, brain and heart), leading to multiple organ failure, known as fat embolism syndrome. To facilitate the diagnosis of FES, certain criteria are followed, including Gurd's criteria (see Table 20.2). However, limitations of Gurd's criteria include the following:

1. Petechiae, the objective criteria incidence rate in the original study by Gurd and Lindeque varies between 39% and 57% in patients with suspected FES (Figure 20.1).
2. Under sedation or general anaesthesia, respiratory insufficiency is a subjective criterion and can be altered by positive pressure ventilation. Cerebral involvement is not a useful criterion for patients under anaesthesia.
3. The minor criteria may be a common finding in other clinical disorders.

Schonfeld et al. proposed a quantitative measure to diagnose FES (Table 20.3). The advantage of Schonfeld's criteria over Gurd's criteria is "Petechiae" gains the maximum points; therefore, this criterion alone is enough for diagnosis of FES.

According to Lindeque et al., FES can be diagnosed based on respiratory system involvement alone (Table 20.4). The advantages of Lindeque's criteria over Gurd's criteria are:

1. Early recognition is possible as blood gas levels are done as a routine procedure.
2. Early resuscitation is adopted without delay.

Etiopathogenesis of FES

According to the current understanding, FES is classified into three phases:

Mechanical phase – The fat globules enter into circulation at the time of injury and can embolize in the lung and other vital organs.

Latent phase – Circulation distress occurs because of droplets.

Chemical phase – The free fatty acid induces a chemical influence in the lung parenchyma. Inflammatory cells infiltrate focally, resulting in tissue oedema, epithelium damage and bronchial obstruction. Finally, tissue fibrosis occurs because of focal inflammation and collagen deposition and smooth muscle action leading to narrowing of the vessel lumen and vessel wall thickening. This results in a ventilation–perfusion mismatch.

DOI: 10.1201/9781003291619-22

Table 20.1: Differential Diagnosis of Desaturation in Long Bone Fracture

ABCDE		Clinical Findings	Laboratory	Radiology
A	Airway obstruction	Foreign body/blood, Oral secretion/vomitus Stridor, facial injury, neck injury	Hypoxia	Chest X-ray infiltrates, foreign body Fascio-maxillary trauma Head injury
B	Blunt trauma chest	Dyspnoea Chest pain Tachypnoea Flail chest Decreased breath sound	Respiratory acidosis/alkalosis	CT/X-ray chest: rib fracture Lung contusion Pneumothorax Haemothorax Dissection of aorta
	ARDS	Acute onset Breathlessness Tachypnoea Tachycardia Cyanosis	Low PaO_2/FiO_2 Mild: > 200 mmHg but ≤ 300 mmHg Moderate: > 100 mmHg but ≤ 200 mmHg Severe: $PaO_2/FiO_2 \leq 100$ mm	Chest X-ray: Bilateral infiltrates
	Fat embolism syndrome	Axillary or subconjunctival petechiae $PaO_2 < 60$ mmHg Neurological symptoms Tachycardia Pyrexia	Raised ESR Decrease in platelets Fat globules in sputum	Chest X-ray: Diffuse lung infiltrates
C	Shock	Tachycardia Tachypnoea Hypotension Decreased urine output	Low haematocrit Low haemoglobin Hypoxia	Fast scan+ Major bone fracture Pelvis fracture Chest trauma Lung parenchymal changes
	Blunt trauma abdomen	Rigidity Tenderness Abdominal pain	Decreased haemoglobin/haematocrit	e-FAST: Fluid collection CT scan: Viscera injury
D	Head injury	Altered sensorium Confusion Absent airway protection Reflex Tachypnoea	Respiratory acidosis/alkalosis	CT scan: fracture Intra- or extra-axial bleeding/ contusion
	Long bone fracture/ associated pelvis fracture	Hypovolaemic shock FES ARDS		
E	Hypothermia	Shivering Subjective awareness of cold Temperature < 36	Acidosis Coagulopathy Shock	

FES, fat embolism syndrome; ARDS, acute respiratory distress syndrome.

Table 20.2: Gurd's Criteria

Major Criteria
Axillary or subconjunctival petechiae
Hypoxaemia $PaO_2 < 60$ mmHg; $FiO_2 = 0.4$
Central nervous system depression disproportionate to hypoxaemia
Pulmonary oedema
Minor Criteria
Tachycardia < 110 bpm
Pyrexia < 38.5°C
Emboli present in the retina on fundoscopy
Fat present in urine
A sudden inexplicable drop in haematocrit or platelet values
Increasing ESR
Fat globules present in the sputum

Note: Diagnosis of FES requires the presence of at least one major criterion and at least four minor criteria.

Investigations

Detection of fat droplets in sputum, urine and blood. Arterial blood gas analysis shows hypoxia, with a PaO_2 of less than 60 mmHg along with the presence of hypocapnia. An increase in pulmonary shunt fraction and an alveolar-to-arterial oxygen tension difference, especially within 24–48 h of an event, is suggestive of the diagnosis.

Hypofibrinogenaemia, thrombocytopenia, anaemia, and increased erythrocyte sedimentation rate (ESR) with the increase in haematocrit may occur.

A chest radiograph could be normal initially and gradually evolve in generalized interstitial and alveolar opacification over 1 to 3 days, without pleural effusions (Figure 20.2). These radiological changes may remain for three weeks despite the clinical improvement of the patient. On a spiral chest CT for pulmonary embolism (PE), focal areas of ground-glass opacification with interlobular septal thickening are seen.

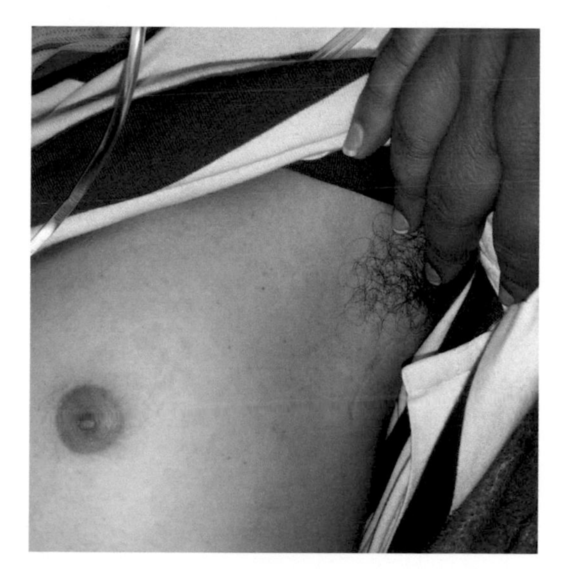

Figure 20.1 Petechial haemorrhage in axillary area and chest wall

Management

Respiratory Care

Continuous pulse oximetry monitoring in high-risk patients helps in early detection of desaturation, allowing early administration of oxygen, decreasing the risk of secondary hypoxic injuries.

Treatment objectives are to ensure good arterial oxygenation and to treat the underlying cause as soon as possible. High-flow oxygen is given to maintain the arterial oxygen tension in the normal range, and adequate maintenance of intravascular volume is important.

The initial management of hypoxia should be with spontaneous ventilation. A face mask with a high-flow gas delivery system can be used to deliver the inspired oxygen concentration

Table 20.3: Schonfeld's Criteria

Petechiae	5
Chest X-ray changes (diffuse alveolar infiltrates)	4
Hypoxaemia (Pa_2 <9.3 kPa)	3
Fever (> 38°C)	1
Tachycardia (> 120 beats/min)	1
Tachypnoea (> 30 bpm)	1
Cumulative score > 5 required for diagnosis	

Note: Diagnosis of FES requires the presence of a score of more than 5.

Table 20.4: Lindeque's Criteria

Sustained $PaO_2 < 8$ kPa
Sustained PCO_2 of > 7.3 kPa or a pH < 7.3
Sustained respiratory rate > 35 breaths/min, despite sedation
Increased work of breathing: dyspnoea, accessory muscle use, tachycardia and anxiety

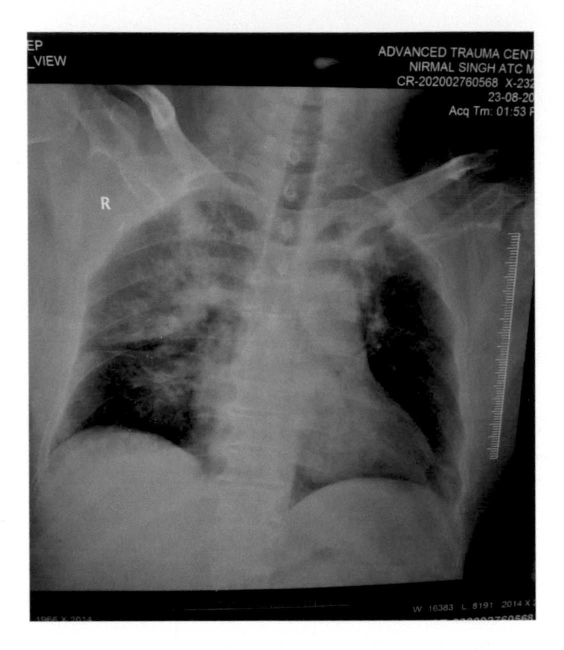

Figure 20.2 Radiograph chest PA view showing bilateral lung field opacities

(FiO_2) of up to 50%–80% to achieve a PaO_2 of more than 60 mmHg. Alternatively, CPAP and non-invasive ventilation may offer improvement in PaO_2 without increasing the FiO_2. Intubation and mechanical ventilation are considered in patients not maintaining saturation > 90% despite high FiO_2 administration, in patients unable to maintain saturation on non-invasive ventilation, and in patients requiring FiO_2 of > 60% and CPAP > 10 cmH_2O to achieve a PaO_2 > 60 mmHg.

Supportive Care

Heparin and corticosteroids have been proposed as treatments. Heparin stimulates lipase activity and therefore may accelerate the clearance of lipids from circulation, but the resultant increase in free fatty acids could exacerbate the underlying proinflammatory physiology and anticoagulation in the setting of trauma, and pre-existing haematologic abnormalities may prove harmful. In cases of fulminant fat embolism syndrome, corticosteroids may be considered.

Corticosteroids have been used prophylactically to decrease the incidence and severity of FES. Methylprednisolone 1.5 mg/kg IV can be administered every 8 h for six doses. It acts as an anti-inflammatory agent, reducing the perivascular haemorrhage and oedema. However, insufficient data supports initiating steroid therapy once FES is established.

Prognosis

Fat embolism syndrome is a self-limiting condition, with a mortality of 10%–20%, relating to the degree of respiratory failure.

ACUTE RESPIRATORY DISTRESS SYNDROME (ARDS)

Etiopathogenesis

Inflammatory injury to the lungs caused by the systemic inflammatory response to external noxious stimuli is defined as acute respiratory distress syndrome (ARDS). Patients with ARDS tends to progress through three pathologic stages:

1. Early exudative stage – The early exudative stage during the first 7–10 days is a non-specific reaction to lung injury. It is characterized by interstitial oedema, acute and chronic inflammation, type II cell hyperplasia, and hyaline membrane formation.
2. Fibroproliferative stage – This stage develops 7–10 days after the early exudative phase, characterized by resolution of pulmonary oedema, the proliferation of type II alveolar cells, squamous metaplasia, interstitial infiltration by myofibroblasts and early deposition of collagen. This stage can last between 2 and 3 weeks.
3. Fibrotic stage – This stage is characterized by obliteration of normal lung architecture, fibrosis and cyst formation.

Diagnosis

The Berlin Definition of ARDS requires that all the following criteria be present for diagnosis:

1. Respiratory symptoms must have begun within 1 week of a known clinical insult, or the patient must have new or worsening symptoms during the past week.
2. Bilateral opacities consistent with pulmonary oedema must be present on a chest radiograph or CT scan (these must not be fully explained by pleural effusion, lobar collapse, lung collapse or pulmonary nodules).
3. A moderate to severe impairment of O_2 must be present, as defined by the ratio of the

arterial oxygen tension to the fraction of the inspire O_2 (PaO_2/FiO_2).

a. Mild ARDS: $PaO_2/FiO_2 > 200$ mmHg but ≤ 300 mmHg
b. Moderate ARDS: $PaO_2/FiO_2 > 100$ mmHg but ≤ 200 mmHg
c. Severe ARDS: $PaO_2/FiO_2 \leq 100$ mmHg

Note: On ventilatory setting PEEP ≥ 5 cmH_2O.

Management

General Care

1. Ensure adequate analgesia for polytrauma patients.
2. Target euthermia by avoiding shivering.
3. Adequate hydration and avoid fluid overload (guided by lactate, urine output and sensorium).
4. Prevention of infection (prophylactic antibiotic) or treat the infection (empirical or culture-based).
5. Maintain adequate nutritional support. Patients with ARDS are intensely catabolic, and nutritional support may help to offset catabolic losses, promote immune responses and mitigate oxidative cellular injury. Enteral feedings are preferred because of lower risk of intravascular infections, less gastrointestinal bleeding and preservation of the intestinal mucosal barrier, which also decreases bacterial translocation across the gut.
6. Provide deep vein thrombosis (DVT) prophylaxis with low molecular weight heparin (LMWH)/heparin if there is no coexisting contraindication. This group of patients are prone to DVT/PE due to prolonged immobility, trauma, activation of the coagulation pathway and predisposing illnesses, such as sepsis, obesity and malignancy.
7. Stress ulcer prophylaxis.

Respiratory Care

1. O_2 supplementation by nasal canula, O_2 mask/non-rebreather mask, high-flow nasal cannula.
2. Non-invasive ventilation with different interfaces like nasal CPAP, full face mask.

These modalities lessen the breathing efforts; help in lung recruitment; and lessen chances of ventilator-associated pneumonia (VAP), ventilator-induced lung injury (VILLI) and mechanical injury to the lung.

Complications: pressure ulcer due to mask, dryness of the mucosa, interference in ventilation during nursing care and feeding, gastric distension.

Contraindications: craniofacial injury, active vomiting, poor sensorium or airway reflexes, claustrophobia.

Invasive Mechanical Ventilation

Invasive mechanical ventilation is by far the most used management strategy to deal with any form of ARDS to improve saturation and reduce the work of breathing.

Various modes of ventilations are being utilized for oxygenation that varies from CPAP/PSV, SIMV, controlled modes of ventilation, and advanced modes like APRV and PRVC in ICUs.

Lung protection ventilatory strategies should be used to prevent volume trauma and barotrauma. This involves ventilation using a low tidal volume of 4–6 ml/kg with permissive hypercarbia, plateau pressure under 30 and avoiding high driving pressure (plateau pressure – total PEEP).

These patients need deep sedation with occasional neuromuscular blockers for ventilator synchronization and decreased O_2 consumption. Using sedation scales such as the Richmond Agitation-Sedation Scale (RASS) may help clinicians meet sedation goals more effectively, decreasing the likelihood of over- or undersedation. Most patients are kept comfortable awake or under light sedation (e.g. RASS of 0 or –1), although some patients with more severe lung injury or poor tolerance of mechanical ventilation may need deeper sedation.

Lung Therapies for Refractory Hypoxia

1. Prone ventilation – Improvement of V/Q that facilitate recruitment of the dependent lung alveoli together with mobilizing secretions.
2. Recruitment manoeuvres – A recruitment manoeuvre (RM) is a transient sustained increase in transpulmonary pressure in an attempt to open previously collapsed alveoli and thus increase lung compliance and improve gas exchange.
3. Extracorporeal membrane oxygenation (ECMO) – Extracorporeal membrane oxygenation is a useful mechanism employed to improve oxygenation in patients with severe ARDS with refractory hypoxia. The most common ECMO configuration used in ARDS is veno-venous ECMO, in which blood is withdrawn from a catheter placed in a central vein, pumped through a gas exchange device known as an oxygenator and returned to the venous system via another catheter. Indicated when the risk of

mortality is 80% or greater ($PaO_2/FiO_2 < 100$ on $FiO_2 > 90\%$).

ORTHOPAEDIC CARE IN DESATURATING PATIENT WITH LONG BONE FRACTURE

The principle of long bone fracture care is to stabilize the fracture so as to control further damage and allow easy nursing care. As and when the patient's general condition allows, target for early definitive fixation or early conversion osteosynthesis.

In the case of established FES and patients requiring ICU care, a damage control procedure should be done to ensure fracture stabilization. The rationale of long bone fracture stabilization is to reduce fat globule shower into the system. The preferred approach is to apply external fixation or intramedullary nailing following Pepe's criteria.

Tips for Safe Fracture Fixation

1. Timing – Definitive fixation of the long bone fracture should be attempted in a safe period within the first 24 h after trauma or wait for 5–7 days. Damage control or external fixator should be the preferred method of fracture stabilization to prevent further fracture movement and embolization of the fat globules in between the safe period.
2. Surgical technique – Surgical techniques to reduce fat embolization are:
   a. Venting – Drill holes in the cortex to reduce intramedullary pressure while reaming.
   b. Lavage bone marrow before fixation to reduce marrow for embolization.
   c. Use of tourniquets to prevent embolization have been attempted.
3. Selection of implant – Pepe's criteria gives an appropriate guide for the most appropriate method for fracture fixation. However, in case a definitive fixation is planned, reamed or un-reamed intramedullary nails are equally safe. Reamed intramedullary nailing allows early rehabilitation and more stable fixation of the fracture, therefore less risk of late fracture-related complications. Alternately, an internal fixator may be used in high-risk cases, specifically with chest trauma.

SUGGESTED READING

1. American College of Surgeons. Committee on Trauma. *Advanced Trauma Life Support: Student Course Manual*. Tenth edition. Chicago, IL: American College of Surgeons; 2018.
2. Gurd AR, Wilson RI. The fat embolism syndrome. *J Bone Joint Surg Br*. 1974;56B:408–16. PMID: 4547466.
3. Schonfeld SA, Ploysongsang Y, DiLisio R, Crissman JD, Miller E, Hammerschmidt D, et al. Fat embolism prophylaxis with corticosteroids. A prospective study in high-risk patients. *Ann Intern Med*. 1983;99:438–43. PMID: 6354030.
4. Lindeque BG, Schoeman HS, Dommisse GF, Boeyens MC, Vlok AL. Fat embolism and fat embolism syndrome. A double-blind therapeutic study. *J Bone Joint Surg Br*. 1987;69:128–31. PMID: 3818718.
5. Kumar V, Fausto N. *Abbas A. Robbins and Cotran's Pathologic Basis of Disease*. Seventh ed. Philadelphia, PA: Elsevier Saunders; 2005:137.
6. Worthley LI, Fisher MM. The fat embolism syndrome treated with oxygen, diuretics, sodium restriction, and spontaneous ventilation. *Anaesth Intens Care*. 1979;7:136–42. PMID: 41462.
7. Tachakra SC, Potts D, Idowu A. Early operative fracture management of patients with multiple injuries. *Br J Surg*. 1990;77:1194. doi.org/10.1002/bjs.1800771040.
8. Staub NC. Pulmonary oedema due to increased microvascular permeability. *Annu Rev Med*. 1981;32:291–312. PMID: 7013669.
9. Matthay MA, Zimmerman GA. Acute lung injury and the acute respiratory distress syndrome: four decades of inquiry into pathogenesis and rational management. *Am J Respir Cell Mol Biol*. 2005;33:319–27. PMID: 16172252.
10. Scheiermann C, Kunisaki Y, Jang JE, Frenette PS. Neutrophil microdomains: linking heterocellular interactions with vascular injury. *Curr Opin Hematol*. 2010;17:25–30. PMID: 19923987.
11. Ferguson N, Fan E, Camporota L, Antonelli M, Anzueto A, Beale R et al. The Berlin definition of ARDS: an expanded rationale, justification, and supplementary material. *Intens Care Med*. 2012;38:1573–82. doi: 10.1007/s00134-012-2682-1.
12. Jacobi J, Fraser G, Coursin D, Riker R, Fontaine D, Wittbrodt E et al. Clinical practice guidelines for the sustained use of sedatives and analgesics in the critically ill adult. *Crit Care Med*. 2002;30:119–41. PMID: 11902253.

13. Tsai HC, Chang CH, Tsai FC, Fan PC, Juan KC, et al. Acute respiratory distress syndrome with and without extracorporeal membrane oxygenation: a score matched study. *Ann Thorac Surg.* 2015;100:458–64. PMID: 26116481.

14. Anwar IA, Battistella FD, Neiman R, Olson SA, Chapman MW, Moehring HD. Femur fractures and lung complications: a prospective randomized study of reaming. *Clin Orthop Relat Res.* 2004;422:71–6. PMID: 15187836.

SECTION III

SUBSPECIALITY TRAUMA CARE

21 Paediatric Mild Head Injury

Apinderpreet Singh, Chandrasekhar Gendle and Sushant K Sahoo

LEARNING OBJECTIVES

- Know the paediatric Glasgow Coma Scale according to age
- Learn classification of severity of head injury
- Know the indication of the required radiological investigation

INTRODUCTION

Paediatric head injuries always remain a reason for concern since children usually sustain injuries because of frequent domestic falls, sports and recreational activities, and sometimes due to child abuse. Moderate to severe head injuries are dreaded and might lead to serious complications, while minor to mild head injuries sometimes remain unnoticed for a long period. Many reasons could be attributed to such delay. Initial symptoms might be mild enough to get ignored or there may be no symptoms at all. Many times the parents are not even aware of a mild injury because of the inability of children to communicate. Early diagnosis and management remain the key to avoid secondary insult. The initial investigation of choice for any patient of head injury is the CT scan of the brain. It has the advantage of diagnosing most traumatic intracranial bony and parenchymal pathologies and can be obtained quickly. The delay in diagnosis sometimes may result in serious consequences, with many intracranial injuries needing no further intervention. In such cases of mild head injury patients, the decision for performing a CT scan becomes difficult. To avoid such dilemma, many researchers have attempted to bring forward certain guidelines to categorize high-risk and low-risk patients requiring further radiological investigations.

MEASURING THE GLASGOW COMA SCALE IN CHILDREN

The Glasgow Coma Scale (GCS) is used most commonly for assessing the neurological status of the patients in trauma and comprises of three components: best eye response, best verbal output and best motor response. It is an easier scale to remember and provides a quick assessment of the neurological status. In children above 5 years of age, the adult version of GCS can be used, but in younger age groups, it becomes difficult to assess by standard method, as they are unable to provide adequate verbal response or obey the given command. Various timely modifications have been done for the paediatric age group. These are summarized next:

Children of age < 2 years (preverbal)

Best eye response

1. No eye opening to any stimuli
2. Eye opening only to painful stimuli
3. Eye opening to sound
4. Eye opening is spontaneous

Best verbal response

1. No verbal response
2. Moaning in response to pain
3. Crying in response to painful stimuli
4. Irritability/crying
5. Coos and babbles

Best motor response

1. No motor response
2. Abnormal extension to pain (decerebrate posturing)
3. Abnormal flexion to pain (decorticate posturing)
4. Withdrawal to painful stimuli
5. Withdraws to touch
6. Moves spontaneously and purposefully

Children of age >2 years (verbal)

Best eye response

1. No eye opening to any stimuli
2. Eye opening only to pain
3. Eye opening to sound
4. Eyes open spontaneously

Best verbal response

1. No verbal response
2. Incomprehensible sounds
3. Incomprehensible words
4. Confused
5. Orientated, appropriate

Best motor response

1. No motor response to any stimuli
2. Abnormal extension to pain (decerebrate posturing)
3. Abnormal flexion to pain (decorticate posturing)
4. Withdrawal to pain
5. Localizes to painful stimuli
6. Obeys commands

DOI: 10.1201/9781003291619-24

CLASSIFICATION OF HEAD INJURY ACCORDING TO SEVERITY

Before we go into the details of indications of CT scan and the challenges, the classification of severity of head injury needs to be known. This classification involves the clinical status of the patient assessed by the GCS and may be defined as:

Mild – injury with a GCS of 13–15

Moderate – injury with a GCS of 9–12

Severe – injury with a GCS of 8 or less

This classification is based on the conscious status of the patient at the time of presentation to the emergency department, but sometimes this doesn't depict the severity of an underlying brain injury, particularly in children who present with usually a higher GCS score.

ROLE OF CT SCAN

A non-contrast CT scan of the brain remains the investigation of choice for ruling out any bony or parenchymal injury at the time of admission.

Indications of CT Scan in Mild Head Injury

Children sometimes harbour significant intracranial injuries in spite of a good GCS score. Henceforth, declaring a patient safe merely on the basis of the GCS is not right. On the other hand, an unnecessary CT scan in a child who is a low-risk patient for head trauma carries the risk of unwanted radiation exposure. Many authorities like the Children's Head injury Algorithm for the prediction of Important Clinical Events (CHALICE), Canadian Assessment of Tomography for Childhood Head injury (CATCH), Pediatric Emergency Care Applied Research Network (PECARN), and the National Institute of Health and Care Excellence (NICE) have attempted to lay some guidelines in risk stratification of children harbouring any significant intracranial injury. Summarizing these few guidelines, broader recommendations can be drawn (Tables 21.1 and 21.2). In addition, few other findings like gradually worsening headache; evidence of intoxication; evidence of trauma above the clavicles; and the presence of other significant injuries suggesting dangerous mechanism of injury like intra-abdominal injuries, long bone fractures and degloving injuries should also raise the suspicion of intracranial injury requiring an early CT scan.

If more than one of the aforementioned factors are present, a CT scan within the first hour of admission is required. If any of the factors is present alone, we can observe the patient clinically and perform a CT scan only in case of additional findings, as listed earlier.

INDICATIONS FOR MAGNETIC RESONANCE IMAGING (MRI) IN HEAD INJURY

In spite of the superiority of MRI over CT scan in identifying the structural abnormality in the brain, routine use of MRI in management of

Table 21.1: Indications of Underlying Brain Injury Warranting CT Scan

GCS < 15 for infants and < 14 for older children

Injury without evidence of any accident

History of seizures after injury (with no prior history of epilepsy)

Tense fontanelle

Any evidence or suspicion of open or depressed fracture

Features of skull base fractures like blackish discolouration around eyes (panda sign), hemotympanum, bleeding or CSF leak form ear, nose or throat, battle's sign (bruises across the back of ears)

Presence of any bruise or laceration > 5 cm in an infant

Note: Presence of any of these factors requires a CT, preferably within first hour of admission.

Table 21.2: Indications for CT Scan If the Patient Is Conscious and Alert (GCS 15)

In a patient of GCS 15, the presence of the following signs should arouse of underlying brain injury requiring a CT scan.

- Any loss of consciousness more than 5 minutes.
- The child is drowsy or sleepy.
- Anterograde or retrograde amnesia for more than 5 minutes (not applicable to children < 5 years).
- Multiple episodes of vomiting (> 3 episodes).
- Any trauma indicative of dangerous mechanism of injury.

acute traumatic brain injury (within first week) is currently not recommended. The long time taken to acquire an MRI, issues of compatibility of the patient for an MRI, lack of bony details, and the lack of MRI-compatible life support equipment in unstable patients are amongst the few reasons.

An MRI can be considered as an adjunct in certain situations like unexplained persistent decreased sensorium with no obvious finding on CT (conditions like diffuse axonal injury), mild head injury with persistent deficits, suspecting child abuse and to quantify the degree of insult particularly in medicolegal cases.

CHILD ABUSE/NON-ACCIDENTAL TRAUMA

Of all the causes of paediatric head injuries, child abuse needs special attention, as it is one of the common causes of injuries in children and is often overlooked. Other causes of non-accidental trauma could be "shaken infant syndrome" and "battered baby syndrome". Any trauma to the child not corroborating with the history, overconcern of the attendants, any evidence of psychiatric disease among the family members and any unexplained injury should arouse the suspicion of abuse. The degree of force required to cause bony fractures and deep injuries in children usually is quite high because of the flexibility in bony and tissue architecture. History of trivial falls, or a minor trauma while playing or a domestic fight between children with such injuries should indicate abuse and should instigate the examiner to look for other evidence of abuse or non-accidental trauma. A few of the findings seen in such injuries are:

- Evidence of rib fractures, corner fractures, diaphyseal fractures.
- Multiple cutaneous bruises of different healing stages.
- Evidence of retinal haemorrhage.
- Presence of subdural hematoma, subarachnoid haemorrhage, diffuse axonal injury. The subdural and other hematomas of different ages on a scan are very peculiar of child abuse because of repeated injuries (acute, subacute and chronic bleed at a same time).
- Evidence of fracture healing in a fresh trauma (indicating old injury).
- Different patterns of skull fracture like multiple eggshell fractures and fractures crossing the sutures.
- Sometimes injury to the viscera can also be seen.

Any suspicion of non-traumatic injury should be investigated with a CT scan and a thorough body skeletal and soft tissue survey for potential injuries. The outcome of such patients usually remains poor because of delayed reporting to hospital, repeated injuries and improper care after discharge from hospital.

CLEARING THE PATIENT FOR DISCHARGE OR TRANSFER

There are no clear guidelines for period of observation of patients with normal initial CT scan, as in some cases delayed deteriorations have happened in spite of normal initial radiology. Even with minor contusions or bleeds, no universal consensus exists for the period of observation for declaring "no further intervention". However the decision for observation and repeat radiology can be decided according to the initial GCS score, severity of injury on CT (Marshall and Rotterdam CT scores), serial clinical examination and presence of any coagulopathy. The presence of any such severity factor should be taken as a potential factor for deterioration and demands a repeat CT scan after a few hours to 48 hours.

CONCLUSION

The management of mild head injury in children starts from suspecting an injury, particularly in children less than 5 years old because of lack of communication. Formulating guidelines and according risk stratification of the patients will decrease the chances of a "missed injury" as well as will help in avoiding unnecessary investigations and radiation exposure.

SUGGESTED READING

1. Jain S, Iverson LM. Glasgow coma scale. [Updated 2021 Jun 20]. In: *StatPearls* [Internet]. Treasure Island, FL: Stat Pearls Publishing; 2021 Jan. Available from: https://www.ncbi.nlm.nih.gov/books/NBK513298/.
2. Reece RM, Sege R. Childhood head injuries: accidental or inflicted? *Arch Pediatr Adolesc Med*. 2000;154:11–5. PMID: 10632244.
3. Keenan HT, Runyan DK, Marshall SW, Nocera MA, Merten DF. A population-based comparison of clinical and outcome characteristics of young children with serious inflicted and noninflicted traumatic brain injury. *Pediatrics*. 2004;114:633–9. doi: 10.1542/peds.2003-1020-L. PMID: 15342832.

4. Berkowitz CD. Physical abuse of children. *N Engl J Med*. 2017;376:1659–66. doi: 10.1056/NEJMcp1701446. PMID: 28445667.

5. Teasdale G, Jennett B. Assessment of coma and impaired consciousness. A practical scale. *Lancet*. 1974;2(7872):81–4. doi: 10.1016/s0140-6736(74)91639-0. PMID: 4136544.

6. Borgialli DA, Mahajan P, Hoyle JD, Powell EC, Nadel FM, Tunik MG, Foerster A, Dong L, Miskin M, Dayan PS, Holmes JF, Kuppermann N., Pediatric Emergency Care Applied Research Network (PECARN). Performance of the pediatric Glasgow Coma Scale score in the evaluation of children with blunt head trauma. *Acad Emerg Med*. 2016;23:878–84. doi: 10.1111/acem.13014.

7. Reilly PL, Simpson DA, Sprod R, Thomas L. Assessing the conscious level in infants and young children: a paediatric version of the Glasgow Coma Scale. *Childs Nerv Syst*. 1988;4:30–3. doi: 10.1007/BF00274080. PMID: 3135935.

8. Davis T, Ings A, National Institute of Health and Care Excellence. Head injury: triage, assessment, investigation and early management of head injury in children, young people and adults (NICE guideline CG 176). *Arch Dis Child Educ Pract Ed*. 2015;100:97–100. doi: 10.1136/archdischild-2014-306797.

9. Easter JS, Bakes K, Dhaliwal J, Miller M, Caruso E, Haukoos JS. Comparison of PECARN, CATCH, and CHALICE rules for children with minor head injury: a prospective cohort study. *Ann Emerg Med*. 2014;64:145–52, 152.e1–5. doi: 10.1016/j.annemergmed.2014.01.030.

22 Early Management of Adult Head Injury

Karthigeyan M, Pravin Salunke and Sunil K Gupta

LEARNING OBJECTIVES

- Knowledge of the concepts of primary and secondary brain injury
- Evaluation of adult head injury in the emergency department
- The rationale of imaging in head injury patients
- Management principles of post-traumatic seizure and raised intracranial pressure

INTRODUCTION

Although a wide range of definitions exist, traumatic brain injury (TBI) is considered "an alteration in brain function, or other evidence of brain pathology, caused by an external force". Consistent with global data, the TBI/head injury (HI) disease burden in India has been a major public health issue and contributes to significant morbidity and mortality. In India, road-traffic accident-related injuries are quite common, particularly in younger ages, and remain a major cause of death.

> Following an insult, the brain incurs injury at two levels: primary and secondary.
>
> Early HI management intends at minimizing secondary brain injury.

Primary brain injury owes to the damage caused by direct impact during the initial injury mechanism, while the secondary injury is a cascade of events that follow to produce further insults. The latter include phenomenon like hypotension, hypoxia, hypo-hypercapnia, seizures and elevated intracranial pressure (ICP) that can cause secondary brain damage. Hence, early HI management aims at minimizing the secondary injury in the at-risk brain. For this, timely resuscitation and appropriate management by an early organized trauma care is considered to be the key.

CLASSIFICATION OF HEAD INJURY

Most patients sustain mild HI constituting about 80% of all injuries, with moderate and severe accounting for 10%–15% each.

On the basis of the Glasgow Coma Scale (GCS), HI is classified as:

> - Mild HI: GCS 13–15
> - Moderate HI: GCS 9–12
> - Severe HI: GCS 3–8
> - Critical HI: GCS 3–4, unreactive pupils and absent/decorticate motor response

ASSESSMENT IN THE EMERGENCY DEPARTMENT

Initially, HI patients are assessed by following the standard Advance Trauma Life Support (ATLS) protocol.

Initial Patient Assessment

A) ***Airway maintenance with cervical spine protection***

i) Intubation should be carried out in comatose patients (GCS < 8) and those who are unable to maintain their airway.

> Presume associated spine injury until it is ruled out.

ii) Every HI patient should be presumed to have a cervical spine injury until proven otherwise. This is specifically for those in comatose state or under alcohol influence/drug intoxication. Therefore, a cervical collar has to be applied until the time a spine injury is ruled out by clinical examination and imaging. While securing the airway, perform *manual in-line stabilization* and avoid excessive spinal movements (hyperextension/hyperflexion).

B) ***Breathing and ventilation***

i) Ventilate to maintain oxygen saturation > 98%.

ii) As a temporizing ICP-reduction measure, maintain $PaCO_2$ around 30–35 mmHg. Prophylactic prolonged hyperventilation (< 30 mmHg) is not recommended, as profound hypocarbia has been associated with cerebral vasoconstriction and impairment of cerebral perfusion pressure.

C) ***Circulation with haemorrhage control***

i) Isotonic crystalloid (normal saline/Ringer's lactate) is the preferred resuscitation fluid.

DOI: 10.1201/9781003291619-25

ii) Maintain blood pressure (SBP $>$ 100 mmHg).

iii) Hypotension causes decreased cerebral perfusion pressure and can result in an altered level of consciousness; the source of bleeding and hypotension has to be promptly identified and controlled.

> Head injury per se does not cause hypotension unless associated with a terminal brainstem failure or spine injury. Hence, other systemic injuries have to be excluded.

D) ***Focused neurological examination***

Once airway, breathing and circulation of the patient is addressed, perform a rapid and focused neurological examination (GCS, pupillary light response and lateralizing signs) followed by a secondary survey.

CLINICAL EVALUATION

Evaluation of an HI patient includes clinical (history, physical examination, GCS and neurological) and relevant imaging.

A) ***History***

This includes questions regarding mode of injury, loss of consciousness, vomiting, seizures, amnesia, limb weakness/other neurological deficits and alcohol consumption. Also, details of any associated medical comorbidities and anticoagulant intake has to be obtained.

> In unconscious patients with unknown mechanism, a possibility of non-traumatic aetiology such as stroke, aneurysmal bleed (not uncommon in our set-up when CT shows subarachnoid haemorrhage) and intoxication should be borne in mind.

B) ***Physical examination***

i) In unconscious HI patients, a collar has to be fit in until spin -injury is excluded clinically and by appropriate imaging.

ii) Scalp inspection for laceration/depressed fracture, which may be a significant source of bleed. Look for underlying dural laceration and exposed brain tissue.

iii) Presence of tachycardia and hypotension in an HI patient should alert the possibility of systemic injuries; hypotension is only a rare phenomenon which may be seen with profound scalp haemorrhage, more common in children. Cushing's reflex, i.e. hypertension and bradycardia, indicates raised ICP, while hypotension and bradycardia suggest spinal cord injury.

C) ***Glasgow Coma Scale***

Introduced by Teasdale and Jennet in 1974, the GCS is a practical scale used to describe the depth of coma and is commonly used in TBI evaluation (Table 22.1).

> The adult GCS can be used for HI victims $\geq$ 5 years of age; a modified version is available for paediatric assessment.

Methods such as pressure over the nail bed, trapezius muscle or supra-orbital area (not recommended if there is suspicion of facial fracture) are used to evoke deep pain in comatose patients. The GCS score ranges between 3 and 15. The response should be recorded on a total score of 15 mentioning individual components. Whenever an asymmetric motor response is noted between the upper and lower or right and left limbs, the patient's best response should be used to calculate the score. However, the actual response on both sides and upper and lower limbs needs to be documented.

> Be aware of factors influencing GCS.

i) Factors such as hypotension, hypoxia, intoxication, sedation, muscle relaxants and alcohol influence can alter the patient's sensorium. The timing of GCS assessment potentially determines the scores obtained. Therefore, post-resuscitation GCS is considered more appropriate and predicts the overall outcome.

ii) The GCS has certain confounding factors that render some of its components untestable. For example, the eye and verbal responses can be affected by local orbital injury/swelling, and intubation, respectively. Likewise, limb and spinal injuries can affect the motor scale. In such

Table 22.1: Adult Glasgow Coma Scale

Response	Score
Eye Opening	
Spontaneous	4
To speech	3
To pain/pressure	2
No response	1
Verbal Response	
Oriented	5
Confused, but able to answer questions	4
Inappropriate words	3
Incomprehensible sounds	2
No response	1
Motor Response	
Obeys commands	6
Localizes pain	5
Withdraws in response to pain (normal flexion)	4
Abnormal flexion (decorticate posturing) in response to pain	3
Extension (decerebrate posturing) in response to pain	2
No response	1

circumstances, it is preferable to mention the reason why a particular component could not be assessed. For instance, in a patient with eye swelling/ptosis, mention the eye component as "C". In intubated patients, a verbal score of 1 is usually assigned, which often leads to overestimation of injury severity. Hence, it is more appropriate to note the verbal scale as "T" in those who are intubated or tracheostomised.

D) *Pupillary assessment*

> Commonly, optic nerve or third cranial nerve involvement affects pupillary size and reactivity.

A change in pupillary size and reactivity in HI patients commonly indicates optic nerve or third cranial nerve dysfunction, and less commonly drug-induced dysfunction (intoxication or iatrogenic). An optic nerve injury causes impairment of both the direct and indirect light reflex, and may manifest fixed or sluggish pupils, with spontaneous fluctuations. On the other hand, in a patient with unilateral third-nerve palsy, the pupil is mydriatic and shows an impaired direct light response, however with preservation of the consensual light reflex (i.e. constriction of the opposite pupil in response to bright light). Although an oculomotor nerve dysfunction can occur anywhere along its path, it is frequently seen in conditions of raised ICP secondary to its compression over the tentorial free edge. A primary orbital injury can also cause third-nerve palsy and may be associated with other extraocular muscle paresis.

E) *Imaging in head injury*

Plain computed tomography (CT) remains the investigation of choice for identifying clinically important HI. Many clinical decision rules are in place to identify the HI patients at higher risk for intracranial complications and those requiring CT imaging. Their basis has been to pick up potential lesions that need neurosurgical intervention or observation, while at the same time minimize unnecessary CT radiation hazard. The following guideline is based on the National Institute for Health and Care Excellence (NICE) recommendations for performing CT scan in adult HI. Some other frequently used and validated protocols include the New Orleans Criteria, NEXUS II and Canadian CT Head Rules. Of note, these criteria aid CT decision-making, with clinical acumen likely warranting additional imaging.

The NICE guideline recommends a CT when any of the following risk factors are present:

- GCS < 13 on initial assessment in the emergency department (ED)

- GCS < 15 at two hours after injury on assessment in ED
- Suspected open/depressed skull fracture, penetrating injuries
- Signs of basal skull fracture, such as haemotympanum, periorbital ecchymoses (black/panda) eyes, cerebrospinal fluid otorrhoea/rhinorrhoea, retroauricular ecchymoses (Battle's sign)
- Occurrence of seizure
- Focal neurological deficit
- > 1 vomiting episode
- Patients on anticoagulant treatment

A CT is also recommended with any of the following risk factors with some loss of consciousness or amnesia since the injury:

- Age ≥ 65 years
- History of bleeding or clotting disorders
- Dangerous injury mechanism (a pedestrian or cyclist struck by a motor vehicle, an occupant ejected from a motor vehicle, or a fall from height of > 1 metre or five stairs)
- > 30 min retrograde amnesia for events immediately before HI

OBSERVATION OF ADMITTED PATIENTS

> Minimum observation parameters: GCS, pupil size and reactivity, limb movements, respiratory rate, heart rate, blood pressure, temperature and blood oxygen saturation

For patients admitted with HI, the aforementioned parameters are documented.

i) Record observations half-hourly until a GCS of 15 has been achieved.

ii) The minimum recommended observation frequency for patients with GCS 15 is half-hourly for 2 hours, then hourly for 4 hours, and 2 hourly thereafter.

iii) If the patient with GCS 15 deteriorates at any time after the initial 2-hour period, observations should revert to half-hourly frequency.

iv) In a patient with a normal CT scan but with no improvement in GCS 15 after 24 hours of observation, a further CT or MRI scan should be considered.

v) Close observation for potential neurological deterioration.

> Features indicative of neurological worsening:
>
> - Agitation or abnormal behaviour
> - Drop in GCS score (especially a drop in the motor response)
> - Increasing headache or persisting vomiting
> - New neurological symptoms or signs, such as pupil inequality or asymmetrical limb movement

SEIZURES IN HEAD INJURY

Following HI, seizures are classified as:

i) Immediate seizures that occur < 24 hours after injury

ii) Early seizures that manifest < 1 week

iii) Late seizures that occur beyond a week

> Antiepileptic drugs prevent early post-traumatic seizures.

Early seizures are known to occur in 2%–17% of HI patients and are more frequent after severe HI. Approximately 50% of the early seizures occur within the first 24 hours. Apart from the typical convulsions, post-traumatic seizures can also be present in a non-convulsive form and can be detected only by electroencephalography monitoring.

There are certain risk factors that have been identified for early seizures and include young age (< 5 years), intracranial haematoma, acute subdural haematoma, diffuse cerebral oedema, subarachnoid haemorrhage, intracranial foreign body, focal neurologic deficits, depressed/linear skull fractures, loss of consciousness > 30 minutes, and post-traumatic amnesia > 24 hours. Studies have shown that antiepileptic drugs are effective in preventing early post traumatic seizures.

The Brain Trauma Foundation recommends phenytoin prophylaxis to reduce the incidence of early post-traumatic seizures. The loading dose is 18 mg/Kg with an IV infusion rate no faster than 50 mg/min followed by maintenance of 5 mg/kg/day in two to three divided doses (usually 100 mg 8 hrly).

MANAGEMENT PRINCIPLES IN RAISED ICP

Clinically, an elevated ICP/cerebral herniation is indicated by sudden deterioration in sensorium, new onset pupillary asymmetry and hemiparesis, and Cushing's reflex. After the following initial ICP-reduction measures, the patient is shifted for either ICU management or surgical intervention depending upon the clinical and imaging findings.

i) ABCDE assessment

ii) General measures like elevating head end to 30 degrees

iii) O_2 supplementation to avoid hypoxia (SaO_2 > 90%)

iv) Short-term hyperventilation ($PaCO_2$ 30–35 mmHg)

v) Mannitol: 20% mannitol bolus at dose of 1g/kg, followed by 0.25 g/kg 6 hourly

- Avoid indiscriminatory use, and preferably reserved for clinical features of raised ICP.
- This has to be avoided in hypotensive patients (< 90 mmHg).
- Hypertonic saline (3% to 23.4%) is also used to reduce ICP; however, its superiority over mannitol is controversial.

vi) Early neurosurgical consult for possible surgery

SUGGESTED READING

1. American College of Surgeons. Committee on Trauma. *Advanced Trauma Life Support: Student Course Manual.* Tenth edition. Chicago, IL: American College of Surgeons; 2018.

2. Carney N, Totten AM, O'Reilly C, Ullman JS, Hawryluk GW, Bell MJ, et al. Guidelines for the management of severe traumatic brain injury: fourth edition. *Neurosurgery.* 2017;80(1):6–15.

3. Ding K, Gupta PK, Diaz-Arrastia R. Epilepsy after traumatic brain injury. In: Laskowitz D, Grant G, editors. *Translational Research in Traumatic Brain Injury.* Boca Raton, FL: CRC Press/Taylor and Francis Group; 2016. Chapter 14. Available from: https://www.ncbi.nlm.nih.gov/books/NBK326716/.

4. Dinsmore J. Traumatic brain injury: an evidence-based review of management. *Continuing Educ Anaesth Crit Care Pain.* 2013;13(6):189–95. https://doi.org/10.1093/bjaceaccp/mkt010.

5. Foks KA, van den Brand CL, Lingsma HF, van der Naalt J, Jacobs B, de Jong E, et al. External validation of computed tomography decision rules for minor head injury: prospective, multicentre cohort study in the Netherlands. *BMJ.* 2018;362:k3527. https://doi.org/10.1136/bmj.k3527.

6. Karthigeyan M, Gupta SK, Salunke P, Dhandapani S, Wankhede LS, Kumar A, et al. Head injury care in a low- and middle-income country tertiary trauma center: epidemiology, systemic lacunae, and possible leads. *Acta Neurochir.* 2021;163(10):2919–30. doi: https://doi.org/10.1007/s00701-021-04908-x.

7. Moppett IK. Traumatic brain injury: assessment, resuscitation and early management. *Br J Anaesth.* 2007;99(1):18–31. https://doi.org/10.1093/bja/aem128.

8. National Clinical Guideline Centre (UK). *Head Injury: Triage, Assessment, Investigation and Early Management of Head Injury in Children, Young People and Adults.* London: National Institute for Health and Care Excellence (UK); 2014 Jan. (NICE Clinical Guidelines, No. 176). Available from: https://www.ncbi.nlm.nih.gov/books/NBK248061/. Accessed July 20, 2021.

9. NSW Government Health. *Closed Head Injury in Adults: Initial Management.* NSW Ministry of Health. 2012. https://www1.health.nsw.gov.au/pds/ActivePDSDocuments/PD2012_013.pdf.

10. Teasdale G, Maas A, Lecky F, Manley G, Stocchetti N, Murray G. The Glasgow Coma Scale at 40 years: standing the test of time. *Lancet Neurol.* 2014;13(8):844–54. doi: 10.1016/S1474-4422(14)70120-6.

23 Management of Acute Burn Injuries

Tarush Gupta

LEARNING OBJECTIVES

- Management of burns at the site of the injury
- Resuscitation of burn wound patient in the triage area and assessment of depth of the wound
- Recognizing early the wounds that will heal with dressing and which will require surgery
- Recognizing early the complications like compartment syndromes as well as the importance of splinting for different body regions involved

INTRODUCTION

- Burn injury is a serious public health problem in India. A burn is an injury to the skin or other organic tissue primarily caused by heat or radiation, radioactivity, electricity, friction or chemical contact.
- Around 7 million people suffer from burn injuries every year in India, with 1.4 lakh deaths and 2.4 lakh people suffering from a disability.

TYPES OF BURNS

1. Thermal burns
   a) Flash and flame burns: most common cause in adults
   b) Scalds: most common cause in children
   c) Contact burns: common in epileptics, alcoholics or drug abusers
2. Electrical burns
   a) Low-voltage: household electricity with < 1000 V
   b) High-voltage: outside home electricity with > 1000 V
   c) Flash burns
   d) Lightning burns
3. Chemical burns
4. Radiation burns
5. Friction burns
6. Cold injuries

MANAGEMENT OF BURN PATIENT AT THE SITE OF INJURY

- When a patient suffers from a burn injury, all of his burnt clothes should be removed immediately at the site of injury.
- The thermal wound injured part should be washed with running water, with a water temperature of around 15 degrees Celsius till the burning sensation is reduced considerably. Ice-cold water should not be used.
- Shift the patient to the hospital as soon as possible.

MANAGEMENT OF BURN PATIENT ONCE BROUGHT TO THE TRAUMA CENTRE

- Once the patient comes to the trauma centre, if he is still wearing burnt clothes, those should be removed immediately.
- Initial management and resuscitation of major burn patients on arrival to the trauma care centre should be as per the Advanced Trauma Life Support (ATLS) guidelines (Table 23.1).

Assessment of TBSA in a Burn Patient

The most common method to assess the total body surface area (TBSA) of the burnt wound is via the Wallace rule of nines, represented in Figure 23.1.

Admission Criteria

Table 23.2 enumerates the admission criteria for burn injury patients.

Burn Wound Depth Assessment

- There are various methods to assess the depth of the burn wound, but most important is a serial clinical assessment. It is important to know and follow the depth of the wound serially, as our main aim is to identify the deep wounds and aggressively treat those which may require intervention, with the aim that all wounds heal within three weeks.
- Majority of burns which present to the hospitals are a mixture of various depths of burns.
- Burn wounds are classified based on the depth of skin involvement (Figure 23.2).
- Other methods to measure the burn wound depth are:
  a) Laser doppler: monitors microcirculation of the blood flow in the dermis
  b) Indocyanine green fluorescence
  c) Punch biopsy for histological evaluation

DOI: 10.1201/9781003291619-26

Table 23.1: Major Burn Injury Management Sequence in the Trauma Centre

Initial Assessment and Management of a Major Burn	
1.	Primary survey (ABCDEF). A: Airway with cervical spine control B: Breathing C: Circulation D: Disability (neurological) E: Exposure with environmental control F: Fluid resuscitation
2.	Assess burn size and depth.
3.	Establish intravenous access with two wide-bore 16-G cannula or central line or interosseous access (esp. in children) and start intravenous fluids.
4.	Give adequate analgesia, opioid analgesics/NSAIDS.
5.	Catheterize.
6.	Take baseline blood investigations.
7.	In electrical injury: • 12 lead electrocardiography • Cardiac enzymes (high-voltage electrical injuries) • Serum potassium levels

8.	When suspecting inhalational injuries, proceed as follows:
	• Look for clinical signs
	  • Full thickness or deep dermal burns to face, neck or upper thorax in closed room burn injury
	  • Signed nasal hair
	  • Carbonaceous sputum or carbon particles, in oropharynx
	  • Progressive change in voice, hoarseness, stridor or wheeze
	• Chest X-ray
	• Arterial blood gas analysis

9.	After completion of the primary survey, a secondary survey should assess the depth and total body surface area (TBSA) burnt, reassess and exclude or treat associated injuries.
10.	Arrange safe transfer to specialist burns unit.

d) Non-contact ultrasonography
e) Thermography
f) MRI

Fluid Resuscitation of Burn Patient

- Early and aggressive fluid resuscitation of burn patients form the most important part of patient treatment.
- In adults, intravenous fluid resuscitation is usually necessary for burns involving >20% TBSA. In infants, resuscitation should be started for > 10% TBSA and in older children with burns > 15% TBSA. Ringer's lactate (RL) solution is the most commonly used fluid for burn resuscitation.
- Clinically, urine output should be used to measure renal perfusion with a target of 0.5–1 ml/kg/hour.
- Crystalloids are the resuscitation fluid of choice. Colloids can be given along with crystalloids, but albumin is contraindicated in the first 24 hours post burn.
- Parkland formula has been renamed the consensus formula, as it is the most widely used resuscitation formula. Half of the fluid calculated from the formula is given in the first 8 hours, and the next half is given in the next 16 hours from the time of burn injury.
- Table 23.3 describes the various fluid resuscitation formulas.

Management of Burn Wounds

Topical Ointments

1) Silver sulfadiazine: Most commonly used, has intermediate wound penetration and good antibacterial spectrum. Used twice a day but may cause transient leucopenia.
2) Mafenide acetate: Excellent eschar penetration and bacteriostatic action. It may cause metabolic acidosis.
3) Dakin solution: 0.25% sodium hypochlorite.
4) 0.5% Silver nitrate.
5) 0.25% Acetic acid: In pseudomonas infection.
6) Povidone-iodine solution.

Wound Dressing

1) Biological dressings: fresh or frozen human cadaveric split thickness skin graft

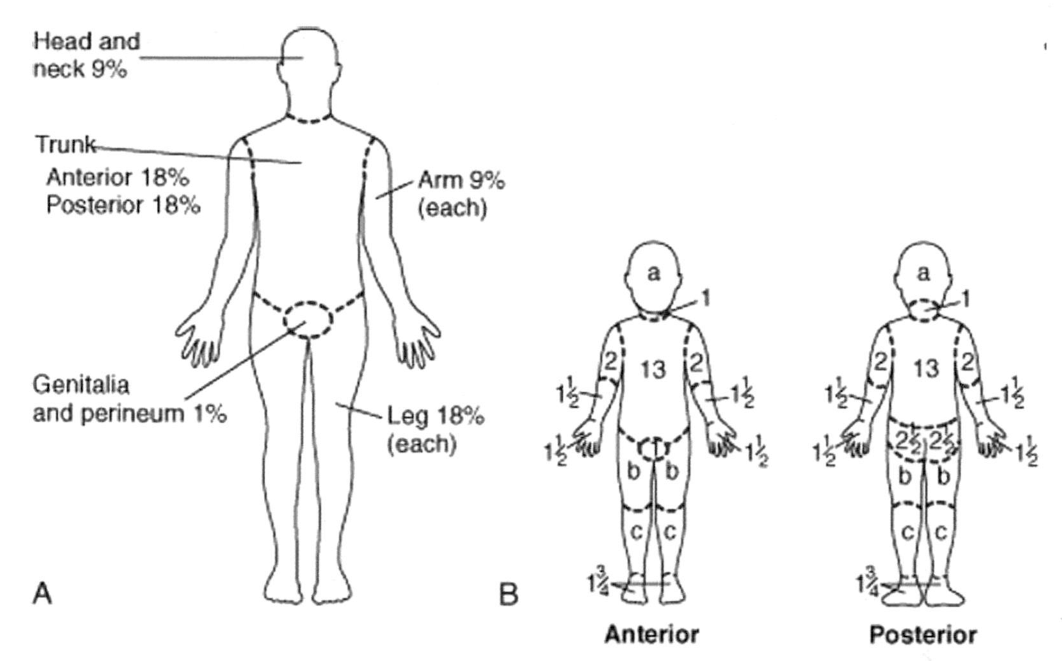

Relative percentage of body surface area (% BSA) affected by growth

Body Part	Age				
	0 yr	1 yr	5 yr	10 yr	15 yr
a = 1/2 of head	9 1/2	8 1/2	6 1/2	5 1/2	4 1/2
b = 1/2 of 1 thigh	2 3/4	3 1/4	4	4 1/4	4 1/2
c = 1/2 of 1 lower leg	2 1/2	2 1/2	2 3/4	3	3 1/4

Figure 23.1 (a) Wallace rule of nines with each area allocated a surface area in multiples of nine. (b) In children, TBSA is measured with the Lund and Browder method. Reprinted with permission from Diller, K.R. (1985). Analysis of Skin Burns. In: Shitzer, A., Eberhart, R.C. (eds) *Heat Transfer in Medicine and Biology*. Springer, Boston, MA. https://doi.org/10.1007/978-1-4684-8285-0_3.

Table 23.2: Admission Criteria for Burn Injury Patients in the Burn Care Unit

1	Partial thickness burns, adult > 10% TBSA burns and patient requiring burn shock resuscitation
2	Face, hand, feet, genitalia, perineum or major joints involvement
3	Deep partial thickness burns and full thickness burns of any age
4	Circumferential burns in any age group
5	Electrical burns, including lightning injury
6	Inhalational burns
7	Chemical burns
8	Any burn patient with concomitant trauma (such as fractures, head injuries)
9	Suspected non-accidental injury
10	Diseases associated with burns, such as toxic epidermal necrolysis, necrotizing fasciitis, staphylococcal scalded child syndrome

2) Physiological dressings: consist of synthetic material such as polyethylene or silicone

Figure 23.3 describes the algorithm showing the approach to the management of burn wounds.

NUTRITION

- A burns is a hypermetabolic state, where the energy requirement is much higher than a normal person for proper recovery and for wound healing.

Depth of burn	Skin involvement	Signs	Sensation	Healing time	Scarring	Figures depicting the corresponding depth of burns
Superficial Burns	Epidermis	Dry and red, blanches with pressure, no blisters	Maybe painful	Within 7 days	No scarring	
Partial thickness burns-Superficial	Epidermis and part of papillary dermis	Pale pink with fine blistering, blanches with pressure	Usually extremely painful	Within 14 days	Can have colour match defect. Low to moderate risk of hypertrophic scarring	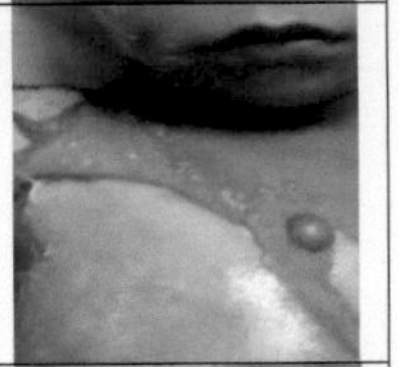
Deep partial thickness burn	Epidermis, papillary dermis, down to reticular dermis	Dark pink to blotchy red, maybe large blisters, no capillary refill- sluggish to none	Maybe painful or reduced/absent sensation	14 days- over 21 days	Moderate to high risk of hypertrophic scarring	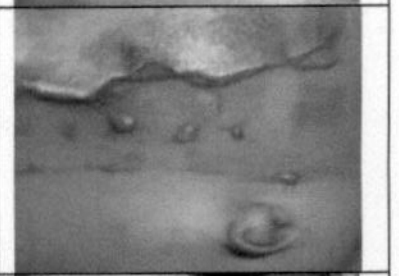
Full thickness burn	Entire thickness of the skin and deeper structures	White, waxy or charred, no blisters, no capillary refill. May be dark lobster red with mottling in child	No sensation	Does not heal spontaneously	Will scar	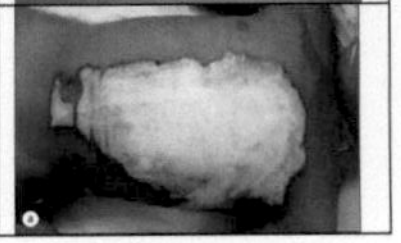

Figure 23.2 Classical signs associated with each depth of burn, along with a representative photograph and the expected number of days it will take to heal

Table 23.3: Fluid Resuscitation Formulas for Burns

Formula	Electrolyte	Colloid	Glucose
Colloid Formula			
Brooke	RL at 1.5 ml/kg/%TBSA burn	0.5 ml/kg/%TBSA burn	2L 5% Dextrose
Evans	0.9% NaCl at 1 ml/kg/% TBSA burn	1 ml/kg/% TBSA burn	2L 5% Dextrose
Crystalloid Formula			
Parkland formula (also known as consensus formula)	RL at 4 ml/kg/% TBSA burn	—	—
Modified Brooke's	RL at 2 ml/kg/% TBSA burn	—	—
Hypertonic Saline			
Monafo	Maintain U/O at 30 ml/h, fluid contains sodium 250 mmol/l	—	—

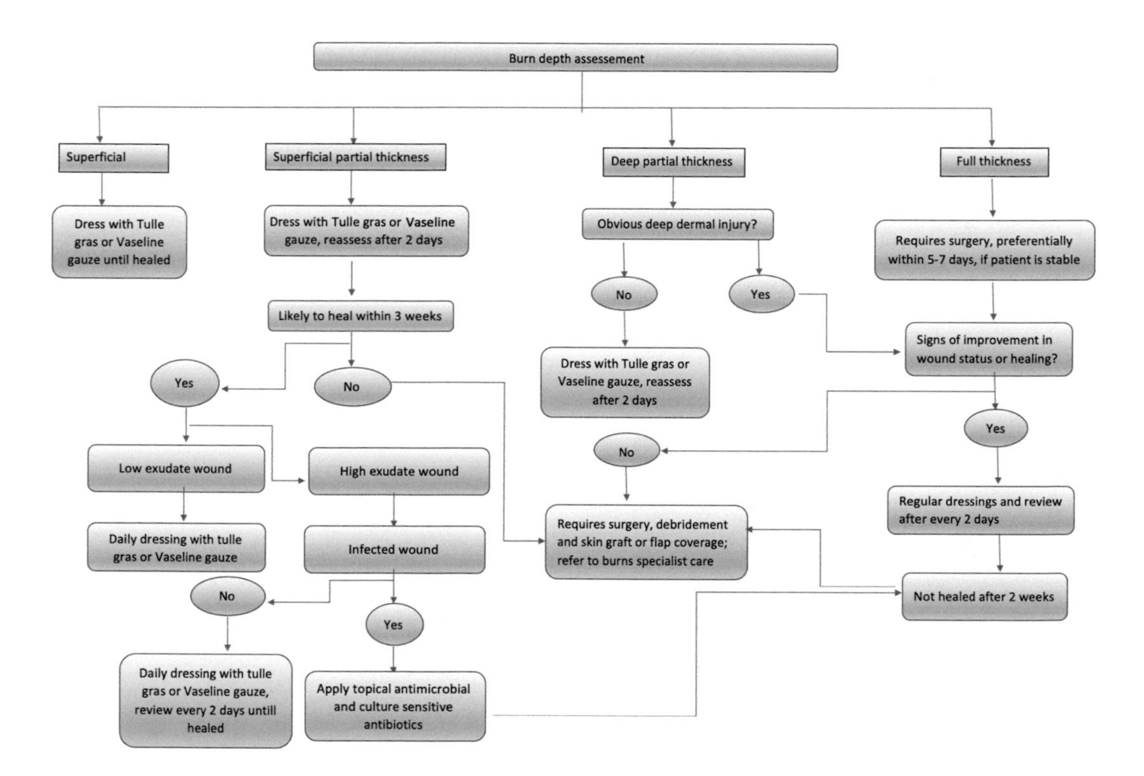

Figure 23.3 Algorithmic approach in managing burn wound patients. The goal is to achieve early burn wound healing, preferably within three weeks. Superficial wounds generally heal with regular dressings, but deep wounds mostly require surgical intervention to achieve early wound healing

- The goal of treatment is to start early enteral nutrition, which can relieve gastrointestinal damage and prevent intestinal mucosal damage.
- A nasogastric tube is placed in any patient with > 20% TBSA burn injury.
- Parenteral nutrition is started in those in whom early enteral feeding cannot be started.
- Table 23.4 describes modified Harris-Benedict formula to calculate the daily calorie requirement of burn patients.

Table 23.4: Modified Harris-Benedict Formula to Calculate the Daily Calorie Requirement of Burn Patient

Modified Harris-Benedict Formula	Calories (Kcal) per Kg (Multiply the Calculation by 1.5 for Age < 40 Years and by 2 for Age > 40 Years)	Protein
Male	[66 + (13.7 × Weight in kg) + (5 × Height in cm) – (6.8 × Age)]	1.5 gm × Weight in kg (< 40 Years of Age)
Female	[655 + (9.6 × Weight in kg) + (1.7 × Height in cm) – (4.7 × Age)]	2 gm × Weight in kg (> 40 Years of Age)

Table 23.5: Position for Anti-Contracture Splint Application in Burn Wound Patients

Region	Position of the Splints
Neck	Hyperextension, no rotation
Shoulder	Abduction 90 degrees, slight horizontal flexion
Elbow	Full extension, supination
Wrist	Extension at 20–30 degrees
Fingers	Metacarpophalangeal joint extension at 70 degrees, interphalangeal (IP) joints full extension
Thumb	40–50 degree abduction, IP joints extension
Hip	20 degree abduction, extension, no rotation
Knee	Full extension
Ankle/foot	Neutral ankle, neutral toes

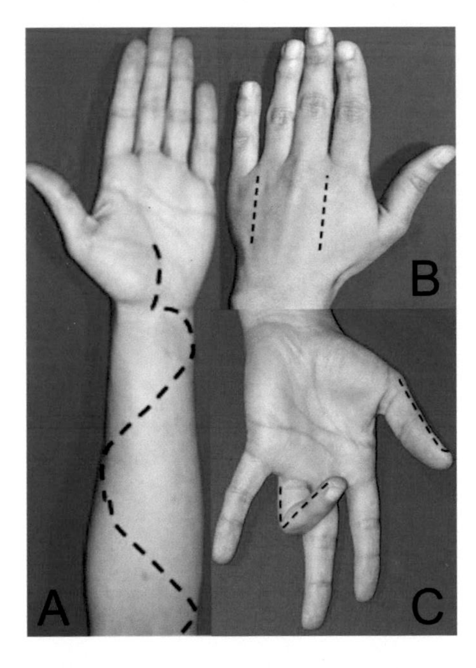

Figure 23.4 Fasciotomy incisions of forearm, hand and fingers. (A) Preferred incision of fasciotomy of the forearm. (B) Dorsal hand incisions used to release the dorsal, volar and adductor compartment of the thumb. (C) Incision for the digit fasciotomies. Digits are released at the mid-lateral line on the ulnar side, while the thumb is released at the radial side

SPLINTS

- Use of splint forms is an integral part of burn wound management.
- Splints help in reducing the pain and oedema, maintain or improve range of motion, and prevent development of joint contractures, which can complicate the management of burn wounds and delay rehabilitation of patients (Table 23.5).

COMPARTMENT SYNDROME

- Compartment syndrome occurs when the tissue pressure within an enclosed space is elevated to the extent that there is decreased blood flow within the space, decreasing the tissue oxygenation and impairing metabolic functions.
- In extremities, there is impaired capillary refill, paraesthesia and increased passive movement pain, which develops earlier than impaired palpation of pulsation.
- Emergency escharotomies, fasciotomies or both are required for the release of compartment syndrome.
- Figure 23.4 illustrates the incisions to release compartment syndrome of the upper limb.

SUGGESTED READING

1. Neligan P. *Plastic Surgery*. Fourth edition. Elsevier; 2017: Volume 4.

2. Sood R. *Achauer and Sood's Burn Surgery: Reconstruction and Rehabilitation*. Elsevier; 2006.

3. Herdon D. *Total Burn Care*. Fifth edition. Elsevier; October 2017.

4. Özkan A, Şentürk S, Tosun Z. Fasciotomy procedures on acute compartment syndromes of the upper extremity related to burns. *Eur J Gen Med*. 2015;12:326–33. doi.org/10.15197/ejgm.01410.

24 Pelvic Trauma

Diagnosis and Management

Sandeep Patel and Shahnawaz Khan

LEARNING OBJECTIVES

- Evaluating a case of pelvic injury
- Classification of pelvic injuries
- Management of pelvic injury in an emergency set-up

INTRODUCTION

Pelvic trauma is always a result of high-velocity trauma. It is one of the leading causes of death among youngsters and accounts for one-third of intensive care unit (ICU) admissions. Pelvic injuries account for 3% of traumatic skeletal injuries. The injuries can range from minor closed injuries to open injuries to life-threatening shock-like conditions. The pelvic cavity contains some vital organs (urogenital structures and hindgut structures), blood vessels (both arteries and veins) and nerves. The injuries to any of these can lead to significant morbidity. The injuries in children is severe as compared to adults due to greater plasticity of the immature pelvic ring, which requires very high velocity forces to disrupt the pelvic ring. Pelvic injuries are often associated with injuries to other body parts like the thorax, abdomen, spine and head injuries.

EVALUATION

The initial evaluation of a patient is done as per the primary survey of the Advanced Trauma Life Support (ATLS) protocol in the order of ABCDE.

Primary Survey

- A: Airway and cervical spine protection
- B: Breathing and ventilation
- C: Circulation
- D: Disability
- E: Exposure and environmental control

Assessment of haemorrhage and adequate control of bleeding is crucial for pelvic trauma patients. The stability of the pelvis should be assessed during the primary survey, as gross instability will give an idea of a severe unstable fracture with the potential for massive blood loss. Stability can be assessed by firmly holding the iliac crest with both hands and gently compressing and distracting. The pelvic compression test is done only once and should not be repeated due to the risk of dislodgement of the thrombus. Of late, the pelvic compression test has shown no added benefit and lacks sensitivity and specificity.

Secondary Survey

During the secondary survey period, a thorough head-to-toe examination is performed.

Symptoms

- Localized pain
- Inability to bear weight
- Numbness and weakness over the dorsum of the foot

Signs – The following clinical signs should raise suspicion of pelvic injury:

- Abnormal positioning of limbs (exaggerated external rotation)
- The anterosuperior iliac spines are not at the same level
- Limb-length discrepancy
- Ecchymosis over the flanks
- Scrotal, labial or perineal hematoma
- Perineal lacerations
- Gross visible haematuria
- Blood at the tip of the urethra (suspect urethral injury)
- Neurological examination (L5 and S1 are most commonly injured)
    - Sensation loss over the dorsum of the foot
    - Loss of perianal sensations
    - Lax anal sphincter

A pelvic examination is never complete without a digital rectal examination and examination of the vagina and urethra. An open pelvic fracture and those with rectal and vaginal injuries have poor outcomes and high mortality, and have different management wherein they will undergo a diversion colostomy as an emergency procedure (Figure 24.1).

DOI: 10.1201/9781003291619-27

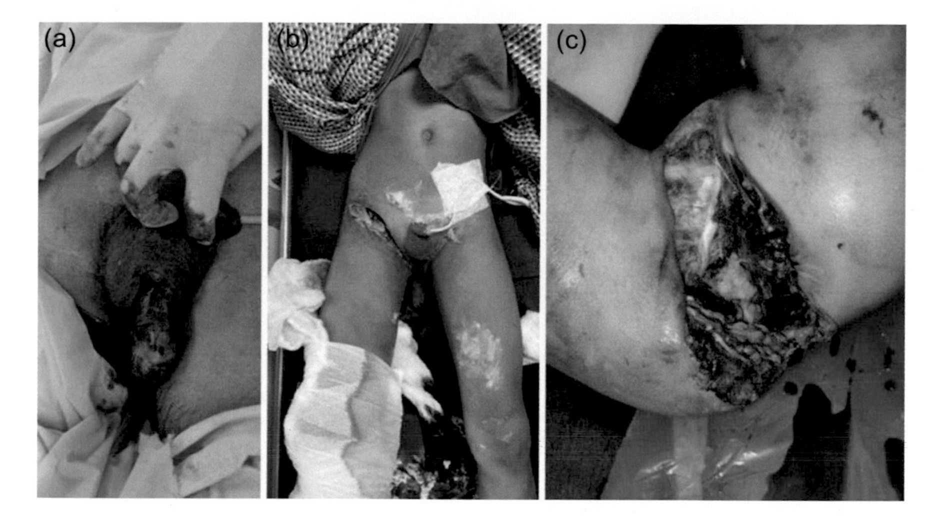

Figure 24.1 Open fractures of the pelvis: (a) open scrotal injury with testis exposed; (b) open injury in the groin extending to scrotum and perineum; (c) open injury involving the perineal floor, vagina and anal opening

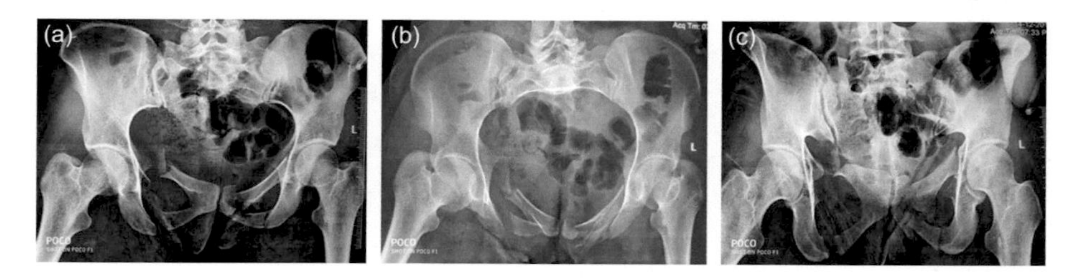

Figure 24.2 Radiographs of pelvis: (a) anteroposterior view of pelvis with both hips and proximal femur; (b) an inlet view of the pelvis with both hips; (c) an outlet view of the pelvis with both hips

Investigations

Blood investigations – The following blood investigations are for primary shock management:

- Haemoglobin
- Serum lactate
- Arterial blood gas
- Coagulation profile
- Thromboelastography (TEG)

Imaging

- FAST/eFAST: An easy technique that uses ultrasonography to identify free fluid in body cavities. This can be performed immediately in the resuscitation area of a trauma centre.
- Radiographs (Figure 24.2)
  - Anteroposterior (AP) view: The initial management of pelvic fractures needs only AP view and is mandatory in all trauma patients. One must look for asymmetry, rotation or displacement of both hemipelves.
  - For definitive fixation, additional pelvic radiographic views and CT scan are required to plan the fixation strategies.
  - Additional views
    - Inlet view: The X-ray beam is angled 40 degrees caudally. This view helps in identifying anterior and posterior translation of the hemipelvis along with its rotation, sacral fractures and sacroiliac joint opening.
    - Outlet view: The X-ray beam is angled 40 degrees cephalad. This view helps in identifying the translation of the hemipelvis in the vertical plane. It is also useful in identifying flexion or extension of

the hemipelvis, the integrity of the sacral foramen and sacral fractures.

- CT scan: A CT scan helps in identifying comminution and posterior ring injuries.

CLASSIFICATION

There are various classification systems available for the classification of pelvic fractures and the most commonly used ones are the Tile classification and Young and Burgess classification. It is important to understand the Young and Burgess classification as it gives an idea of the mechanism of injury and thereby predicting the patterns of injury and displacements. It also guides in initial and definitive treatment (Table 24.1).

1. Anterior–posterior compression (APC) injury – This usually results from an anterior direct blow, thereby opening up the pelvis by external rotation force (usually referred to as an open book injury). These injuries lead to a significant increase in the pelvic volume and are usually associated with significant haemorrhage. In these types of injuries, there is a high risk of venous bleed.
2. Lateral compression (LC) injury – This usually results from side-impact injuries sustained in motor vehicle accidents and leads to internal rotation forces of one hemipelvis leading to fracture of the anterior part of the pelvic ring (pubic rami) and ipsilateral sacral ala compression fractures. As the injury force increases, there can be more injury posteriorly with iliac fractures (crescent fractures, LC2), and with progressive internal rotation force, the opposite hemipelvis opens up as in APC (LC3). These patients typically have blunt trauma chest and solid organ abdominal injuries due to the impact.
3. Vertical shear (VS) – This injury usually results from a fall from height or motor vehicle accident. The hallmark of injury is the vertical displacement of the hemipelvis due to bony and/or ligamentous disruption. These injuries require skeletal traction to counter the deforming forces.
4. Combined mechanism (CM) – The patterns which do not fit the aforementioned three mechanisms and have features of more than one are classified in this group.

World Society of Emergency Surgery (WSES) classification. This classification is a recent classification which is based on the fracture stability and haemodynamic stability of the patient. It helps in clinical classification and management of patients in trauma centres (Table 24.2).

CAUSE OF BLOOD LOSS IN PELVIC TRAUMA

- *Venous bleed*
    - Source: Pre-sacral venous plexus.
    - Most common source of blood loss.
    - Mechanism: Shearing forces lead to disruption of pelvic venous plexus.
- *Fracture itself*
    - The pelvic bone is cancellous and is highly vascular. Fractured bone surface is a significant source of blood loss.

Table 24.1: Young and Burgess Classification of Pelvic Injuries

Anterior–Posterior Compression (APC) Injuries	
I	• Pubic symphysis opening less than 2.5 cm.
II	• Pubic symphysis opening more than 2.5 cm. • Anterior sacroiliac joint opening. • Sacrospinous and sacrotuberous ligaments are disrupted.
III	• Anterior and posterior sacroiliac ligaments are disrupted. • Sacrospinous and sacrotuberous ligaments are disrupted.
Lateral Compression (LC) Injuries	
I	• Oblique or transverse fracture of pubic ramus with ipsilateral anterior sacral ala fracture.
II	• Pubic rami fracture with ipsilateral posterior ilium fracture dislocation.
III	• Ipsilateral LC injury with APC injury on the opposite side.
Vertical Shear (VS)	
	• The hemipelves are not at the same level. • Disruption of pelvic floor ligaments. • Highest mortality rate.

Table 24.2: World Society of Emergency Surgery (WSES) Classification of Pelvic Trauma

Severity	WSES Grade	Fracture Pattern	Hemodynamic Status	Examples
Minor	I	Stable	Stable	APC-I, LC-I
Moderate	II	Unstable	Stable	APC-II, III; LC-II and III
	III	Unstable	Stable	VS and CM
Severe	IV	Stable/unstable	Unstable	Any pattern

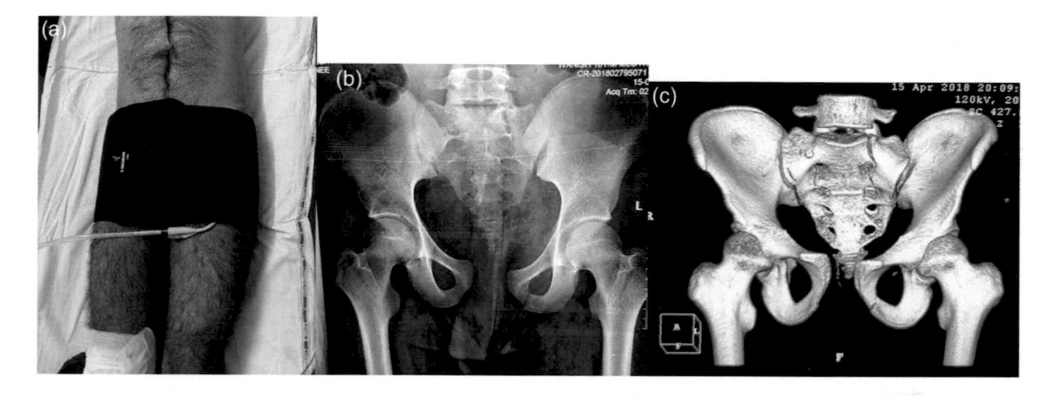

Figure 24.3 Pelvic binder application: (a) pelvic binder application in a pelvic ring injury patient; (b) AP view radiograph of the patient before pelvic binder application (note the pubic diastasis); (c) 3D CT image of the same patient after binder application (note the decreased opening of the diastasis compared to before binder application)

- *Arterial bleed*
    - Superior gluteal artery is the most common source in APC-III injury and posterior ring disruption.
    - Obturator artery.
    - Internal pudendal artery.

MANAGEMENT

Successful management requires a multidisciplinary team approach involving an anaesthetist, an emergency trauma surgeon, an orthopaedic surgeon, a urologist and a general surgeon.

Resuscitation, bony stability and haemorrhage control are the three main goals of early management.

Resuscitation

- Two large-bore cannulas are inserted, and two units of crystalloid are transfused immediately.
- Transfusion of blood products: PRBC, platelet and FFP should be transfused in the ratio of 1:1:1.
- Pelvic binder (Figure 24.3)
    - A pelvic binder application is done as the initial management of unstable pelvic injuries.
    - It reduces the volume of the pelvis and creates a tamponade effect which reduces bleeding.
    - The binder is centred over the greater trochanter of the femur.
    - Applied as soon as the primary survey is over.
    - Risk and complications of using a pelvic binder:
        - Pressure sores and skin necrosis.
        - Overcompression of the pelvis can mask pelvic injuries in radiographs.
        - In lateral compression injuries with transforaminal sacral fractures, there is a risk of neural and visceral injury.

Surgical Management

Emergency surgical management is indicated when the patient continues to be haemodynamically unstable despite resuscitation. The goal of emergency surgery is to stop ongoing bleeding and achieve haemodynamic stability. The three main sources of bleeding are bony bleed, venous bleed and rarely arterial bleed.

The three surgical steps involved are directed to:

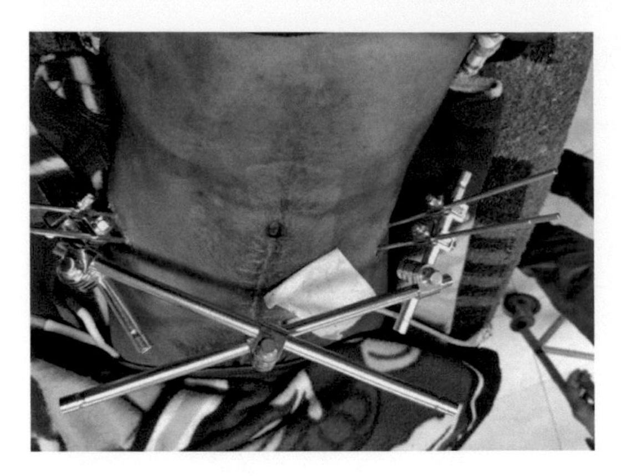

Figure 24.4 Pelvic exfix with a healed midline laparotomy wound with suprapubic catheter in situ

1. Provide bony stability and decrease pelvic volume
2. Control venous bleed (pelvic packing)
3. Control arterial bleed (angioembolization)

Approximately 80%–90% of patients respond to steps 1 and 2, and rarely do we need angioembolization.

Patients with pelvic injury can be managed by:

1. Skeletal stabilization: Bony stability is achieved to reduce the pelvic cavity volume and can be done by three methods: external fixation, pelvic C-clamp or posterior iliosacral screws.
    - External fixation (Exfix) (Figure 24.4).
        - Exfix also reduces the pelvic cavity and stabilizes bones.
        - Conventional exfix can be applied by inserting pins in the superior aspect of the iliac blade or supra-acetabular region.
        - Risks and complications include:
            - Opens up posterior ring injuries.
            - Pin tract infections.
            - Perforation of the inner table of pelvis can injure pelvic organs.
    - Pelvic C-clamp: Useful in posterior ring injuries.
    - Iliosacral screws: This is more of a definitive procedure. However, it's an easy, fast and reproducible procedure that can be attempted in the operation theatre with good fluoroscopy. The procedure is becoming popular these days and can be used for emergency management.
2. Pelvic packing: This is done to control the venous bleeding.
    - Steps of surgery.
        - Performed using a midline incision.
        - Skin and subcutaneous tissues are opened in the midline.
        - The bladder is retracted away.
        - Three laparotomy pads are placed in retroperitoneal space on either side towards the iliac vessels. Hence, a total of six pads are used.
        - Packs are left in situ for 24 to 48 hours.
    - Advantages.
        - Can be performed rapidly.
        - Can be performed at a peripheral health centre before transfer to a level 1 trauma centre.
        - Decreases mortality from haemorrhage and need for transfusion.
        - Rescue procedure in case of failed embolization.
        - Can be performed at centres where angiography is not available.
    - Disadvantages.
        - Infections have been reported in 15% to 33% of cases mostly due to retained gauze pieces.
3. Angioembolization: It is considered in patients with pelvic injury with an arterial bleed. The most commonly embolized vessels include the internal iliac artery and the superior gluteal artery followed by the internal pudendal artery and rarely the lateral sacral arteries. In the majority of cases, the catheter is introduced into the body through the femoral artery and following identification of the bleeding site, an absorbable gelatin foam is injected. This procedure is followed by a repeat angiogram just to ensure no dye leakage or bleeding at the site of procedure. This procedure is, however, not free of complications. Complications like severe haemorrhage, embolism and perforation of viscera have been reported.

The algorithm that should be followed for management of pelvic trauma is depicted in Figure 24.5.

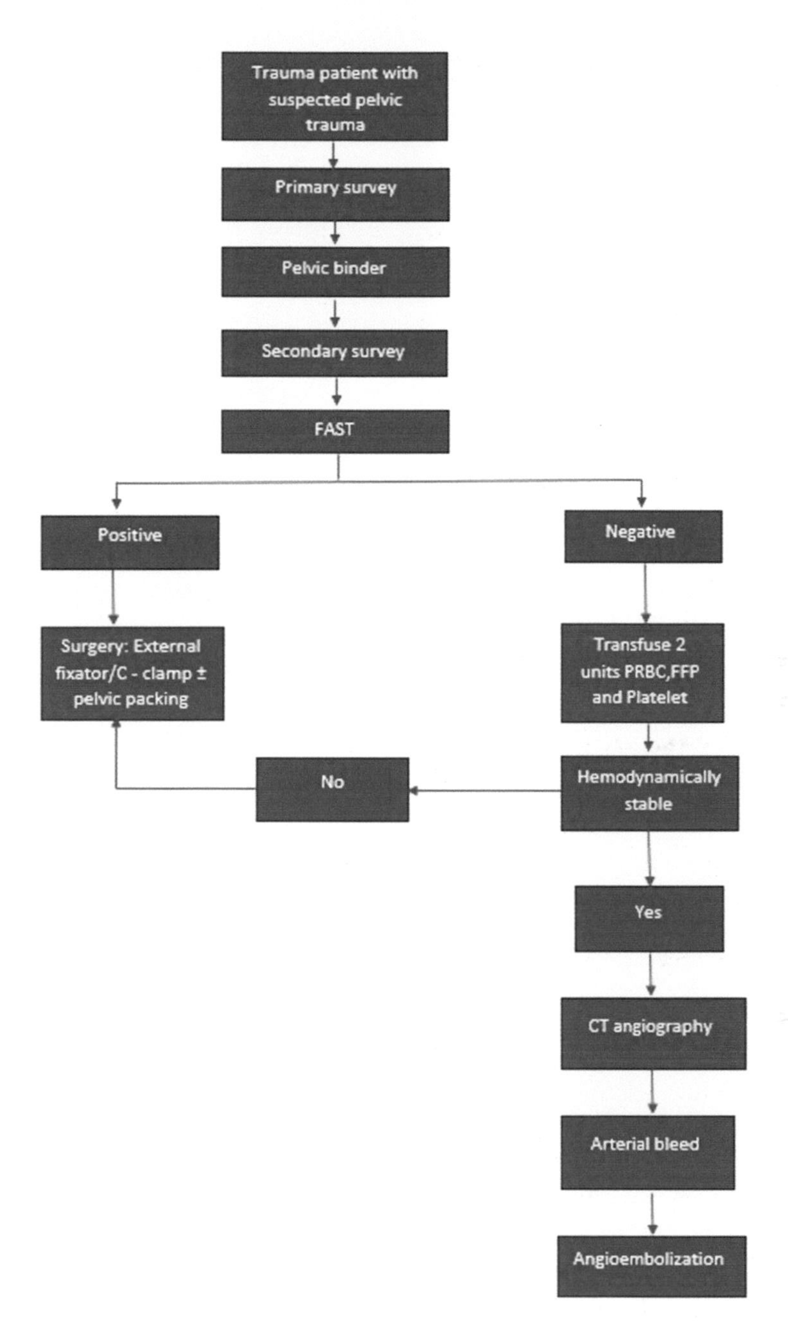

Figure 24.5 Algorithm for management of pelvic trauma

SUGGESTED READING

1. Tullington JE, Blecker N. Pelvic trauma. In: *StatPearls*. Treasure Island, FL: StatPearls Publishing; 2021. Available from: http://www.ncbi.nlm.nih.gov/books/NBK556070/.

2. Mackenzie EJ, Rivara FP, Jurkovich GJ, et al. The National study on costs and outcomes of trauma. *J Trauma*. 2007;63(6 Suppl):S54–67; discussion S81–86.

3. Grotz MRW, Allami MK, Harwood P, Pape HC, Krettek C, Giannoudis PV. Open pelvic fractures: epidemiology, current concepts of management and outcome. *Injury*. 2005;36(1):1–13.

4. Black EA, Lawson CM, Smith S, Daley BJ. Open pelvic fractures: the University of Tennessee Medical Center at Knoxville experience over ten years. *Iowa Orthop J*. 2011;31:193–8.

5. Burgess AR, Eastridge BJ, Young JW, et al. Pelvic ring disruptions: effective classification system and treatment protocols. *J Trauma.* 1990;30(7):848–56.

6. Tile M. Pelvic ring fractures: should they be fixed? *J Bone Joint Surg Br.* 1988;70(1):1–12.

7. Coccolini F, Stahel PF, Montori G, et al. Pelvic trauma: WSES classification and guidelines. *World J Emerg Surg WJES.* 2017;12:5.

8. Ben-Menachem Y, Coldwell DM, Young JW, Burgess AR. Hemorrhage associated with pelvic fractures: causes, diagnosis, and emergent management. *AJR Am J Roentgenol.* 1991;157(5):1005–14. doi: 10.2214/ajr.157.5.1927786. PMID: 1927786.

9. Demetriades D, Karaiskakis M, Toutouzas K, Alo K, Velmahos G, Chan L. Pelvic fractures: epidemiology and predictors of associated abdominal injuries and outcomes. *J Am Coll Surg.* 2002;195(1):1–10. doi: 10.1016/s1072-7515(02)01197-3. PMID: 12113532.

10. Li P, Liu F, Li L, et al. Effectiveness of pelvic packing in hemodynamically unstable patients with pelvic fracture: a meta-analysis. In Review; 2020. Available from: https://www.researchsquare.com/article/rs-42238/v1.

11. Filiberto DM, Fox AD. Preperitoneal pelvic packing: technique and outcomes. *Int J Surg Lond Engl.* 2016;33(Pt B):222–4. doi: 10.1016/j.ijsu.2016.05.072.

12. Vaidya R, Waldron J, Scott A, Nasr K. Angiography and embolization in the management of bleeding pelvic fractures. *J Am Acad Orthop Surg.* 2018;15;26:e68–76. doi: 10.5435/JAAOS-D-16-00600. PMID: 29351135.

25 Managing Blunt Abdominal Trauma

Ajay Savlania, Venkata Vineeth Vaddavalli and Kishore Abuji

LEARNING OBJECTIVES

- Aetiology of blunt abdominal trauma
- Evaluation and management strategies in a patient with blunt abdominal trauma
- Knowledge of various investigations that can aid in diagnosis and further management
- Commonly associated organ and vessel injuries in patients sustaining blunt abdominal trauma

INTRODUCTION

The abdomen is frequently injured in road traffic accidents and requires the care of a trauma care team. Eighty percent of the patients with abdominal injuries have blunt abdominal trauma, with the majority of these being due to roadside accidents. With the advancements in critical care management, surgical techniques and the multidisciplinary team approach, the outcome in blunt abdominal trauma has improved significantly. However, most of them are being managed conservatively. Knowledge of management strategies of various injuries of blunt abdominal trauma is important for a successful patient outcome.

EVALUATION AND MANAGEMENT OF BLUNT ABDOMINAL TRAUMA

In a patient from a roadside accident, history should be asked regarding vehicle speed, type of collision, whether the seat belt was in use, deployment of airbags and the patient's position in the vehicle.

- For patients sustaining a fall from height, the height of fall is essential information.
- A primary survey (airway, breathing, circulation, disability, and exposure) is done for all patients.
- A detailed examination should be done in haemodynamically stable patients by fully undressing the patient for proper inspection. Anterior and posterior abdominal walls, lower chest, flank and perineum should be inspected for any contusions or abrasion.
- Blood at the meatus indicates urethral injury, which might be due to pelvic fracture. The pelvic binder should be applied centred on the greater trochanters.
- The goals of rectal examination in a patient with blunt abdominal trauma are to assess for sphincter tone, rectal mucosal integrity and to palpate for any pelvic fractures.

Investigations

An abdominal ultrasound is considered as an adjunct to primary survey in Advanced Trauma Life Support (ATLS). FAST (focused assessment with sonography for trauma) evaluates the pericardium, hepatorenal pouch, splenorenal pouch and the pouch of Douglas. If free fluid is present, it indicates blunt abdominal trauma. If FAST is unavailable, diagnostic peritoneal lavage can be used as per ATLS guidelines. Peritoneal aspiration revealing bile, GI contents or more than 10 ml of gross blood suggests operative intra-abdominal trauma. Neither an abdominal ultrasound or diagnostic peritoneal lavage (DPL) can evaluate the retroperitoneum, which may be the source of bleeding. With the increased availability of CT scans, it has become the primary method of comprehensive workup for a patient with blunt trauma.

Management

After initial resuscitation, management is based on the patient's haemodynamic status (Figure 25.1). For haemodynamically unstable patients, an exploratory laparotomy should be done. To provide adequate exposure, the abdomen is opened from the xiphoid process to the pubic symphysis. When the injuries are identified, they are repaired. The development of physiological compromise prompts the need to abbreviate the operation and proceed with the damage control method. For haemodynamically stable patients, a detailed evaluation is done with an abdominal CT. If there is a perforated hollow viscus, it should be operated upon. Haemodynamically stable patients with solid organ injury should be monitored at timely intervals with serial abdominal examinations, vital monitoring and checking for haemoglobin drop.

SPLENIC INJURY

The spleen, in alternation with the liver, is the most common organ injured in blunt abdominal trauma. The non-operative management in splenic trauma has increased from 40% to 70%, with an associated decrease in mortality among higher grades of injury. The success rate

DOI: 10.1201/9781003291619-28

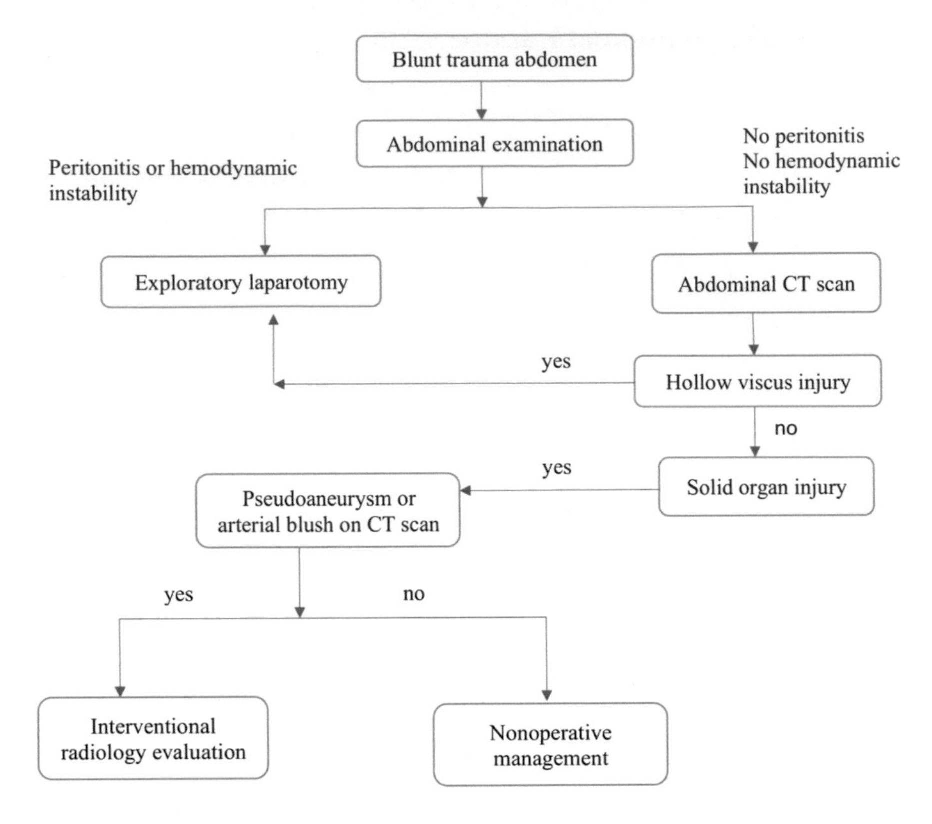

Figure 25.1 Management algorithm of blunt abdominal trauma

of non-operative management in high-volume centres is 90%.

Patients with abdominal trauma who are haemodynamically stable or respond to initial resuscitation must undergo further evaluation with abdominal CT with IV contrast administration. CT scan is the gold standard for abdominal trauma, with sensitivity and specificity of nearly 96%–100%. Splenic injuries are characterized by the American Association for the Surgery of Trauma (AAST) injury scoring scale, which grades injuries based on the presence of vascular involvement, and parenchymal or subcapsular abnormality (Table 25.1).

Management

After initial resuscitation, haemodynamically stable patients with no signs of peritonitis are considered for non-operative management. The patient should be admitted to the intensive care unit and kept nil per oral for at least 24 hours with serial haemoglobin level monitoring every 6 hourly. Patients are usually observed for 1–3 days. In imaging studies, patients with higher-grade splenic injuries (> grade III) or active extravasation of contrast or pseudoaneurysm are evaluated by angiography and embolization. Patients who become haemodynamically unstable during non-operative management should be operated.

Haemodynamically unstable patients (SBP < 90 mmHg, HR > 120 bpm, peripheral vasoconstriction, altered mental status, dyspnoea) who do not respond to initial resuscitation should be considered for operative management. In low-volume trauma centres where critical care monitoring is unavailable, even stable patients with > grade III splenic injuries undergo operative management. Splenectomy is the preferred operative management.

Post-splenectomy, immediate increase in platelets and white blood cells (WBCs) is normal. Beyond postoperative day 5, a WBC count of > 15000/cc and a platelet/WBC ratio of < 20 indicate sepsis.

Complications following splenectomy include subphrenic abscess, which should be managed with percutaneous drainage, and iatrogenic injury to the tail of the pancreas, which might result in pancreatic ascites or pancreatic fistula. Overwhelming post-splenectomy sepsis is rare and caused by *Streptococcus pneumonia*, *Haemophilus influenzae* and *Neisseria meningitides*. In patients undergoing splenectomy, vaccination is provided against these bacteria, optimally at > 14 days post injury.

Table 25.1: AAST Splenic Injury Scale (2018)

Grade	Imaging Criteria
I	Subcapsular haematoma < 10% surface area Parenchymal laceration < 1 cm depth Capsular tear
II	Subcapsular haematoma 10%–50% surface area Parenchymal laceration 1–3 cm Intraparenchymal haematoma < 5 cm
III	Subcapsular haematoma > 50% surface area Parenchymal laceration > 3 cm Intraparenchymal haematoma > 5 cm
IV	Any injury in the presence of splenic vascular injury or active bleeding confined within the splenic capsule Parenchymal laceration involving segmental or hilar vessels producing > 25% devascularization
V	Any injury in the presence of splenic vascular injury with active bleeding extending beyond the spleen into the peritoneum Shattered spleen

AAST, American Association for the Surgery of Trauma.

HEPATIC INJURY

The posterior portion of the right lobe is commonly injured in blunt abdominal trauma. The most common cause of injury is motor vehicle collision. Liver injury should be suspected when there is trauma involving the right upper quadrant, right rib cage or right flank. Physical findings associated with hepatic injury include right upper quadrant or generalized abdominal tenderness, haematoma, or abdominal wall contusion.

Haemodynamically stable patients should undergo a contrast-enhanced CT scan for a detailed evaluation of the organ involved. Typical findings on imaging include disruption of liver parenchyma with perihepatic blood or haematoma and haemoperitoneum. The American Association for the Surgery of Trauma – Organ Injury Scale (AAST-OIS) can be used to categorize liver injury based on parenchymal involvement and the presence of vascular injury (Table 25.2).

Management

In haemodynamically stable patients who respond to initial resuscitation, non-operative management is considered the standard of care. In non-operative management, the patient is observed with serial clinical examination, vital monitoring and haemoglobin levels. If there is active contrast extravasation or pseudoaneurysm on imaging, it should be managed using angioembolization.

Complications associated with non-operative management are bleeding, abdominal compartment syndrome, biliary complications (bile leak, bilioma, haemobilia, biliary fistula, and biliary peritonitis) and liver necrosis. Haemobilia is managed by embolization of the vessel communicating with the biliary tree. Biliomas and abscesses are drained percutaneously using CT or ultrasound. Endoscopic retrograde cholangiopancreatography (ERCP) might be necessary to decompress the biliary tree and promote the healing of bile leaks. Biliary ascites not amenable for percutaneous drainage might require laparotomy. Patients who have uncomplicated hospital courses can resume usual activity within 3–4 months, as most of the lesions heal by that time, and patients should be advised to consult in case of severe abdominal pain, nausea or vomiting.

Operative management is considered in haemodynamically unstable patients or those with other internal organ injuries that require operative management. The minor bleeding at laparotomy can be controlled using compression or electrocautery, bipolar devices, topical haemostatic agents, argon beam coagulation, or omental packing. For those at risk of abdominal compartment syndrome or needing a relook laparotomy, temporary abdominal closure can be considered.

In those with major bleeding, perihepatic packing and the Pringle manoeuvre should be done along with intraoperative resuscitation to reverse the lethal triad. In case of injury to the hepatic artery is found intraoperatively, attempts should be made to repair it primarily. If it is not possible, selective arterial ligation should be considered. A cholecystectomy should be done to avoid gallbladder necrosis in case of right or common hepatic artery ligation.

If bleeding persists despite the Pringle manoeuvre, retrohepatic caval or hepatic vein injury should be suspected. Perihepatic packing is the best method for venous injuries. Vascular isolation with shunting procedures

Table 25.2: AAST Liver Injury Scale (2018 Revision)

Grade	Imaging Criteria on CT
I	Subcapsular haematoma < 10% surface area Parenchymal laceration < 1 cm depth Capsular tear
II	Subcapsular haematoma 10%–50% surface area Intraparenchymal haematoma < 10 cm in diameter Laceration 1–3 cm in depth and < 10 cm in length
III	Subcapsular haematoma > 50% surface area Ruptured capsular or parenchymal haematoma Intraparenchymal laceration > 10 cm, laceration > 3 cm depth Any injury in the presence of a liver vascular injury or active bleeding contained within liver parenchyma
IV	Parenchymal disruption involving 25%–75% of a hepatic lobe Active bleeding extending beyond the liver parenchyma into the peritoneum
V	Parenchymal disruption of > 75% of a hepatic lobe Juxtahepatic venous injury to include retrohepatic vena cava and central major hepatic veins

AAST, American Association for the Surgery of Trauma.

Table 25.3: Classification of Blunt Aortic Injuries

Type of Aortic Injury	Definition
Absent External Contour Abnormality	
Intimal tear	No aortic external contour abnormality; tear and/or associated thrombus is < 10 mm
Large intimal flap	No aortic external contour abnormality; tear and/or associated thrombus is > 10 mm
Present External Contour Abnormality	
Pseudoaneurysm	Aortic external contour abnormality, contained
Rupture	Aortic external contour abnormality, contained; not contained, free rupture

can be considered if bleeding persists despite packing. Isolation of the liver with an atriocaval shunt and Pringle manoeuvre theoretically allows repair of the vena cava or hepatic veins with minimal blood loss.

Damage control surgery is often required, as most patients are already physiologically deteriorated. Control of bleeding is obtained surgically by perihepatic packing followed by resuscitation post-operatively to reverse hypothermia, coagulopathy and metabolic acidosis. After the patient has been stabilized, the abdomen can be re-explored and packs removed.

Angioembolization is considered for patients with uncontrolled bleeding after emergency laparotomy and for those with primary operative haemostasis with evidence of active bleeding on contrast-enhanced CT scans.

AORTIC INJURY IN BLUNT TRAUMA

Vascular injury is uncommon after blunt abdominal trauma but has significant mortality of 17%. It can be clinically silent, result in hemodynamic instability or present with acute lower limb ischaemia. In blunt trauma, the incidence of abdominal aortic injury is 0.2%, frequently caused by a steering wheel, seat belt or cycle handlebar impact.

The endovascular technique has moved from elective settings for haemodynamically compromised patients. This has significantly decreased morbidity and mortality from blunt abdominal trauma. The classification of blunt abdominal aortic injuries by Starnes et al. is depicted in Table 25.3.

Management

Patients with minimal aortic injuries, intimal tear < 10 mm can be safely observed by starting B blockers. Those with large intimal flaps should be observed; if there is a progression on repeat CT scan within 72 hours, then intervention is needed. If the patient is likely to survive, then all pseudoaneurysms should be treated with endovascular repair. Open intervention is required for those who present with free rupture, thrombosis or acute limb ischaemia. In a systematic review, 90% of blunt abdominal aortic injuries were managed conservatively. Of the rest, the majority underwent endovascular intervention and only a few needed open repair.

RETROPERITONEAL HAEMATOMA

In traumatic retroperitoneal injury, 44%–80% of cases are blunt trauma. The colon, kidney,

Table 25.4: Zones of Retroperitoneum

Zone	Extent	Organs
Zone 1	Central retroperitoneum extending from diaphragm superiorly to bifurcation of aorta inferiorly	Aorta, inferior vena cava, origins of renal and major visceral vessels, a portion of duodenum and pancreas
Zone 2	Lateral paranephric areas of upper retroperitoneum extending medially from renal vessels till lateral reflection of the posterior parietal peritoneum	Adrenal glands, kidneys, renal vessels, ureters, and ascending and descending colon
Zone 3	Inferior to the aortic bifurcation	Bilateral internal and external iliac vessels, distal ureter, distal sigmoid colon, and rectum

duodenum, pancreas, urinary bladder and rectum are commonly injured. The zones of the retroperitoneum are depicted in Table 25.4.

Mechanism of Injury

In blunt trauma, direct transfer of energy causing organ compression, adjacent rib fracture causing organ puncture or shear force from deceleration are the mechanisms of injury.

Evaluation

After resuscitation, contrast-enhanced CT is the imaging study of choice in haemodynamically stable patients.

Management

Stable patients are managed conservatively by pain control, serial abdominal examination, haemoglobin monitoring and follow-up imaging, as needed. If active contrast extravasation is noted on imaging, angioembolization should be done. For blunt trauma, based on the zone of injury, the management is as follows:

Zone 1: Explore, as there is a chance for major vascular injury.

Zone 2: Exploration should be done for expanding haematoma or for bleeding not controlled by angioembolization.

Zone 3: Exploration should not be done. Alternative methods like preperitoneal packing or angioembolization should be used.

GASTROINTESTINAL INJURY

In blunt trauma, gastrointestinal injury is due to crushing of the bowel between the solid structures such as the spine and steering wheel or seat belt. The incidence of gastrointestinal injuries in patients with blunt abdominal trauma is 3.1%, with the small bowel (jejunum/ileum) most commonly injured.

Haemodynamically stable patients should be evaluated. FAST in patients with gastrointestinal injury reveals free peritoneal fluid. Abdominal X-ray (erect) and computed tomography reveal free air under the diaphragm or retroperitoneal air.

Haemodynamically unstable patients and those with perforations should be explored. Mesenteric haematoma identified on CT that is not associated with active contrast extravasation or signs of bowel ischaemia can be managed non-operatively, as most of them resorb spontaneously.

SUGGESTED READING

1. American College of Surgeons. *Committee on Trauma. Advanced Trauma Life Support*. Tenth ed. Chicago: American College of Surgeons; 2018.

2. Rotondo MF, Schwab CW, McGonigal MD, et al. 'Damage control': an approach for improved survival in exsanguinating penetrating abdominal injury. *J Trauma*. 1993;35:375–82. PMID: 8371295.

3. National Clinical Guideline Centre. *Major Trauma: Assessment and Initial Management*. NICE guideline NG39. London. National Clinical Guideline Center; 2016. Available from: https://www.nice.org.uk/guidance/ng39/evidence/full-guideline-2308122833.

4. Nishijima DK, Simel DL, Wisner DH, Holmes JF. Does this adult patient have a blunt intra-abdominal injury? *JAMA*. 2012;307:1517–27. doi: 10.1001/jama.2012.422. PMID: 22496266.

5. Osgood MJ, Heck JM, Rellinger EJ, et al. Natural history of grade I–II blunt traumatic aortic injury. *Journal of Vascular Surgery*. 2014;59:334–41. doi: 10.1016/j.jvs.2013.09.007. PMID: 24342065.

6. Olthof DC, Van Der Vlies CH, Joosse P, Van Delden OM, Jurkovich GJ, Goslings JC. Consensus strategies for the nonoperative management of patients with blunt

splenic injury: a Delphi study. *J Trauma Acute Care Surg*. 2013;74:1567–74. doi: 10.1097/TA.0b013e3182921627.

7. Carter JW, Falco MH, Chopko MS, Flynn WJ, Wiles Iii CE, Guo WA. Do we rely on fast for decision-making in the management of blunt abdominal trauma? *Injury*. 2015;46:817–21. doi: 10.1016/j.injury.2014.11.023.

8. Tinkoff G, Esposito TJ, Reed J, et al. American Association for the Surgery of Trauma organ injury scale I: spleen, liver, and kidney, validation based on the National trauma data bank. *J Am College Surg*. 2008;207:646–55. doi: 10.1016/j.jamcollsurg.2008.06.342.

26 Special Concerns in Pregnant Trauma Patients

Aashima Arora

LEARNING OBJECTIVES

- How management of pregnant trauma victims is different
- Approach to trauma during pregnancy
- Knowledge of anatomical and physiological changes of pregnancy affecting trauma assessment/management
- Imaging concerns during pregnancy
- Role of resuscitative hysterotomy

INTRODUCTION

- Trauma affects 5%–8% of all pregnancies.
- Trauma is the most common non-obstetric cause of morbidity and mortality during pregnancy.
- Common causes of trauma in pregnancy: motor vehicle accidents, falls, assault, burns.
- Blunt trauma is more common in pregnancy than penetrating injuries.
- Fetal loss rate: 40%–50% in life-threatening maternal trauma and 1%–5% in minor injuries. However, 60%–70% fetal losses follow minor injuries, as 90% of trauma cases during pregnancy lead to minor injuries.
- For any trauma during pregnancy, the patient must visit a physician.
- A multidisciplinary team approach is a must for severe trauma cases in pregnancy. This team must comprise a cardiac arrest team, a maternity crisis team and a neonatal crisis team.

APPROACH TO TRAUMA DURING PREGNANCY

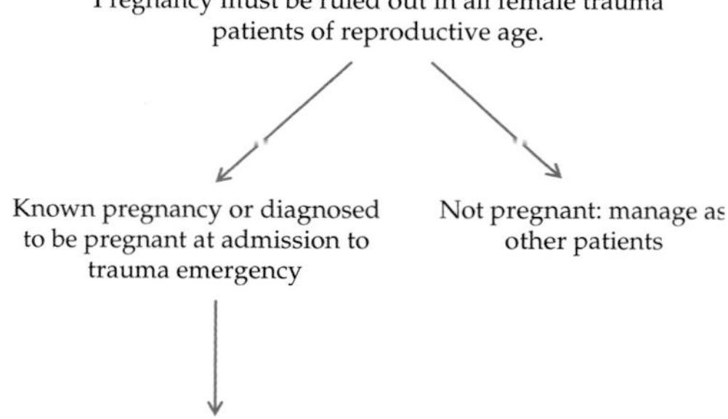

PLACE OF MANAGEMENT

For major trauma, pregnant patients are to be managed in trauma emergency irrespective of period of gestation (POG).

In minor trauma and POG > 26 weeks, pregnant patients are to be managed in the maternity unit.

The abdominal portion of anti-shock garment must not be inflated during transfer.

PRIMARY SURVEY AND STABILIZATION

Must focus on pregnant woman and not on fetus.

Follow ABCDEF protocol with F being fetus.

Airway: Keep low threshold of intubation; early placement of nasogastric tube to prevent aspiration.

Breathing: Target saturation is 95%.

Circulation: Administration of fluid and blood products as per standard trauma protocols.

Target haematocrit: 30%.

Vasopressors decrease utero-placental perfusion; to be used only if hypotension is fluid unresponsive.

Uterine displacement must be done to facilitate resuscitation if uterine size above umbilicus or POG > 24 weeks.

REASONS WHY MANAGEMENT OF PREGNANT TRAUMA PATIENTS IS DIFFICULT

1. Anatomical and physiological changes of pregnancy make assessment difficult.
2. It is difficult for emergency non-obstetric resident doctors to identify pregnancy-specific complications.
3. Trauma in pregnancy is a less common condition than non-pregnant patients.
4. Injury to both mother and fetus needs assessment.
5. There is fear of radiation/drug exposure to fetus.

ANATOMICAL AND PHYSIOLOGICAL CHANGES OF PREGNANCY AFFECTING TRAUMA ASSESSMENT/MANAGEMENT

The anatomical and physiological changes of pregnancy affect the assessment and management of a woman when she is received in a

DOI: 10.1201/9781003291619-29

Table 26.1: Anatomical and Physiological Changes of Pregnancy Affecting Trauma Assessment/Management

System	Changes	Effect
Cardiovascular	• Mild hypotension • Tachycardia • Peripheral vasodilatation • Hypervolaemia • Rotation of heart around its long axis • Mild cardiomegaly may be normal	• Vital signs are poor markers of maternal and utero-placental circulation • Delayed detection of hypovolaemia as vital signs show gross change only after 1.5 to 2 L blood loss • ECG: left axis deviation
Gastrointestinal	• Delayed gastric emptying • Oesophageal sphincter relaxation • Decreased bowel motility	• Increased risk of aspiration • Penetrating injuries of upper abdomen may cause bowel injury • Guarding and rigidity may be less apparent
Respiratory system	• Airway oedema • Increased oxygen requirement • Increased tidal volume • Decreased tidal volume • Physiological hyperventilation with respiratory alkalosis and metabolic compensation	• Difficult intubation • Low threshold for respiratory insufficiency • Rapid worsening of acidosis in case of hypoperfusion/hypoxia
Urogenital system	• Increased renal blood flow and glomerular filtration rate (GFR) • Decrease in serum creatinine • Compression of ureters	• Renal dysfunction possible with normal creatinine • Urine output poor indicator of shock
Others	• Pituitary gland enlargement • Splenic engorgement • Hypercoagulable state • Weight gain with increased lordosis	• Pituitary more prone to ischaemia/necrosis • Spleen more prone to rupture leading to intra-abdominal haemorrhage • Increased risk of thromboembolism • Increased predisposition to consumptive coagulopathy • Unstable gait with predisposition to falls

trauma emergency. Hence, clinicians attending to these women must be well appraised with changes in various organ systems in the body. These changes are shown in Table 26.1.

Seek urgent obstetric consultation for any of the following:

1. Uterine contractions
2. Suspicion of abruption (pain or uterine tenderness or vaginal bleeding)
3. Suspicion of traumatic uterine rupture
4. Rupture of membranes (suggested by history of leaking per vaginum)
5. POG more than 26 weeks

OBSTETRIC MANAGEMENT OF TRAUMA PATIENT

1. Obstetrician must quickly assess POG, details of present pregnancy to be reviewed if available and obstetric history to be taken. Quick obstetric examination should be done.
2. Common obstetric complications following trauma include placental abruption, preterm labour, rupture of membranes, uterine rupture, feto-maternal haemorrhage.
3. Occasional uterine contractions may occur in up to 40% of trauma cases; these resolve spontaneously in 90% of cases.
4. All pregnant women > 26 weeks POG must have electronic fetal monitoring of fetus for at least 4 hours after trauma. For women < 26 weeks, only presence or absence of fetal heart rate (FHR) needs to be documented.
5. Observe for at least 24 hours if any of the following adverse factors present: uterine tenderness, significant abdominal pain, vaginal bleeding, sustained contractions after 4 hours, rupture of membranes, abnormal FHR pattern, deranged coagulation, high risk mechanism of injury.
6. Urgent obstetric ultrasonography (USG) must be done if BPV is present or POG is unknown. USG must not replace electronic fetal monitoring.
7. Steroids for fetal lung maturity must be given if POG is between 26 and 34 weeks, and delivery is imminent.
8. Anti D must be given to all Rh negative pregnant women (exception being very minor limb injuries). If facility is available, a Kleihauer–Betke (KB) test must be done in

all pregnant trauma patients to assess feto-maternal haemorrhage.

9. Around 5% of maternal trauma cases require urgent Caesarean delivery; hence simultaneous preparation must be done for same.

CONCERNS IN IMAGING OF PREGNANT TRAUMA PATIENT

- Imaging studies are extremely beneficial in pregnancy to exclude injuries or to detect injuries that can be managed non-operatively as laparotomy has high chances of preterm labour (varying from 25% to 80% depending on POG).
- Ultrasound is the first-line imaging modality to detect intra-abdominal injuries with a sensitivity of 61%–83% and specificity of 94%–100% during pregnancy.
- Target must be to keep radiation exposure to a minimum by avoiding multiple imaging. However, no imaging which is required for management of pregnant lady must be deferred due to concern of fetal radiation exposure.
- Fetal anomalies are not reported below 50 mGy. Radiation exposure of each radiological procedure is well below 50 mGy, except extended fluoroscopic examination or intervention of pelvis.
- Intravenous iodinated contrast can be used when required information cannot be acquired by non-contrast studies or when imaging findings are expected to affect management.

ROLE OF PMCD/RESUSCITATIVE HYSTEROTOMY

In case of maternal cardiac arrest secondary to trauma, if return of spontaneous circulation (ROSC) is not achieved after 4 minutes of correctly performed CPR, a perimortem Caesarean delivery (PMCD) must be undertaken to assist maternal resuscitation in a patient with > 24 weeks of gestation or if uterine fundus is above the level of umbilicus.

- No need to check for fetal viability before performing PMCD.
- CPR and left uterine displacement must be continued uninterrupted during the PMCD.
- PMCD must be performed at the site of arrest for all cases of in-hospital maternal arrest.
- PMCD must be performed by the person with the most surgical experience present at the site, preferably an obstetrician. In an emergency, a general surgeon may also need to perform it.
- There is no standard surgical technique for performing PMCD. The surgeon must use the technique with which he/she is most familiar and fastest.
- If maternal resuscitation leads to ROSC after delivery of fetus, the patient must be shifted to the operation theatre (OT) immediately.
- In cases of major trauma of obvious fatal nature, performing PMCD does not need to be delayed for 4 minutes of CPR and may be undertaken immediately.

SUGGESTED READING

1. Murphy NJ, Quinlan JD. Trauma in pregnancy: assessment, management, and prevention. *Am Fam Physician*. 2014;90:717–22. PMID: 25403036.
2. Argent LD, Verelst S, Sabbe M. Management of the pregnant trauma patient: a literature study. *Open J Trauma*. 2020;4:38–46.
3. Jain V, Chari R, Maslovitz S, et al. Guidelines for the management of a pregnant trauma patient. *J Obstet Gynaecol Can*. 2015;37:553–74. doi: 10.1016/s1701-2163(15)30232-2. PMID: 26334607.
4. Raptis CA, Mellnick VM, Raptis DA, et al. Imaging of trauma in the pregnant patient. *Radiographics*. 2014;34:748–63. doi: 10.1148/rg.343135090. PMID: 24819793.

27 Managing Crush Injuries on Arrival

Sarvdeep Singh Dhatt and Deepak Neradi

LEARNING OBJECTIVES

- Always suspect the possibility of crush syndrome in patients with blunt injury to any muscle compartment
- Blood investigations (increased serum creatinine kinase) and urine for myoglobulin are the keys for diagnosis
- Early aggressive fluid resuscitation is the key to the successful management of crush syndrome
- Always keep the 5 Ps in mind (pain, pallor, paraesthesia, pulselessness and paralysis) to detect compartment syndrome

INTRODUCTION

Crush syndrome, or Bywaters syndrome (first described by Seigo Minami and Eric Bywaters), is a "reperfusion injury" secondary to crushing and rupture of muscle cells. When the contents of muscle cells are released into circulation, they cause systemic effects (Figure 27.1). A few are enumerated next below:

1. Shock is due to injury to blood vessels and subsequent loss of blood.
2. Activation of the nitric oxide system causes vasodilation, which worsens hypotension.
3. Response to ischaemia leads to swelling of the affected limb further compromising blood supply.
4. Extracellular fluid may penetrate injured muscles (third spacing) and can lead to depletion of intravascular fluid, hypovolaemic shock and cardiac arrest.
5. Replacement/restoration of local blood supply causes muscles to absorb sodium chloride, which leads to swelling and rhabdomyolysis and release of degradation products (K^+, myoglobulin, lactate, creatine) into circulation.
6. Myoglobulin is excreted in urine (leading to brown-coloured urine), but after crossing threshold levels, it precipitates in the distal convoluted tubules of the kidneys leading to obstruction and acute tubular necrosis (manifesting as oliguria and uraemia). Precipitation of myoglobulin is enhanced with the acidity of urine.
7. Lactate causes metabolic acidosis, and its levels correspond with muscle ischaemia time.
8. Potassium released from muscles can cause interference with cardiac conduction leading to arrhythmias.
9. Cytokines like TNF-α released from immune cells in response to injury cause a systemic inflammatory immune response, shock, acute respiratory distress syndrome (ARDS) and multi-organ failure.
10. Crush injury victims are susceptible to sepsis due to immunocompromised state (acute renal failure and catabolic state from injury) and increased exposure to pathogens from wounds, catheters, etc.

Muscle injury can occur during the initial crushing, during ischaemia and during reperfusion. Irreversible damage to muscle cells usually takes around 4–6 hrs, but this can vary with the crushing force. The initial injury is now considered to be due to pressure-stretch myopathy. Na^+, Cl^-, Ca^{+2} and water enter the cell when crushing pressure is applied on the stretched cell membrane. This results in loss of ATP (makes cells prone to ischaemic injury) and swelling of myocytes. Intracellular swelling combined with interstitial oedema (due to shifting of water from the vascular compartment) in tight fascial compartments results in compartment syndrome. Maximum damage to muscle takes place during the reperfusion stage. Xanthine oxidase plays a key role in generating free radicals from oxygen during reperfusion. Generated free radicals cause damage to muscle and other organs. Damage to microvasculature from free radicals leads to increased permeability, which worsens oedema and compartment syndrome. During reperfusion, calcium accumulates in the cell due to sodium–calcium pump-driven exchange with accumulated intracellular sodium. Increased intracellular calcium causes muscle contracture, inhibits ATP formation, and activates a cascade of events leading to autolysis and free radical generation (Figure 27.2).

MANAGEMENT

Release of crushing force can cause sudden haemodynamic collapse and cardiac arrest due to reperfusion injury, which can be prevented

DOI: 10.1201/9781003291619-30

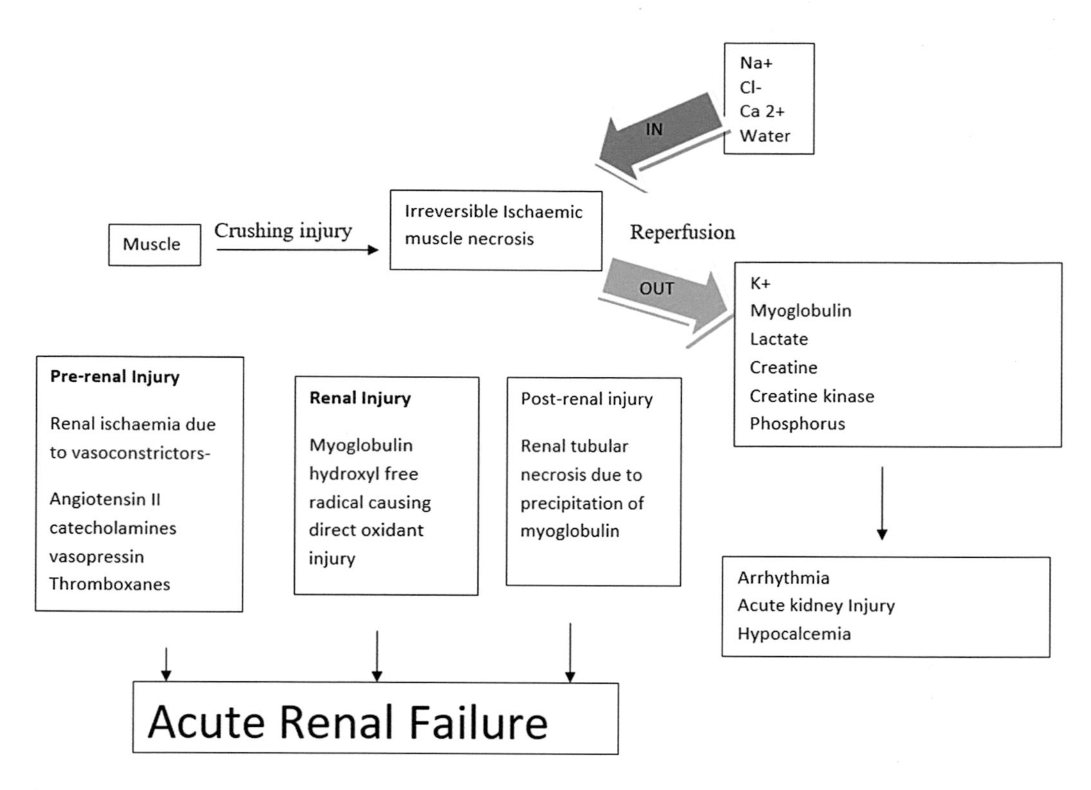

Figure 27.1 Pathogenesis of crush syndrome leading to acute renal failure

by initiating resuscitation/monitoring with the patient still trapped. Basic life support should be provided at the earliest, and the patient should be transported to a definitive medical care facility as quickly as possible. Patients with crush injury should be monitored for basic observations (blood pressure, respiratory rate, heart rate, temperature, oxygen saturation). Urine output and continuous cardiac monitoring should be started as early as possible. Blood electrolytes and gases should be measured every 6 hrs. Hyperkalaemia, hypocalcaemia and oliguria are early signs which can precipitate arrhythmias and cardiac arrest. Venous bicarbonate < 17 mmol/L in presence of myoglobinuria is associated with the development of acute renal failure (ARF). Due to the high risk of hypothermia in crush victims, aggressive rewarming should be achieved with warm IV fluid administration, warm air blankets, warmers, bladder/peritoneal lavage, warm enemas, etc. Slow rewarming is associated with a sevenfold increase in mortality in trauma patients. Blood loss should be replaced by transfusion of whole blood or blood components in a 1:1:1 ratio of packed red blood cells:plasma:platelets. Various principles of management of crush injuries are depicted in Table 27.1.

Management of crush syndrome consists of adequate rehydration of the patient and alkalinization of urine. The condition of the patient can deteriorate quickly due to acute kidney injury from crush syndrome, and requires immediate and vigorous fluid replacement in the short window period to increase their chances of survival. Fluid replacement should be continued till myoglobinuria has disappeared. Forced alkaline diuresis can prevent dialysis even if fluid resuscitation is delayed. Sodium bicarbonate is administered to help correct metabolic acidosis and reduce myoglobulin precipitation, thus decreasing injury to kidneys and risk of kidney failure. Urine pH should be maintained at > 6.5 to prevent ARF. Overaggressive use of bicarbonate can cause metabolic alkalosis and metastatic calcification. Acetazolamide can help counter metabolic alkalosis while alkalizing urine. It can be given in metabolic alkalosis if urine pH < 6.5. The use of acetazolamide/bicarbonate should be according to urine output, urine pH and serum pH (Figure 27.3).

Mannitol (osmotic diuretic and free radical scavenger) may be used to treat and prevent ARF. It also helps to reduce compartment pressure by osmotic diuresis and decreasing vascular permeability. However, due to possible

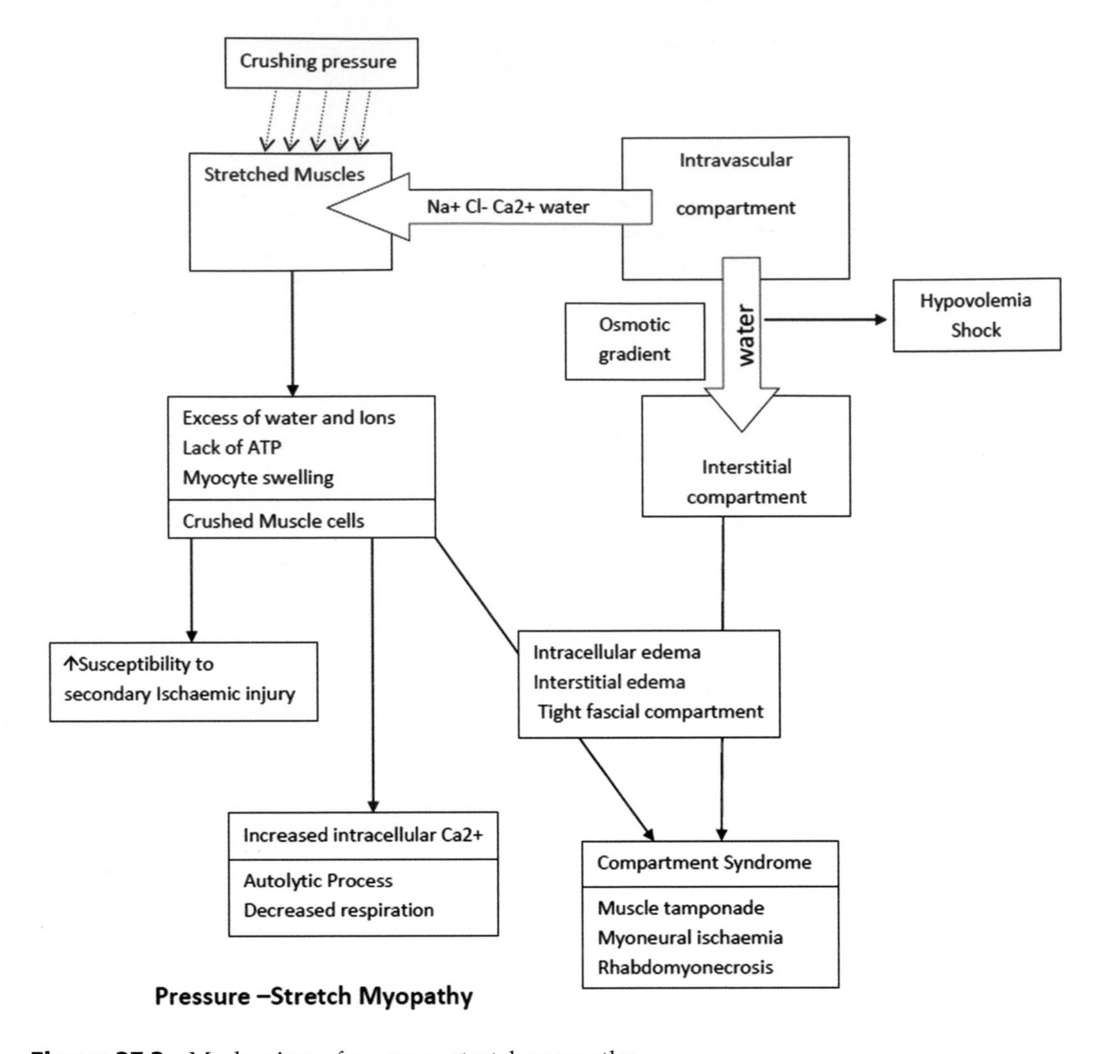

Figure 27.2 Mechanism of pressure-stretch myopathy

complications [nephrotoxicity/congestive heart failure (CHF)], its use is controversial and should be started/titrated according to urine output. Furosemide (loop diuretic) should be avoided, as it acidifies urine and promotes myoglobulin precipitation. Hyperkalaemia is an early sign of cardiac arrhythmia and needs early corrective measures. Early administration of 15 g/day of sodium polystyrene sulfonate (potassium binder) can be used to prevent fatal hyperkalaemia due to reperfusion injury. Correction of hypocalcaemia should be avoided, as administered calcium gets trapped in injured muscles and causes metastatic calcification and rebound hypercalcaemia. Calcium should be used only to prevent hyperkalaemic cardiac arrhythmia. Allopurinol (xanthine oxidase inhibitor) given early may be used to protect from reperfusion injury to ischaemic cells by reducing free radical formation. Dialysis is required in hyperkalaemia/metabolic acidosis resistant to medical therapy, volume overload and uraemia. Dialysis is usually required two to three times daily for 2 weeks to restore renal function. Crush victims are at increased risk of sepsis, systemic inflammatory response syndrome (SIRS) or multi-organ failure; therefore, they require intensive care monitoring, aggressive treatment of open injuries and nutritional supplementation.

Besides the high mortality of crush syndrome, crush victims face high morbidity from crushed limbs. There is a lot of controversy regarding the management of crushed limbs. To minimize morbidity (from amputation), the goal should be to salvage the crushed limb. In cases where amputation is inevitable, amputation at the site of injury may be considered before the release of crushing force as a lifesaving intervention, or to prevent reperfusion

Table 27.1: Principles of Management of Crush Victims by Sever and Vanholder

Principle 1 – All patients with crush injury should be accepted for definitive care because appropriate fluid management may prevent crush-related acute kidney injury (AKI), preventing need for dialysis.
Patients should not be abandoned in unavailability of dialysis as adequate fluid replacement can avoid dialysis in crush injury patients.

Principle 2 – Uniform vigorous fluid administration for all crush victims is an oversimplification.
Although fluid administration is necessary to prevent AKI, it should be individualized based on the following:

1. Time spent under the rubble – If rescue is slightly delayed, more fluid is required. However, if extrication is delayed by days, the approach should be conservative considering the possibility of anuria.
2. Length of extrication procedure – Extrication procedure may take hours in some cases. Immediate fluid resuscitation should be started @ 1000 ml/hr, which should be tapered by at least 50% after 2 hrs.
3. Volume status and urine flow – More fluid should be administered in hypovolemia suggested by symptoms of fluid depletion, bleeding and third spacing. While in anuria and signs of hypervolemia, less fluid should be given.
4. Dimensions of disaster – In mass disaster if close monitoring is not possible, fluids should be restricted to 3–6 L/day.
5. Demographic characteristics of victim – In elderly or children patients with low body mass/mild trauma, less fluid should be given as they may develop hypervolaemia.
6. Environmental conditions – Less fluid should be given in places with low ambient temperature.

Principle 3 – Isotonic saline should be preferred and potassium-containing solutions should be avoided at all costs.
Isotonic saline is the first option, as it provides adequate volume replacement and prevents AKI. Sodium bicarbonate solutions added to half isotonic saline corrects metabolic acidosis and hyperkalaemia and prevents AKI. Solutions containing even a small amount of potassium (like Ringer's lactate) are contraindicated because of high risk of fatal hyperkalaemia.
Use of mannitol is controversial and requires individual consideration. Mannitol use is desirable, as it prevents renal cast deposition, reduces intracompartmental pressure, muscle oedema and pain, and has diuretic, antioxidant and vasodilator effects. But it can cause congestive heart failure and nephrotoxicity, so requires proper monitoring. If required, it should be given after positive urinary response to a test dose.

Principle 4 – An arterial tourniquet should not be applied to prevent crush syndrome and used only for life-threatening bleeding.
Prolonged application of tourniquets may expose the patient to palsy, myonecrosis, thrombosis, rigour, blisters/abrasions/contusions and massive release of degradation products on removal. Tourniquets should be removed at earliest to reduce ischaemic tissue injury.

Principle 5 – Hypocalcaemia should not be treated unless symptomatic.
Crush injury patients develop hypocalcaemia due to shifting of calcium into muscle cells, hyperphosphatemia, parathyroid hormone (PTH) resistance and renal failure. But hypercalcaemia is also common in crush victims during recovery due to mobilization of calcium from muscle return of PTH sensitivity. Risk of hypercalcemia is increased in patients who previously received calcium supplementation; this leads to further cell damage. So hypocalcaemia should be treated only if symptomatic.

Principle 6 – Fasciotomy should be performed only on the basis of well-defined clinical indications or objective compartmental pressure measurements.
Blood supply to muscles is decreased due to increased compartmental pressure in crush injury, which can cause muscle necrosis. Compartmental pressure can be decreased by performing a fasciotomy, but it creates open wounds, which increases the risk of infection, sepsis, amputation and death; hemodynamic instability; and nerve injury. A fasciotomy should be performed only in the following indications:

1. Absence of distal pulses
2. For radical debridement of dead muscle
3. Intracompartmental pressure > 30–40 mmHg (especially without decrease within 6 hrs)
4. Diastolic blood pressure < 30 mmHG

Principle 7 – Amputation should be performed only when clearly indicated.
Amputations are associated with acute deterioration physiologically and psychologically. Amputation should be done only when clearly indicated, like when the limb cannot be salvaged because of life-threatening sepsis or SIRS.

Principle 8 – AKI in crush injuries may require earlier start and more frequent dialysis due to higher chances of life-threatening complications compared to AKI due to other causes.
The role of dialysis in AKI is controversial and may be postponed in absence of volume overload and solute imbalance. Crush-related AKI is usually associated with hypervolaemia, hypercatabolism, acidosis, uraemia and life-threatening hyperkalaemia. To prevent potential complications in crush victims, dialysis may be started earlier/more frequently compared to AKI due to other causes.

Principle 9 – In crush victims, intermittent haemodialysis should be the preferred renal replacement therapy (RRT).
All RRT modalities (continuous RRT, intermittent dialysis and peritoneal dialysis) have been found to be equally efficient in AKI. Intermittent dialysis should be the first choice in crush victims due to efficient clearance of potassium, possibility of treating several patients on the same machine or to minimize anticoagulation.

injury or SIRS. Amputation should be performed in case of life-threatening infection or non-salvageable limb.

Compartment syndrome occurring due to fractures (open or closed) or crush injuries is an acute surgical emergency. The vicious cycle of increasing swelling and pressure within tight fascial compartments due to ischaemia/inflammation and rhabdomyolysis leads to compression of vessels, nerves and lymphatics. If neglected, it leads to muscle necrosis, infection, ARF and systemic crush

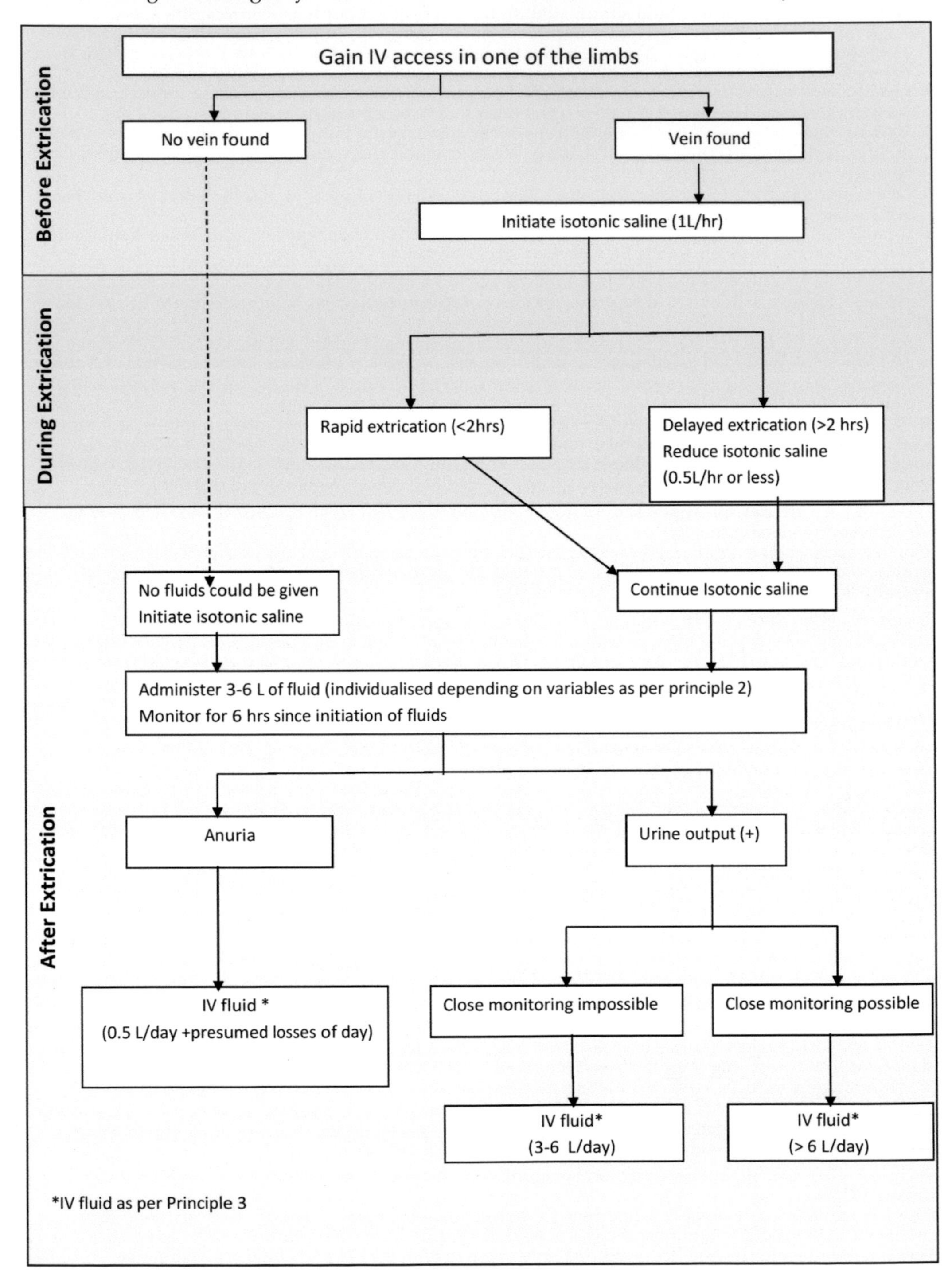

Figure 27.3 Guidelines for fluid resuscitation in crush injury patients

syndrome. Early, extensive fasciotomy with decompression of all limb compartments is the gold standard treatment for compartment syndrome.

Open wounds should be managed with extensive debridement and fasciotomy if needed. Early debridement is incomplete and repeat debridement might be required in the future. For closed wounds, fasciotomy should be performed in case of absent pulses or compartment syndrome. If pulses are intact and have no compartment syndrome, fasciotomy is contraindicated in closed crush injury due to high morbidity and mortality (due to sepsis) associated with fasciotomy. Crushed muscle without restoration of blood supply for the significant duration is already dead and non-salvageable. Fasciotomy in crush injuries is associated with a high risk of life-threatening infections, morbidity and

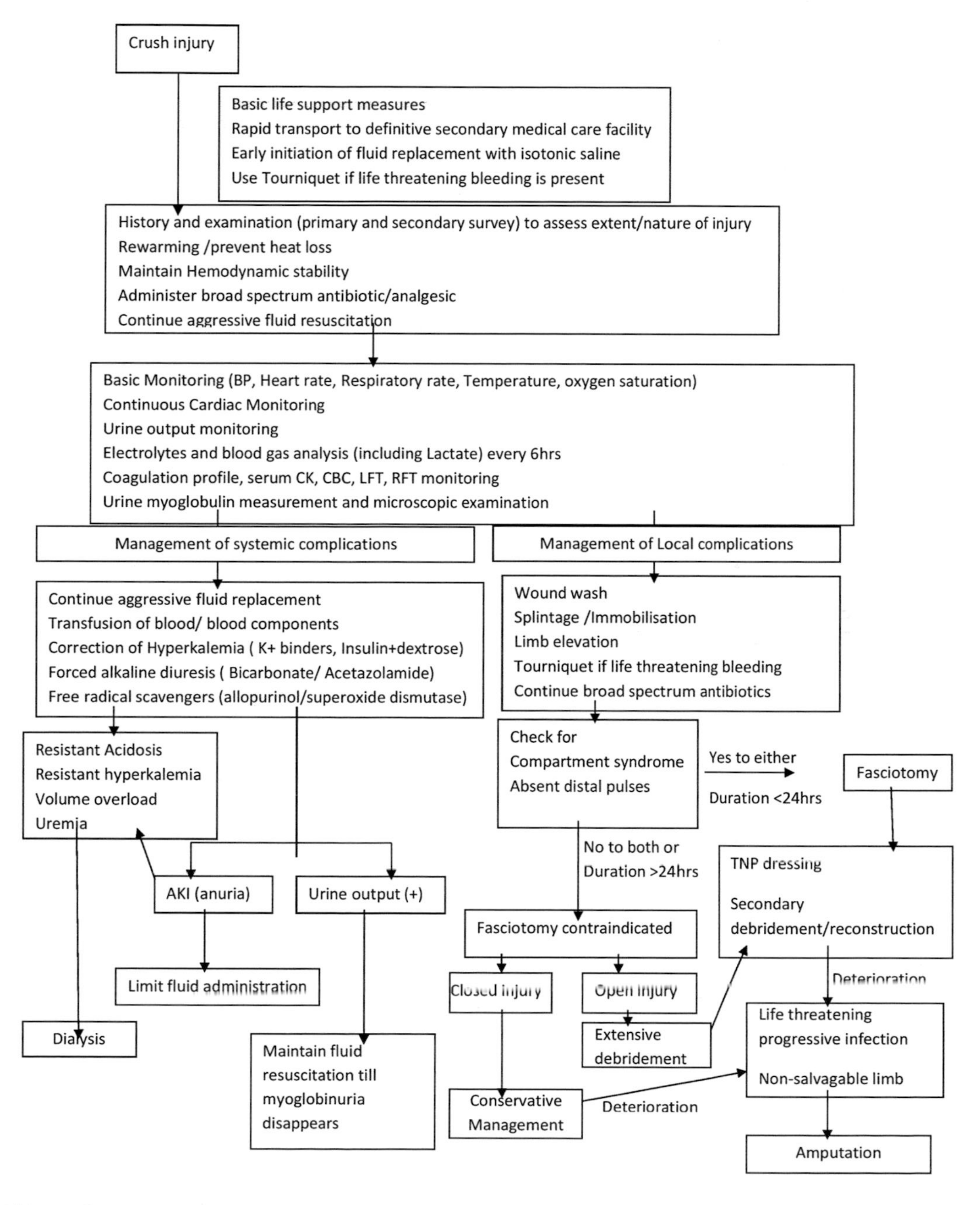

Figure 27.4 Management of crush injury patients

sequelae, requiring surgical intervention due to which there is a lot of controversy regarding whether fasciotomy improves outcome. Despite this, in presence of clinical signs (pain on passive muscle stretch, motor weakness, hypoaesthesia) or objective signs (raised compartmental pressure) of compartment syndrome, fasciotomy should be performed within 6 hrs. After 24 hrs, muscles become necrosed dead and fasciotomy is contraindicated in such cases due to high risk of life-threatening sepsis.

Hyperbaric oxygen therapy increases soluble oxygen in the blood and improves outcomes. Hyperoxia achieves this in crush injury patients by increasing oxygen supply to underperfused tissue, decreasing interstitial oedema (vasoconstriction due to hypoxia), inhibiting free radical formation, facilitating phagocytosis and enhancing wound healing. After fasciotomy, topical negative pressure (TNP) dressings help improve wound healing and minimize infection by reducing oedema, inhibiting local infection and increasing granulation. Management of crush injuries is depicted in a flow chart in Figure 27.4.

COMPLICATIONS

Crush injury predisposes the patient to primary hypothermia (excessive heat loss) and secondary hypothermia (decreased heat production). Any decrease in temperature below 35°C is an indicator of poor prognosis, with temperature < 32°C associated with nearly 100% mortality. Hypothermia prolongs clotting times and inhibits platelet function. Patients with the lethal triad of trauma (hypothermia, coagulopathy and acidosis) have high mortality rates.

CONCLUSION

Crush syndrome can occur in any patient with blunt injury to any muscle compartment. Patients with these kinds of injuries should be monitored closely and are resuscitated as early as possible. There are various options in the management, including fluid resuscitation, alkaline therapy, dialysis and hyperbaric oxygen. Early management is the key to good outcome.

SUGGESTED READING

1. Peiris D. A historical perspective on crush syndrome: the clinical application of its pathogenesis, established by the study of wartime crush injuries. *J Clin Pathol*. 2017;70:277–81. doi: 10.1136/jclinpath-2016-203984.

2. Smith J, Greaves I. Crush injury and crush syndrome: a review. *J Trauma*. 2003;54(Supplement):S226–30. doi: 10.1097/01.TA.0000047203.00084.94. PMID: 12768130.

3. Gonzalez D. Crush syndrome. *Crit Care Med*. 2005;33(Supplement):S34–41. doi: 10.1097/01.ccm.0000151065.13564.6f. PMID: 15640677.

4. Sever MS, Vanholder R. Management of crush victims in mass disasters: highlights from recently published recommendations. *Clin J Am Soc Nephrol*. 2013;8:328–35. doi: 10.2215/CJN.07340712.

28 Traumatic Amputation on Arrival

Akash Kumar Ghosh and Vishal Kumar

LEARNING OBJECTIVES

- Identifying a traumatic amputation
- Management at site of injury
- Management in the triage
- Assessing the salvageability of a severed limb
- Treatment objectives

INTRODUCTION

Traumatic amputation is the accidental loss of an extremity or a part of it. Upper limb amputations account for around 65% of traumatic amputations and usually involve the working and active age bracket of 15–40 years.

A traumatic amputation may be:

- Partial – Distal part attached by a narrow pedicle of muscle/nerve/tendons/vessels or skin (Figure 28.1). Regardless of the amount of injury, partial amputation should be assessed and treated like a complete limb, eligible for reattachment.
- Complete – Distal part is completely dismembered from the proximal part (Figure 28.2). Status of severed part should be enquired for.

Various mechanisms of injury:

- Crush – usually highly contaminated and variable prognosis for reattachment
- Guillotine – clean, sharp cut, suitable for reattachment
- Avulsion – poor prognosis for reattachment

These injuries could be isolated or may be associated with machine cut injuries, farm injuries or crush injuries by rolling machinery; or they could be associated with polytrauma, most commonly due to motor vehicle accidents or blast injuries.

PRE-HOSPITAL MANAGEMENT

Initial management of a traumatic limb amputation is like any other trauma, as per Advanced Trauma Life Support (ATLS) protocols.

Always follow the principle *life before limb* at every step of management.

Immediately call emergency services.

- Follow the sequence airway, breathing, circulation (ABC), as per ATLS guidelines. Secure cervical spine and airway.
- Achieve haemostasis.
  - Make the patient lie down, elevate the affected limb.
  - Wash your hands and remove any visible foreign body on the object, taking care not to rub the stump as it may aggravate bleeding.
  - Apply continuous pressure with a clean cloth. Apply additional cloths as the earlier ones keep getting soaked. *Do not remove the previous layers* as this may dislodge any clots already formed.
  - Continue compression for at least 15 minutes and maintain it throughout transportation.
  - If the bleeding is not controlled by compression, fashion a tourniquet from any available cloth or rubber tubing and apply at a proximal pulse point.
- Splint any partially amputated limb.
- The amputated part, if present, should be washed, covered with a wet gauze or clean cloth and wrapped in a clean, impermeable plastic bag. Place this plastic bag in an ice box containing equal amounts of ice and water.
- Ensure that the amputated part does not directly come in contact with ice. Label and transport the part along with the patient.

MANAGEMENT IN THE EMERGENCY DEPARTMENT

- Follow ATLS guidelines (ABCDE)
  - Secure two wide-bore IV cannulas and start IV fluids (manage as per ATLS shock algorithm).
  - Secure cervical spine and airway, and assess GCS (Glasgow Coma Scale).
  - Once patient is haemodynamically stable, open the dressings (may need to

DOI: 10.1201/9781003291619-31

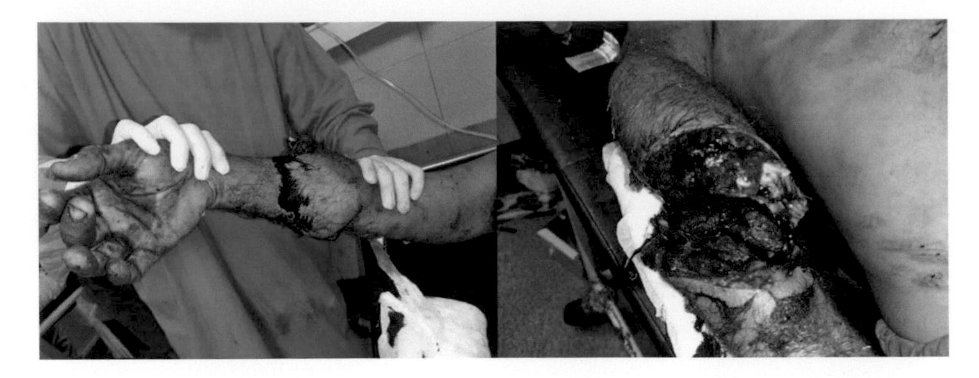

Figure 28.1 Partial amputation of upper limb (guillotine injury)

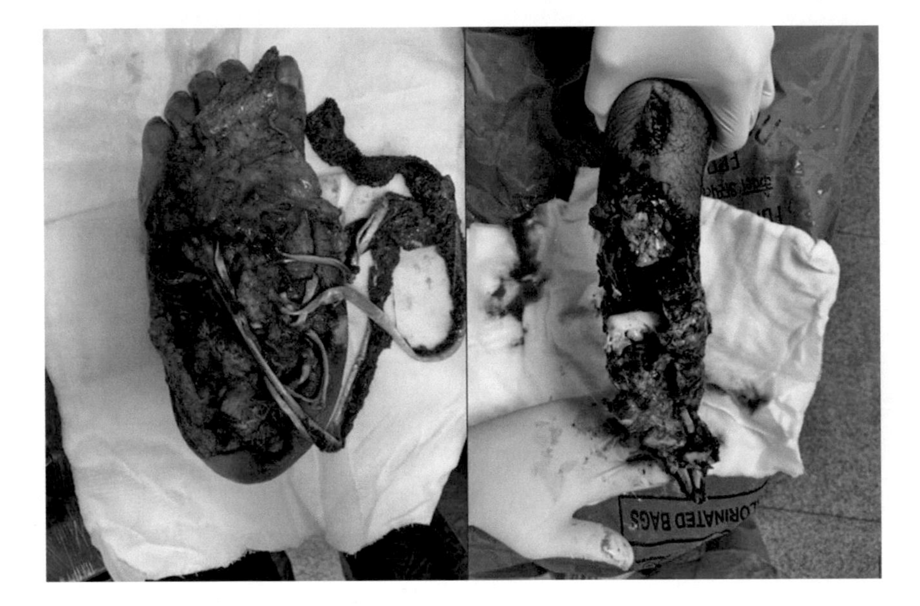

Figure 28.2 Complete amputation of lower limb (avulsion injury)

be done earlier if there is excessive soakage or patient is not responding to fluid therapy).

- Conduct primary survey, look for any other injury and potential sites of bleeding like abdomen, pelvis and long bone fractures.

■ Stump management

- Open dressing slowly, taking care not to dislodge any preformed clots.
- Wash the wounds with copious saline (warm or at room temperature), at least 9–12 L.
- Remove any tourniquet slowly and look for active bleed. For any bleed, first try to achieve haemostasis by continuous compression (15–20 minutes). If patient is planned for replantation, avoid clamping or ligature of vessels, as it crushes the vessel walls. In case patient is planned for a revision amputation, ligate the vessels with a sterile tie.
- In cases of partial amputations, take care not to injure the remaining pedicle.
- When applying compression, do not remove soaked gauze or pad. Keep applying additional gauze or pad on top of it, as removing a soaked pad risks dislodgment of formed clots.
- Apply a sterile compression bandage after achieving haemostasis, followed by adequate splintage if needed (in cases of partial amputation).

- Immediate adjuvants in pharmacotherapy
  - Analgesia
    - Early effective analgesia reduces morbidity and postoperative incidence of phantom pain.
    - Multimodal, round-the-clock perioperative analgesia must be planned in consultation with the anaesthesia team.
  - Commonly used regimens include:
    - Systemic opioids – IV morphine 0.1 mg/kg in children (max = 5 mg), 3–5 mg in adults (can be repeated 6 hourly), IV tramadol (1 mg/kg or 100 mg 12 hourly) after ruling out contraindications.
    - NSAIDs – Inj. paracetamol 10 mg/kg every 6 hourly or 1 g 6 hourly. Avoid inj. diclofenac in patients with traumatic amputations, as the already shock-like state increases predisposition to renal toxicity.
    - NMDA receptor antagonists – IV ketamine (1 mg/kg) can be used with strict monitoring.
    - Local anaesthetic injection around the wound.
  - Regional analgesia – peripheral nerve blocks, epidural analgesia (in consultation with the anaesthetist)
  - Antibiotics
    - Immediately start broad spectrum antibiotics after drug sensitivity testing and collecting appropriate samples for microbiological cultures (in cases of old injuries, > 24 hours).
    - For fresh, clean cut injuries usually a single antibiotic is enough (e.g. inj. cefuroxime 1.5 g IV TDS and STAT 30 to 60 minutes prior to surgery).
    - For farm, blast, highly contaminated or old injuries, consider adding additional anaerobic and gram negative coverage as per institute protocol (e.g. in our institution we add inj. amikacin 1g 24 hourly and inj. metronidazole 800 mg IV TDS).
  - Consider adding inj. penicillin or inj. clindamycin if suspecting gas gangrene, due to their specific antitoxin action
  - Tetanus prophylaxis

    Criteria for tetanus prophylaxis are listed in Table 28.1.
  - Other investigations
    - Radiographs – Of proximal joint and amputated limb, and the amputated part if replantation is planned.
    - Doppler – To be done in cases of partial amputation to assess vascularity.
    - Routine preoperative blood workup.
    - Photography from various angles of the stump and the amputated part. – Essential for surgical planning, communication and medicolegal purpose.

PLANNING TREATMENT

- Addressing a traumatic amputation requires a multimodal team, including orthopaedic surgeon, plastic surgeon, vascular surgeon, anaesthetist, nursing staff and a psychologist/social worker (Figure 28.3).
- Replantation is usually done only for upper limb amputation, as prosthesis acceptance is greater for lower limb amputations. A patient planned for replantation should be shifted to the operating theatre without any delay.
- Replantation of limb has selected few indications (Table 28.2).
- Replantation is, however, not suitable for all traumatic amputations (Table 28.3).
- Partial amputation can be treated as a mangled limb. The definition of a mangled extremity is a limb with an injury to at least three out

Table 28.1: Criteria for Tetanus Prophylaxis

	Clean, Minor Wounds		All Other Wounds	
History of Tetanus Toxoid (Doses)	**Tdap or Td**	**TIG**	**Tdap or Td**	**TIG**
< 3 or unknown	Yes	No	Yes	Yes
≥ 3	No*	No	No	No

*Yes, if more than 10 years since last dose. Tdap, tetanus diphtheria acellular pertussis; Td, tetanus diphtheria; TIG, tetanus immunoglobulin.

Plastic Surgeon
•Replantation, soft tissue reconstruction, wound coverage
Psychologist
•Counselling
Orthopaedic Surgeon
•Amputation, osseous fixation
Multidisciplinary Team
Nursing Staff
•General care, nutrition, assistance
Anaesthetist
•Analgesia, Pre-Operative optimization

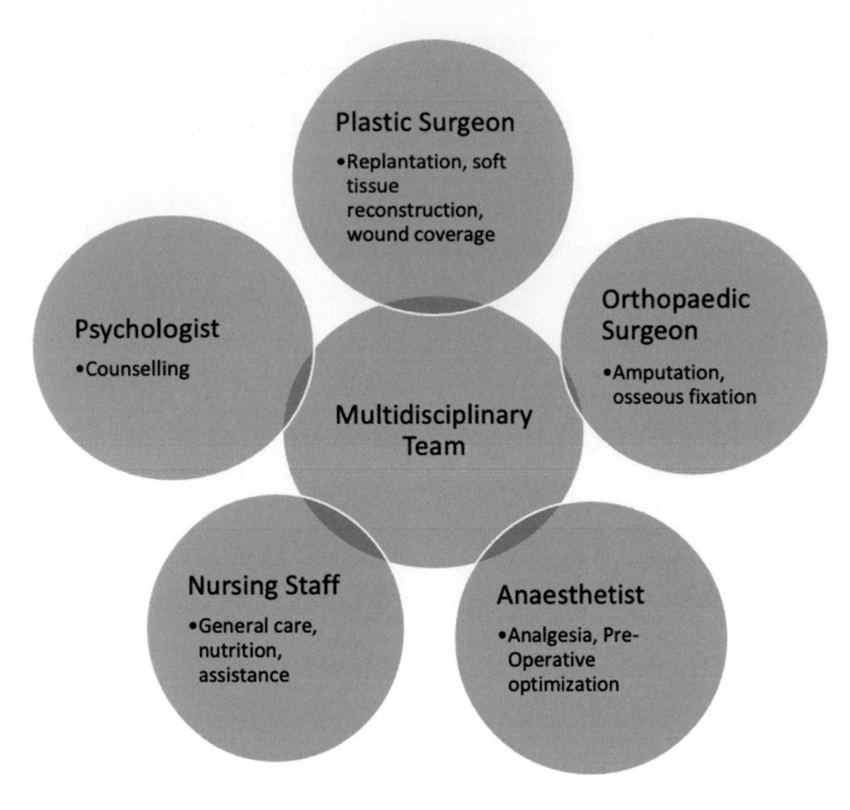

Figure 28.3 Structure and function of multidisciplinary care team for traumatic amputation

Table 28.2: Indications for Replantation of Limb

Indications for Replantation
Injury Factors
Thumb amputation
Multiple digit amputation
Amputation through palm, wrist or forearm
Patient Factors
Any amputation in child

of four systems (soft tissue, bone, nerves and vessels).

- Plan for limb salvage if Mangled Extremity Severity Score (MESS) < 7, amputation if MESS ≥ 7 (Figure 28.4).
- Plan for revision amputation at an appropriate level when complete amputation is unsuitable for replantation.
- In all cases, obtain informed consent from the patient and guardian regarding the possibility of amputation, infection, revision amputation, pain, haemorrhage and permanent disability prior to proceeding for surgery.
- Counsel patient with the help of a social worker regarding availability of prosthetics, rehabilitation services to reduce apprehension prior to surgery.
- A brief overview of management of traumatic limb amputations is illustrated in Figure 28.5.

Table 28.3: Contraindications for Replantation of Limb

Contraindications for Replantation
Haemodynamically unstable patient
Crushed or mangled limb
Avulsion or degloving injuries
Prolonged warm ischaemia time (> 12 hours for a digit and > 6 hours for a muscle-bearing extremity)
Prolonged cold ischaemia time (> 24 hours for a digit and > 12 hours for a muscle-bearing extremity)
Multiple-level amputations of the same extremity

Skeletal / soft-tissue injury
- Low energy (stab; simple fracture; pistol gunshot wound): 1
- Medium energy (open or multiple fractures, dislocation): 2
- High energy (high speed MVA or rifle GSW): 3
- Very high energy (high speed trauma + gross contamination): 4

Limb ischemia
- Pulse reduced or absent but perfusion normal: 1*
- Pulseless; paresthesias, diminished capillary refill: 2
- Cool, paralyzed, insensate, numb: 3*

Shock
- Systolic BP always > 90 mm Hg: 0
- Hypotensive transiently: 1
- Persistent hypotension: 2

Age (years)
- < 30: 0
- 30-50: 1
- > 50: 2

*** Score doubled for ischemia > 6 hours**

Figure 28.4 Mangled Extremity Severity Score (MESS)

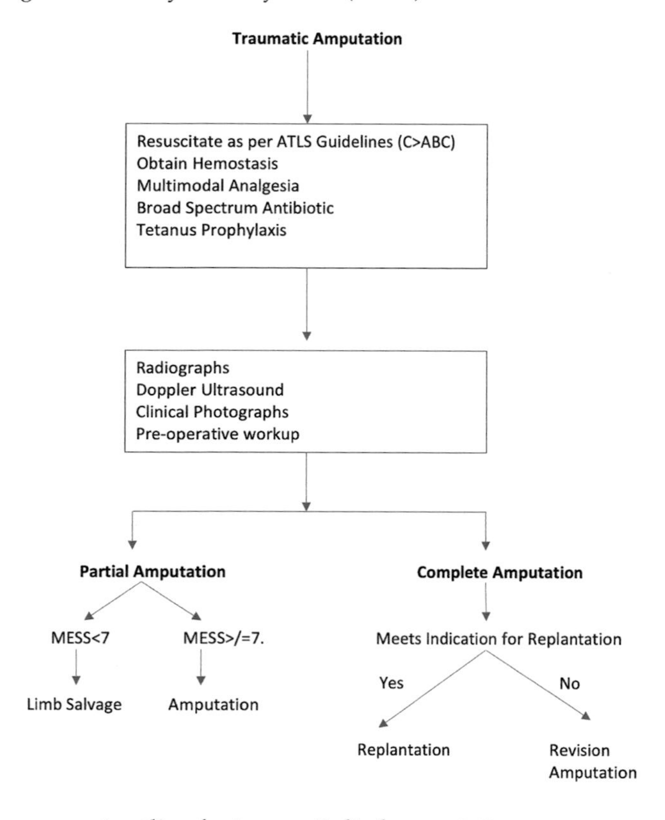

Figure 28.5 Management outline for traumatic limb amputations

SUGGESTED READING

1. Clasper J, Ramasamy A. Traumatic amputations. *Br J Pain*. 2013 May;7(2):67–73. doi: 10.1177/2049463713487324. PMID: 26516502; PMCID: PMC4590129.

2. Cumberworth J, Kieffer W, Harry L, Rogers B. Perioperative management of traumatic limb amputations due to civilian trauma: current practice and future directions. *J Perioper Pract*. 2015 Dec 1;25:262–6. doi: 10.1177/175045891502501203. PMID: 26845788.

3. ATLS Subcommittee, American College of Surgeons' Committee on Trauma, International ATLS Group Working. *Advanced Trauma Life Support: Student Course Manual*. Tenth edition. Chicago, IL: American College of Surgeons; 2018.

4. Win TS, Henderson J. Management of traumatic amputations of the upper limb. *BMJ*. 2014 Feb 10;348:g255. doi: 10.1136/bmj.g255. PMID: 24516069.

29 Basics of CT Scan Head and Trauma Radiographs

Ujjwal Gorsi and Chirag Kamal Ahuja

BASICS OF CT SCAN HEAD LEARNING OBJECTIVES

- To formulate a systematic approach to interpreting head CT scan in trauma
- To know salient features of commonly seen traumatic head lesions

INTRODUCTION

The brain is contained within the skull, a rigid and inelastic container which allows only small increases in volume. Acute pathologies like traumatic contusions and haemorrhages have the potential to cause sudden change in intracranial dynamics. Neuroimaging plays a vital role in the evaluation of neurological trauma and helps to identify treatable injuries, assists in the prevention of secondary damage and provides useful prognostic information. Due to its widespread availability, low cost and good sensitivity in identifying severe injuries, computed tomography (CT) serves as the workhorse for evaluation of head trauma. It is also better compatible with life-support and traction-stabilization devices.

BASICS OF INTERPRETATION

With the current availability of multi-detector CT scanners, CT acquisition takes only a few seconds. The acquired scan should preferably be read on a console in both brain (WW:80, WL:40) and bone (WW:1000, WL:250) windows, or alternately films of both windows should be sought (Figure 29.1). A systematic approach helps not only to not miss out on any important findings but to triage the patients based on injury severity:

- Identify any obvious hyperdensity (extra-axial, parenchymal, cisternal or ventricular), which may indicate haemorrhage. Localize, define, measure and evaluate its consequences (mass effect, adjacent parenchymal compression/distortion, midline shift, herniations).
- Look for any intracranial hypodensity (matching that of air in paranasal sinuses or externally), which may indicate pneumocephalus or pneumoventricle, and evaluate its consequences.
- Assess for parenchymal hypodensity indicating oedema or infarction.
- Actively search for any obvious fractures (on bone window), especially adjacent to hematomas and contrecoup sites.
- Try to search for vascular injury. Direct signs: hyperdensity in the cerebral venous sinuses–sinus thrombosis, prominence of the cavernous sinus and superior ophthalmic (SOV)–carotid-cavernous fistula. Indirect signs: thick blood along the course of vessels, fractures running adjoining major vessels, e.g. close to middle meningeal artery or at skull base close to vertebrobasilar arteries.
- Evaluate extracranial compartments, namely orbit, paranasal sinuses, facial bones and scalp, for any obvious injury or signs of cerebrospinal fluid (CSF) leak.

COMMON TRAUMATIC LESIONS WITH IMAGING CHARACTERISTICS

Traumatic Fractures

Fracture is a breach in the continuity of the bone. It may be linear, depressed or diastatic (which traverses sutures). It may involve the vault or skull base, and may be simple or comminuted. It is best viewed in the bone window settings (Figure 29.2) in multiplanar and volume rendered formats, and should be differentiated from cranial sutures. Some differentiating features between the two are highlighted in Table 29.1.

Acute Subdural Haemorrhage (SDH)

An acute subdural haemorrhage (SDH) is seen as a crescentic blood collection (classically venous) over cerebral hemisphere (Figure 29.3), displacing the cerebral cortex medially and is usually hyperdense (can be mixed due to unclotted blood or torn arachnoid) in nature. It can cross suture (cf. extradural haemorrhage) and can extend into the inter-hemispheric fissure along falx as well as along tentorium.

Extradural Haemorrhage (EDH)

An extradural haemorrhage (EDH) occurs in 1%–3% of admitted patients of traumatic brain injury and results from injury to meningeal arteries. It is seen as a biconvex hyperdense extra-axial blood collection (Figure 29.1) frequently associated with fractures. EDH does not cross sutures, which helps to differentiate it from SDH.

DOI: 10.1201/9781003291619-32

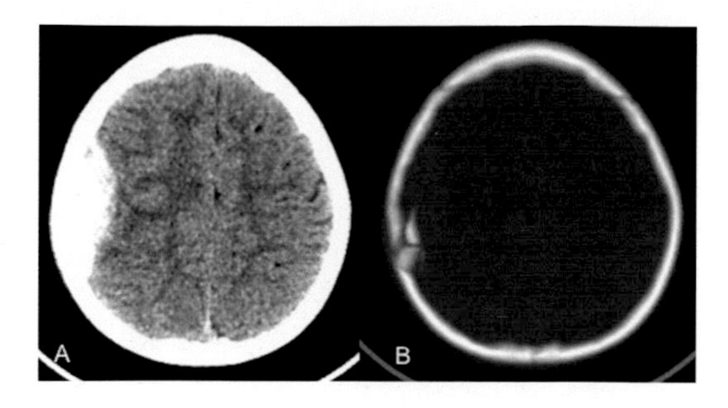

Figure 29.1 Head CT scan axial section (a) brain and (b) bone window settings showing right convexal extradural haemorrhage with overlying depressed fracture, clearly visualized in the bone window setting

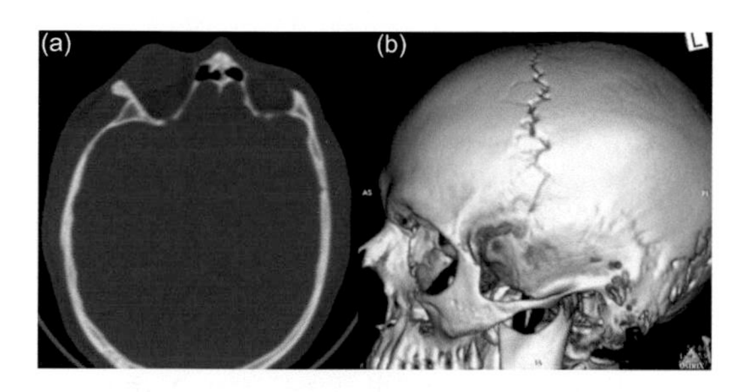

Figure 29.2 Head CT scan axial section in (a) bone window setting demonstrating a break in the continuity of left parietal bone, which is better visualized in the (b) volume rendered image just posterior to the coronal suture

Traumatic Subarachnoid Haemorrhage (SAH)

Trauma is the most common cause of subarachnoid haemorrhage (SAH), which results from tearing of veins in the subarachnoid space as a result of shearing. Rarely it can be arterial in origin due to traumatic aneurysm formation as suggested by large volume bleed and presence along the course of a major vessel. CT angiography is suggested in such patients to map the arterial abnormality for possible intervention. SAH is seen as diffuse hyperdensity in the sulcal and cisternal spaces (Figure 29.4), and is usually associated with cerebral contusion, SDH or other lesions.

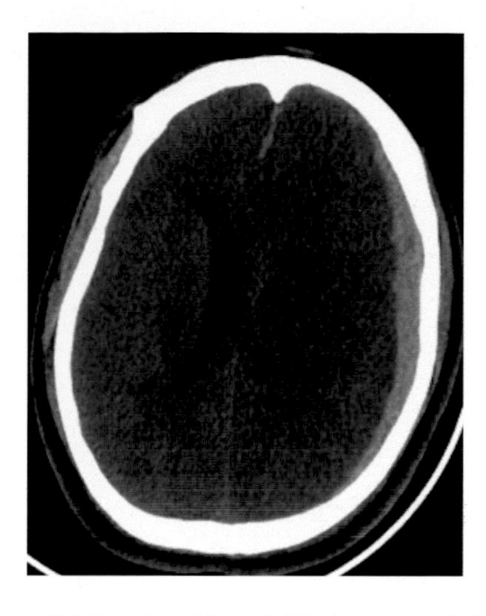

Figure 29.3 Axial head CT depicting left convexal subdural haemorrhage

Cerebral Contusion

Cerebral contusion is the most common parenchymal lesion in head trauma. Contusion results from impact of cerebral gyri to the inner table of the skull, hence seen often in basifrontal and anterior temporal regions due to presence of rough bony edges and ridges. It evolves from small petechiae to small haemorrhages and finally large haematomas over a period of time. Thus, it is important to image contusions at a periodic interval within the first few days to identify haematoma expansion and mass effect. Classical imaging appearance is that of low-density cortex (oedema) mixed with high-density blood (petechial haemorrhage) (Figure 29.5).

Diffuse Axonal Injury (DAI)

DAI results from traumatic deceleration injury with shearing and rotational forces causing microstructural neuronal transection in areas of greater density differential in the brain, e.g. grey–white matter interface, dorsal brainstem and corpus callosum. It can be either haemorrhagic (Figure 29.6) or non-haemorrhagic (the latter is more common), and may be CT occult

Table 29.1: Difference between Fractures and Sutures

Fractures	Sutures
• Greater than 3 mm in width	• Less than 2 mm in width
• Usually run in straight line	• Do not run in straight line
• Have angular turns	• Are curvaceous
• At sites of maximum force	• At specific anatomic sites

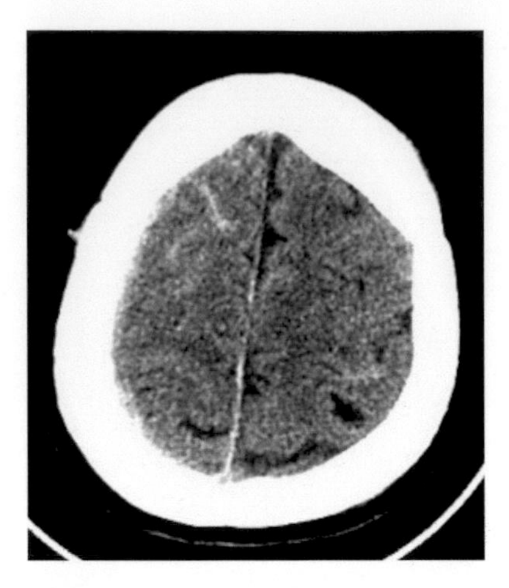

Figure 29.4 Axial head CT showing sulcal subarachnoid haemorrhage

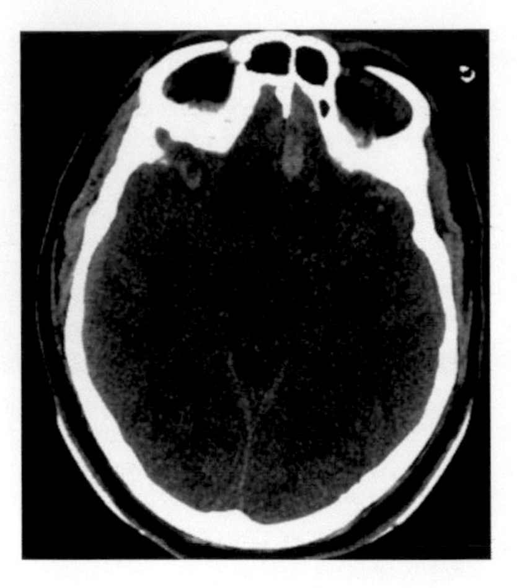

Figure 29.5 Axial head CT scan demonstrating cortical-based haemorrhages in the basifrontal and anterior temporal lobes, which are typical sites of contusions. Also note the diffuse parenchymal hypodensity suggestive of diffuse cerebral oedema

when the lesions are very small and subtle. Lesion number and location predicts prognosis (worst when multiple and in supratentorial location). MRI with susceptibility-weighted imaging is suggested when there is a clinical CT discorrelation, i.e. when the latter is apparently normal while the patient is severely affected.

It is reiterated that in any manifestation of head injury, it is a dictum to evaluate for contralateral midline shift and transcompartmental herniations, e.g. uncal herniation, tonsillar herniation and ascending transtentorial herniation along with corresponding vascular ischaemic effects in the anterior and posterior cerebral territories. There may be late effects of head injury in the form of internal carotid artery injury resulting in carotid-cavernous fistula (Figure 29.7) and CSF rhinorrhoea (Figure 29.8).

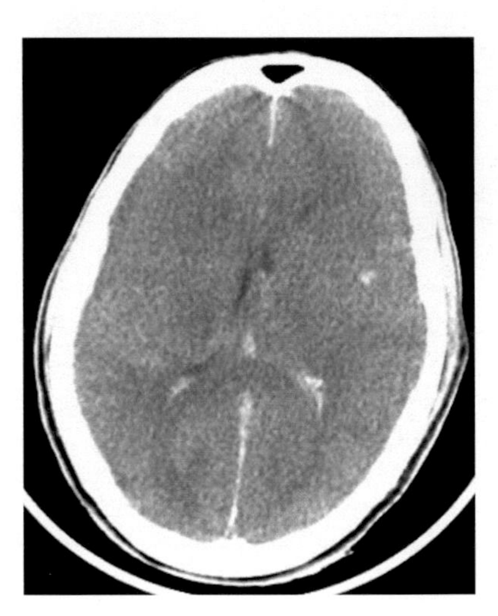

Figure 29.6 Axial head CT scan showing diffuse cortical subcortical hypodensity with small haemorrhages on the left side suggesting diffuse axonal injury. Note also the adjoining oedema and mass effect leading to ventricular compression

BASICS OF CHEST RADIOGRAPHS LEARNING OBJECTIVES

- To know common radiographic findings in thoracic trauma
- To learn systemic approach in interpreting chest radiograph

INTRODUCTION

Chest radiograph is often requested in trauma care of patients arriving in triage. The supine anteroposterior chest radiograph is an invaluable tool, as it can be acquired in the trauma bay with little interruption in ongoing assessment and management of the patient. Chest radiograph assessment includes evaluation of lung parenchymal and extraparenchymal injuries. The position of tubes, lines and associated complications should also be assessed.

LUNG PARENCHYMAL INJURIES

Parenchymal Contusion and Laceration

The most common cause of opacities in lung in chest trauma is contusion. On radiograph, pulmonary contusion is seen as focal or multifocal

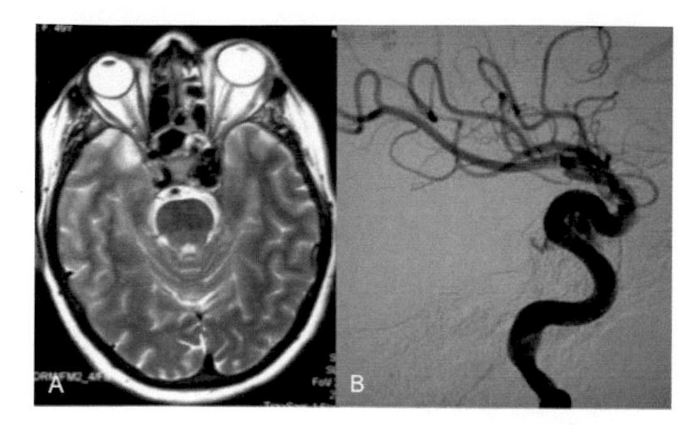

Figure 29.7 (a) Axial T2 weighted MR images depicting the exaggerated flow voids in the left cavernous sinus region indicating arterial flow within the sinus. (b) Left ICA angiogram confirms the presence of carotid-cavernous fistula

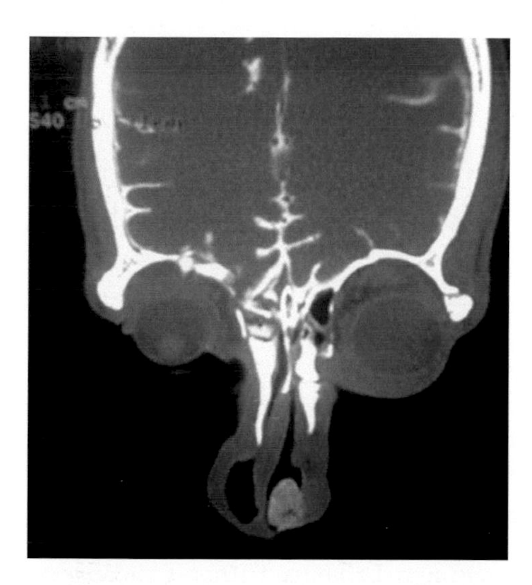

Figure 29.8 Coronal image of CT cisternography showing multiple fractures involving the floor of anterior cranial fossa with contrast stained CSF within the right ethmoid air cell. Also note the contrast staining of cotton pledget placed in the left nostril

areas of consolidation not contained by segmental boundaries. They commonly involve basal segments. After injury, contusions usually develop within 6 hours and resolve over 3 to 10 days. Acute respiratory distress syndrome (ARDS) or secondary infections should be suspected if lung opacities do not clear or increase in this time frame.

Pulmonary lacerations are more severe injuries and represent tears of lung parenchyma. On radiograph, they appear as ovoid or round radiolucencies usually along with surrounding contusions (Figure 29.9).

EXTRAPARENCHYMAL INJURIES

Pneumothorax and Haemothorax

Pneumothorax is second most common injury after rib fracture. Pneumothorax is seen as visualization of the visceral pleural line with non-visible lung markings peripherally (Figure 29.10). In supine patients, air collects in the anteromedial and subpulmonic recesses most commonly. On AP radiograph, a deep sulcus, sharply outlined hemidiaphragm and hyperlucent upper abdomen are features of pneumothorax (Figure 29.11). In haemothorax, blood accumulates in the subpulmonic recess and obscures costophrenic angles and diaphragms on chest radiographs when its volume is approximately 500 ml.

Pneumomediastinum

Pneumomediastinum is seen on radiograph as air surrounding mediastinal structures like oesophagus, trachea and major vessels. The continuous diaphragm sign may also be seen (Figure 29.12). Aetiology of pneumomediastinum is usually rupture of the alveoli, and injury to the oesophagus and tracheobronchial tree.

Chest Wall Injuries

Subcutaneous emphysema on chest radiographs creates radiolucent striations which outline fibres of the pectoralis major (Figure 29.12). Air can also spread to the head, neck and abdomen. Trauma to chest can cause various injuries to the skeleton. Injury to the brachial plexus and great vessels may be seen in association with upper rib trauma. Lower rib fractures may be associated with injuries to upper abdominal organs. Five or more contiguous single fractures or three adjacent segmental rib fractures will lead to flail chest. Respiration can be severely impacted as a result of paradoxical motion during respiration (Figure 29.13). Clavicle fractures are common and usually are not of much clinical significance (Figure 29.14). Sternoclavicular dislocations, scapular and sternal injuries may also be seen. Spinal fractures may cause neurologic and vascular damage.

Diaphragmatic Injury

Disruption secondary to trauma is more common on the left side of the diaphragm. Injuries usually involve muscular posterior and posterolateral portions. Radiograph and CT may show an abnormally coursed nasogastric tube and herniated hollow viscus into the chest. Constriction may be seen at the level of the rent, the so-called "collar sign" (Figure 29.15).

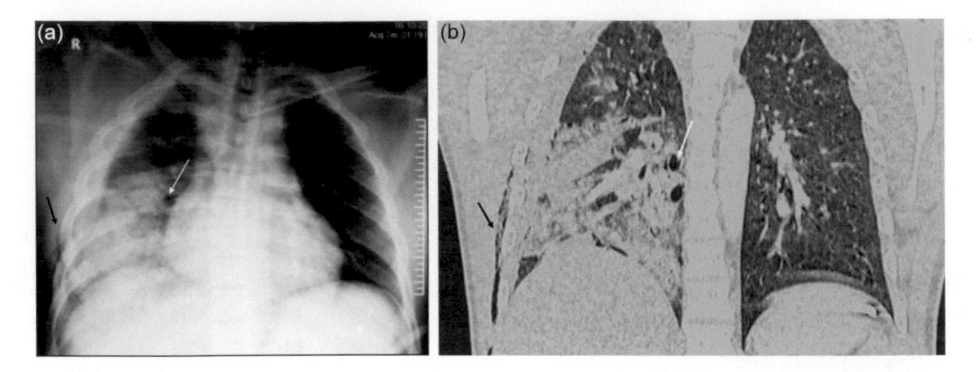

Figure 29.9 a and b: Lung contusion and laceration: Chest radiograph (a) shows confluent area of consolidation in right lower lobe. Small lung laceration is also seen along the medial aspect (white arrow). Findings are confirmed on CT chest. (b) Note there is also subcutaneous emphysema (black arrow in a and b)

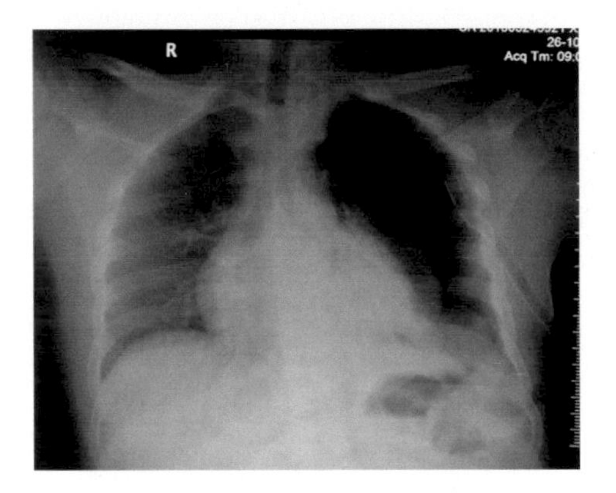

Figure 29.10 Chest radiograph showing left pneumothorax with chest tube in situ

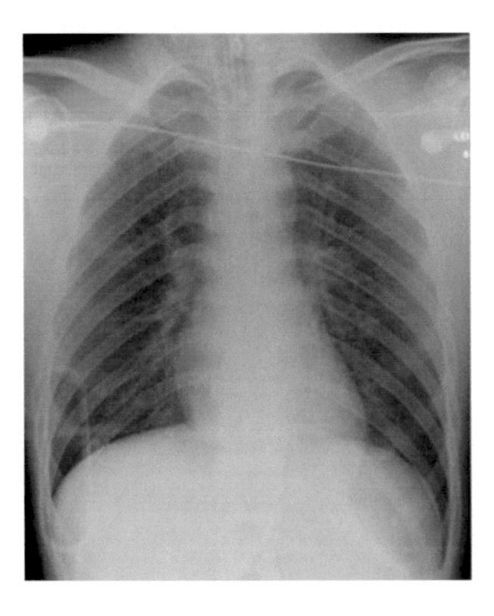

Figure 29.11 Chest radiograph (AP) in supine position shows deep sulcus sign on left side consistent with left pneumothorax

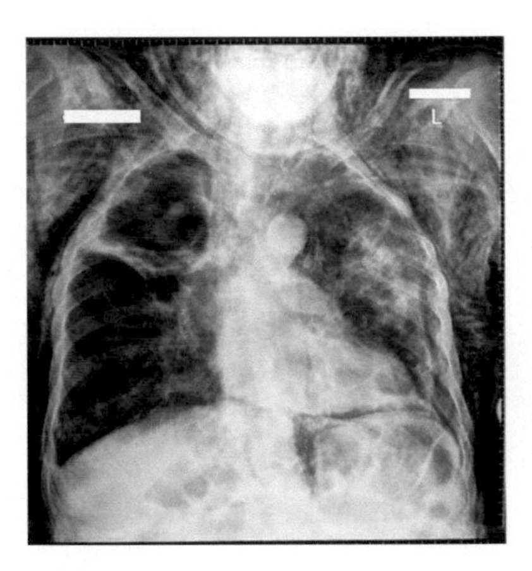

Figure 29.12 Chest radiograph shows pneumomediastinum as evident by continuous diaphragm sign. Left pneumothorax and extensive subcutaneous emphysema is also seen

Aorta

Radiographic features of traumatic injury to the aorta are non-specific and may include widened mediastinum, aortic contour abnormality, loss of aortopulmonary window, depressed left mainstem bronchus, widened paratracheal and paraspinous stripes, left apical pleural cap and haemothorax (Figure 29.16).

Other Injuries

Airway injuries are uncommon. Bronchial tears involve the right side, commonly within 2.5 cm of the carina. Radiographic findings include pneumothorax, pneumomediastinum and subcutaneous emphysema. Radiographic findings which suggest oesophageal injury are left pleural effusion, left lower lobe

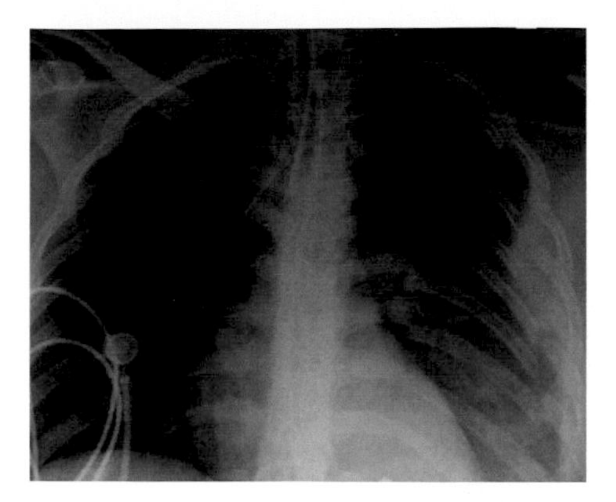

Figure 29.13 Chest radiograph showing multiple segmental rib fractures on left side suggestive of flail chest

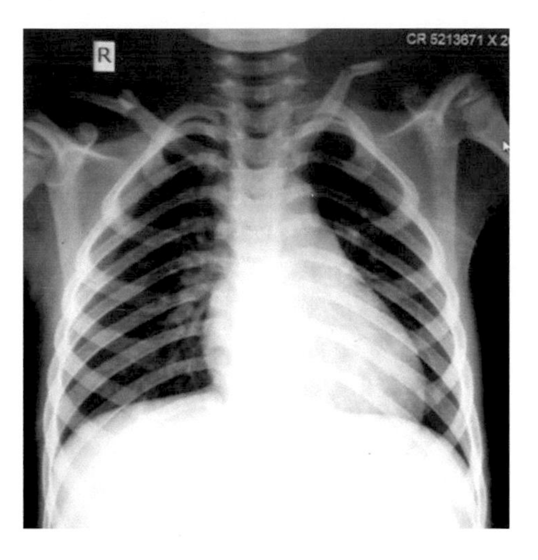

Figure 29.14 Bilateral clavicle fractures in a child with trauma evident on chest radiograph

atelectasis, pneumomediastinum and left pneumothorax. Trauma to heart and pericardium may cause pericardial effusion or pneumopericardium. Radiographic features of effusion include global enlargement of the cardiac silhouette.

Evaluation of Tubes and Lines

Endotracheal tubes should end 5–7 cm above the carina in neutral position of the neck. Position and course of nasogastric tube and central venous catheter should be assessed.

Chest tube may get placed into the fissure with little clinical significance. Placement against mediastinal structures and into lung parenchyma will require repositioning.

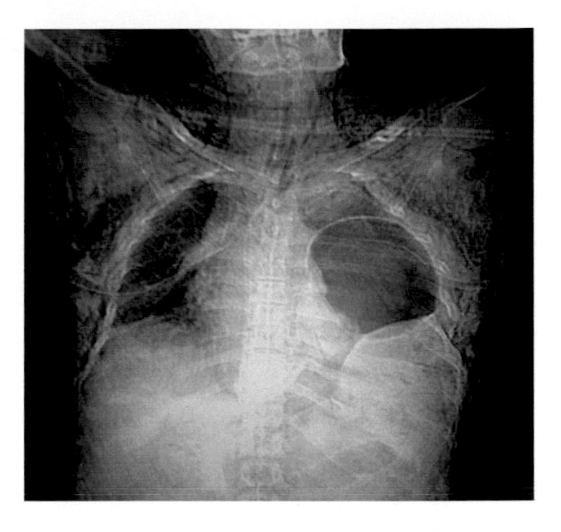

Figure 29.15 CT scanogram showing herniation of stomach in chest with collar sign in a patient of traumatic diaphragmatic injury

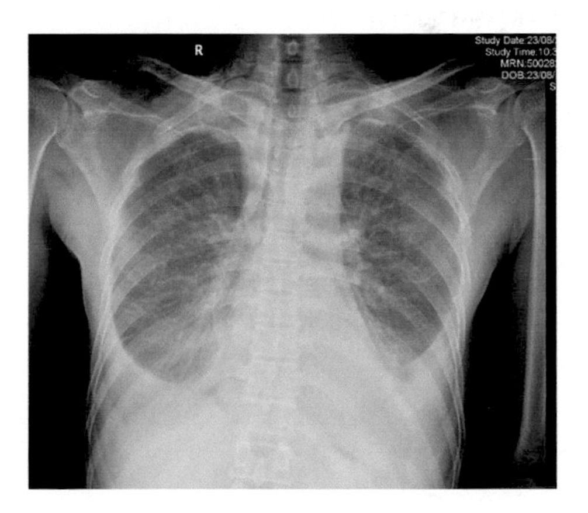

Figure 29.16 Chest radiograph showing mediastinal widening and bilateral pleural effusion in a poly trauma. Patient was found to have traumatic aortic injury on subsequent CT angiography (not shown)

AN APPROACH TO INTERPRET CHEST RADIOGRAPH IN TRAUMA

- Check all lines and tubes, specially the position of the endotracheal tube
- Confirm central position of trachea and patency of airway
- Look for pneumothorax and haemothorax, specially tension pneumothorax
- Exclude flail chest and rib fracture
- Look for size and contour of mediastinum, giving special attention to aortic contour

- Look for pulmonary contusion and laceration
- Check position, outline and contour of diaphragm
- Look for surgical emphysema
- Check for spinal, clavicle, scapular and sternal injuries

SUGGESTED READING

1. Alzuhairy AKA. Accuracy of Canadian CT head rule and New Orleans criteria for minor head trauma: a systematic review and meta-analysis. *Arch Acad Emerg Med*. 2020;8(1):e79.

2. Badhiwala JH, Wilson JR, Fehlings MG. Global burden of traumatic brain and spinal cord injury. *Lancet Neurol*. 2019;18:24–25.

3. Douglas DB, Ro T, Toffoli T, Krawchuk B, Muldermans J, Gullo J, Dulberger A, Anderson AE, Douglas PK, Wintermark M. Neuroimaging of traumatic brain injury. *Med Sci*. 2018;20(7):2.

4. Smith LGF, Milliron E, Ho ML, Hu HH, Rusin J, Leonard J, Sribnick EA. Advanced neuroimaging in traumatic brain injury: an overview. *Neurosurg Focus*. 2019;47(6):E17. doi: 10.3171/2019.9.

5. Costantino M, Gosselin MV, Primack SL. The ABC's of thoracic trauma imaging. *Semin Roentgenol*. 2006;41:209–25.

6. Tocino IM, Miller MH, Fairfax WR. Distribution of pneumothorax in the supine and semirecumbent critically ill adult. *AJR Am J Roentgenol*. 1985;144:901–5.

7. Primack S, Collins J. Blunt nonaortic chest trauma: radiographic and CT findings. *Emerg Radiol*. 2002;9:5–12.

8. Ho ML, Gutierrez FR. Chest radiography in thoracic polytrauma. *AJR Am J Roentgenol*. 2009;192:599–612.

9. Harvey-Smith W, Bush W, Northrop C. Traumatic bronchial rupture. *AJR Am J Roentgenol*. 1980;134:1189–93.

30 Basics of Ventilator Settings

Anjishnujit Bandyopadhyay

LEARNING OBJECTIVES

- How to select ventilator mode based on clinical data
- To learn basic differences between controlled mandatory ventilation, partially spontaneous and fully spontaneous modes
- How to select the initial settings and troubleshoot alarms on the ventilator

INTRODUCTION

Positive pressure ventilation in humans was first reported during the Danish polio epidemic of 1952. During the epidemic, medical students, working in shifts, manually ventilated the patients. This became a huge moment in the history of medical science as it provided the momentum for invention of positive pressure mechanical ventilators. The early positive pressure ventilators were simple yet efficient, but these devices have now been replaced by modern ventilators which are microprocessor controlled. Modern ventilators have multiple modes; various types of flow delivered; and tools to monitor pressures, flow and volume.

In the course of this chapter, we shall only be discussing invasive positive pressure ventilation.

COMMONLY USED MODES OF VENTILATION

1. Controlled modes
   a. Volume-controlled ventilation (VCV)/ volume-targeted ventilation (VTV)
   b. Pressure-controlled ventilation (PCV)/ pressure-targeted ventilation (PTV)
2. Assist/control ventilation (P-ACV/V-ACV)
3. Synchronized intermittent mandatory ventilation (SIMV)
4. Pressure support ventilation (PSV)/assisted spontaneous breathing (ASB)

CHOOSING A MODE AND SETTING THE VARIABLES

Controlled Modes or Continuous Mandatory Ventilation (CMV)

- Do not allow for spontaneous breathing
- Usually used in operation theatre (OT) or intensive care unit (ICU) when muscle relaxants are also being administered concurrently
- Two types: PCV and VCV
- VCV
  - Machine delivers a time-triggered (i.e. after a preset time has elapsed) breath of a preset tidal volume (TV) (volume limited) over a preset time period, after which exhalation starts (time cycled).
  - Inspiratory flow is usually constant, which results in a constant slope in the pressure vs time and volume vs time scalars (Figure 30.1).
  - Clinicians usually set – TV, respiratory rate (RR), fraction of inspired oxygen (FiO_2), inspiratory time (Ti), positive end expiratory pressure (PEEP) or inspiratory flow rate and a maximum inspiratory pressure limit.
  - Advantage – Volume control assures tidal volume delivery despite the changing lung mechanics, thus preventing against hypoventilation.
  - Disadvantages.
    - Volume delivery is assured, but there is no control over the maximum pressure required to deliver that volume. High pressure achieved in a lung with decreased compliance can lead to barotrauma.
    - If the ventilator does not have the ability to compensate for the compressible volume of the circuit tubing (volume lost in the tubing), then adequate tidal volumes may not reach the lungs (important in infants and young children).
  - PCV
  - Machine delivers a time-triggered (i.e. after a preset time has elapsed) breath till a preset inspiratory pressure is reached (pressure limited) over a preset time period, after which exhalation starts (time cycled).
  - The delivered tidal volume usually varies by small amounts amongst the breaths and is determined by the difference of peak inspiratory pressure and PEEP.

DOI: 10.1201/9781003291619-33

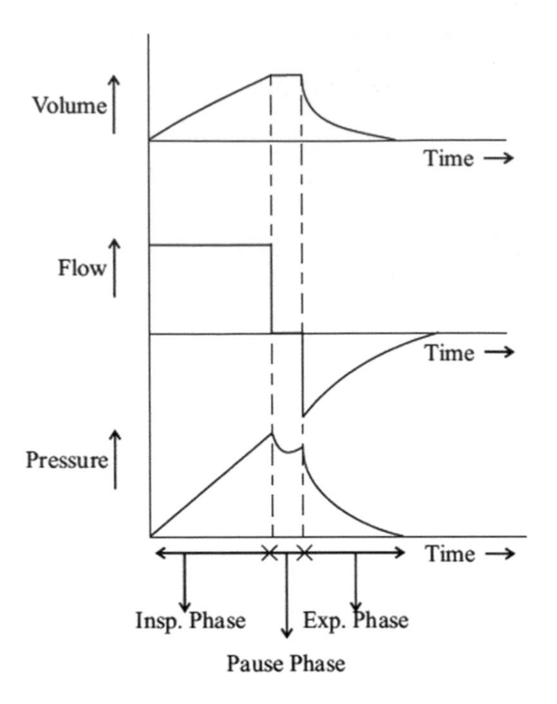

Figure 30.1 Volume vs time, flow vs time and pressure vs time as seen in volume-controlled ventilation

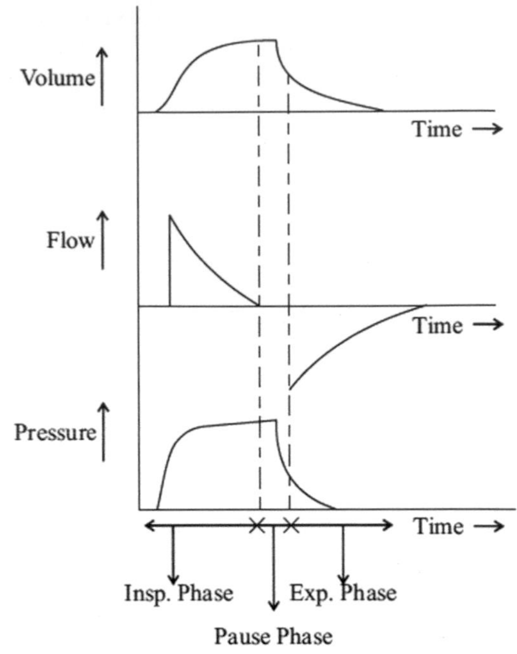

Figure 30.2 Volume vs time, flow vs time and pressure vs time as seen in pressure-controlled ventilation

- A decelerating flow pattern is universal in all pressure modes. In addition, the pressure is maintained for the entire duration of inspiration (Figure 30.2).
- The clinician usually sets inspiratory pressure (Pcontrol/Pc), RR, FiO_2, PEEP, Ti and Trise/ramp speed, which signifies how quickly the set pressure is reached (usually 50–200 milliseconds).
- Advantages.
  - Maximum pressure generated is usually controlled and set by the clinician, lessening chance of inadvertent barotrauma.
- Decelerating flow causes better distribution of ventilation in diseased lung units.
- Disadvantages.
  - Any tube obstruction (secretion or kinking) or sudden change in airway resistance or lung compliance will lead to failure to deliver desired TV and may result in hypoventilation.
  - On the other hand, sudden improvements in lung compliance or resistance may result in delivery of excess TV causing volutrauma.

ASSIST/CONTROL VENTILATION (A/CV)

A/CV allows the patient to initiate a breath which is then assisted to a preset limit variable (pressure or volume). If the patient is unable to generate a breath, then the ventilator delivers control breaths at a preset rate. Hence there are two types of breath: one is patient triggered and the other being time triggered (Figure 30.3). But all breaths whether patient or time triggered have the same set TV (in V-A/CV) or same inspiratory pressure (in P-A/CV). Generally, it works well in patients with reduced respiratory drive by providing adequate ventilator support. But in patients with high respiratory drive leading to frequent breath triggering, it may result in hyperventilation and generation of auto-PEEP due to inadequate time for exhalation.

The mechanism for sensing patient trigger of breath can be based on flow or pressure, with flow being the most common one.

SYNCHRONIZED INTERMITTENT MANDATORY VENTILATION (SIMV)

- In IMV mode, a number of preset mandatory breaths are delivered to the patients,

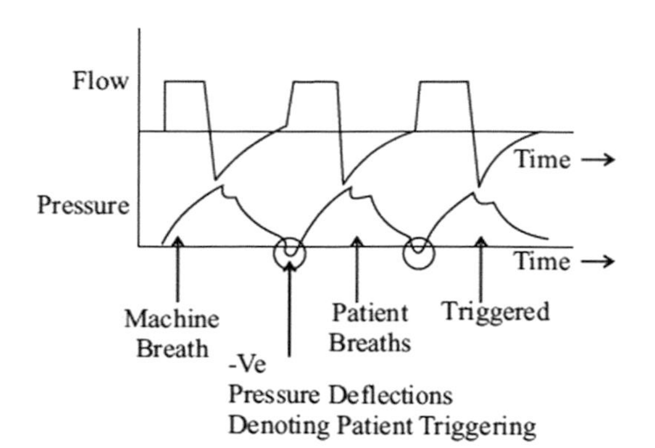

Figure 30.3 Two types of breaths as seen in assist/control modes

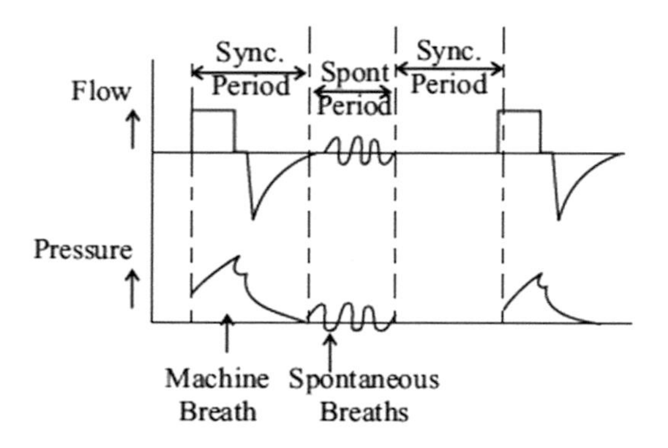

Figure 30.4 Flow vs time and pressure vs time graphs showing types of breaths in synchronized intermittent mandatory ventilation mode

and these breaths can be pressure or volume limited. In between these mandatory breaths, patients can take as many spontaneous breaths as they want. But in this mode, dyssynchrony can still occur if patient inspires or expires during the mandatory breath.

- Thus came the concept of synchronized IMV, which introduced a synchronization window. This is a preset portion of the time interval, in which a patient breath, if it occurs, is supported with the set TV. Any additional breaths are not supported. But if a breath is not taken in this synchronization window, then a mandatory breath is initiated at the preset rate chosen by the clinician (Figure 30.4).
- One of the main disadvantages of this mode is the high work of breathing to inspire via an artificial airway (endotracheal or tracheotomy tube) in the spontaneous breaths. To overcome this, almost all ventilators now only provide SIMV with pressure support instead of SIMV only.
- The level of pressure support is adjusted by the clinician to attain a desired range of TV (4–6 ml/kg).
- In SIMV+PS, the load on respiratory muscles is not relieved completely, so some amount of conditioning can keep taking place.
- The clinician usually sets SIMV rate, TV/Pinsp, FiO_2, PEEP, Psupport, trigger type and threshold (–2 litres/minute usually).
- Once the patient starts getting better, the clinician may sequentially keep reducing the SIMV rate to promote more spontaneous breaths.

PRESSURE SUPPORT VENTILATION (PSV)

- The presence of spontaneous respiratory efforts is a prerequisite for the use of PSV mode.
- All breaths are patient triggered, pressure limited and flow cycled. Flow cycled means that inspiration switches over to expiration when the inspiratory flow touches a specific preset percentage of the peak inspiratory flow (most common default setting is between 20% and 30%). Hence, flow pattern is decelerating in PSV as with most pressure modes (Figure 30.5).
- The percentage of inspiratory flow at which expiration starts is commonly known as the expiratory sensitivity ratio or expiratory trigger sensitivity (Esense or ETS).
- The clinician usually sets PEEP, Psupport, FiO_2, trigger type and threshold, and Esense/ETS.

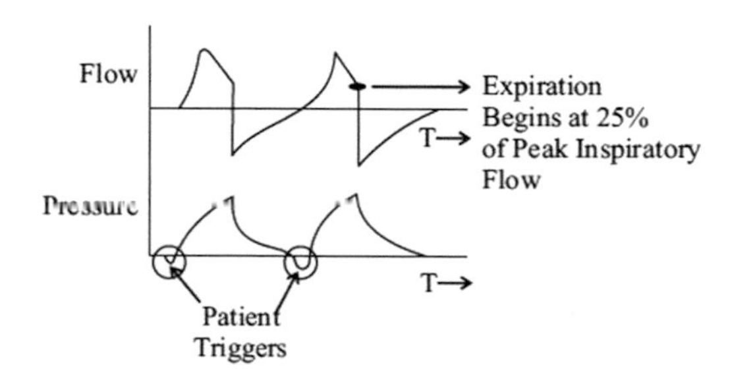

Figure 30.5 Pressure support ventilation mode showing beginning of expiration when inspiratory flow is 25% of the original

- Disadvantages.
  - PSV does not ensure adequate minute ventilation if patient has apnoeic or hypopneic spells. Hence most manufacturers have an apnoea backup built into PSV modes. If a patient does not generate a breath for a certain period of time (apnoea time, set by clinicians), PSV mode is converted to a PCV mode (with predetermined backup settings, set by clinicians).
  - If a circuit leak exists, inspiratory flow may never decrease and the ventilator will not cycle into expiration. To overcome this problem, all new ventilators also have time cycling in PSV modes.

Troubleshooting Alarms

- General principles.
  - All ventilator alarms require clinician attention; never ignore any alarms.
  - Look at the patient first, then follow tubing to the vent to search for any disconnections.
  - If you can't find the problem and the patient is in distress, disconnect the patient from the ventilator and manually ventilate with an Ambu bag with 100% O_2 (and call for help).
- High pressure alarms.
  - Common causes are secretions, kinked or misplaced endotracheal tube (ETT), patient biting the ETT or severe asynchrony, bronchospasm, pneumothorax, decreased compliance as in ARDS.
  - *Word of caution* – If the aforementioned conditions occur in pressure-targeted modes, then instead of high pressure alarms we would get low TV alarms.
- Low pressure alarms.
  - Disconnection from the ventilator or from ETT.
  - Deflated cuff (clue: patient may be able to vocalize).
  - Accidental extubation.
- Low O_2 pressure alarm – Most important, cannot be silenced; immediately inform hospital manifold, disconnect from ventilator and manually ventilate with Ambu bag and 100% O_2 from cylinder.

SUGGESTED READING

1. Holets SR, Hubmayr RD. Setting the ventilator. In: Tobin MJ (ed). *Principles and Practice of Mechanical Ventilation*. Third Edition. New York: McGraw Hill Professional; 2013: 139–58. https://doi.org/10.1186/cc6137.

2. Chatburn RL, Volsko TA. Mechanical ventilators. In: Wilkins RL, Stoller JK, Kacmarek RM (eds). *Egan's Fundamentals of Respiratory Care*. Twelfth Edition. St. Louis: Mosby Elsevier; 2021: 987–1012. https://doi.org/10.1093/med/9780199600830.003.0092.

31 Military Perspective in Trauma Care

Shamik Kr Paul

LEARNING OBJECTIVES

- To understand the differences between combat trauma care and trauma care in the civilian population
- Revisiting the ATLS protocol and modulating in the combat scenario
- Getting acquainted with the MARCHE protocol

INTRODUCTION

The concept of "flying ambulance" in a horse carriage by the Surgeon to the Imperial Guard of Napoleon, Dominique Jean Larrey during the Battle of Rhine was the first kind of medivac of all times. The concept of first aid came up in 1878, developed by medical-stretcher bearers. An aviation accident in rural Nebraska on 17 February 1976 led to the development of the concept of trauma management that was promulgated as Advanced Trauma Life Support (ATLS).

Medical innovations and guidelines were formulated and perfected in various battles and wars. But as time went by, the nature of conflicts changed. Non-conventional warfare, intra-state warfare and global terrorism have overtaken the rules of engaging in battle. There has been constant utilization of the principles of ATLS in the civilian population as well as in military conflicts. Several high-intensity conflicts globally have given us the insight to modify the ATLS philosophy to provide rapid and effective combat casualty care.

In a combat zone, primary trauma care is managed by battlefield nursing assistants or by fellow combatants. A medical officer is present in forward bases covering various combat zones. A specialist is present in a forward surgical centre (FSC) and gives cover to medical officers present in various forward bases. There is always a paradox: the most serious patients at the site of injury are managed by the least experienced medical provider who has to intervene within the platinum 10 minutes or the golden hour. Therefore, there is need for establishing specific guidelines for pre-hospital care in adverse tactical environments to maintain a continuum of care and to salvage as many lives as possible. The challenges faced in combat trauma are presented in Figure 31.1.

According to the Wound Data and Munitions Effectiveness Team (WDMET) study performed during the Vietnam War, it was seen that there are three main causes of preventable deaths during combat: extremity haemorrhage (60%), tension pneumothorax (33%) and obstructed airway (6%).

TACTICAL COMBAT CASUALTY CARE (TCCC)

Inadequacy of applying a civilian trauma model to the tactical situation has long been recognized. Trauma care in the combat scenario is constrained, as shown in Figure 31.1. Due to these peculiarities in combat situations, US forces in 1983 introduced the concept of Tactical Combat Casualty Care (TCCC). ATLS provides the basic foundation on which its guidelines and protocols are formulated.

TCCC guidelines recognize that trauma care in the tactical environment has three goals: (1) treat the casualty, (2) prevent additional casualties and (3) complete the mission. TCCC is divided into three phases as shown in Figure 31.2.

Key elements of the three phases are summarized next:

1. Care Under Fire – CUF refers to care rendered to a casualty at the site of injury during a firefight by the first responder or combatant himself. The following comprises CUF:
   a. Return fire and take cover
   b. Direct or expect casualty to remain engaged as a combatant
   c. Direct or evacuate the casualty to cover
   d. Try to avoid casualty sustaining additional injuries
   e. The most important medical aspect is to stop life-threatening external haemorrhages by self-care, buddy care and by battlefield nursing assistants. The effective use of limb tourniquets is crucial
2. Tactical Field Care – TFC is care rendered by first responder or pre-hospital medical personnel while still in a tactical environment. It follows the MARCHE protocol.

DOI: 10.1201/9781003291619-34

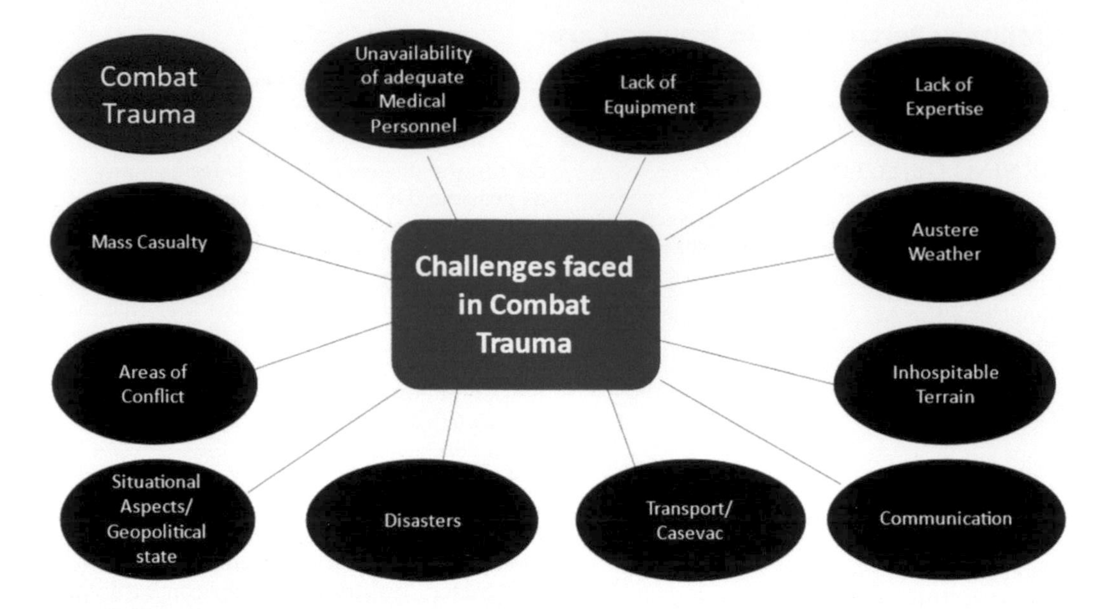

Figure 31.1 Challenges faced in combat trauma

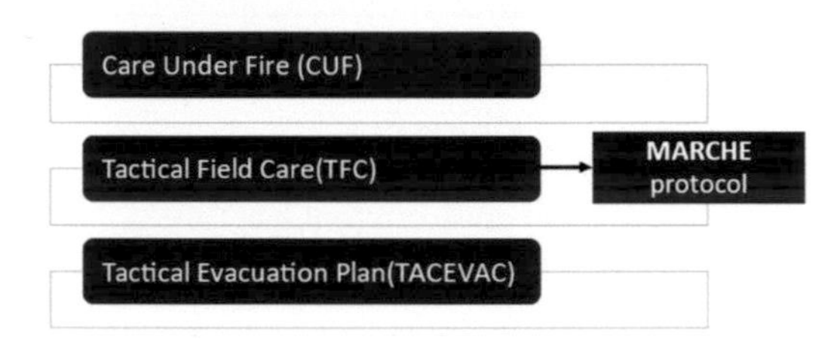

Figure 31.2 Phases of Tactical Combat Casualty Care

MARCHE Protocol

TCCC in the face of inhospitable terrain and extreme temperatures is always a challenge. Delay in the evacuation of casualties from the ongoing theatre of war adds to the complexity of the situation. Timely initiation of the MARCHE protocol is imperative. It consists of:

i. *M*assive haemorrhage: Managed by application of tourniquets, haemostatic dressings and or pressure dressings. In the ATLS algorithm, it is mentioned as "X" (eXanguinating haemorrhage).

ii. *A*irway management by basic skills to keep airway patent, with emphasis on cricothyroidotomy in difficult airways.

iii. *R*espiration and breathing, mainly focused on the identification of tension pneumothorax and its management by needle decompression.

iv. Circulation managed by IV/IO access, judicious fluid administration, early administration of tranexamic acid, blood/blood products and measures to control haemorrhage, which may include damage control resuscitation (DCR) and damage control surgery (DCS).

v. *H*ypothermia prevention, which is often neglected.

vi. *E*verything else (analgesia, antibiotics and monitoring).

3. Tactical Evacuation Care (TACEVAC) – Refers to the care rendered for and en route during the evacuation of the casualty. Follows principles similar to TFC with additional focus on certain advanced procedures.

Medivac and Casevac

Medivac teams have emergency medical services (EMS) personnel in them; in casevac teams, EMS personnel are generally absent. The inventory of transport is also different in these two cases. Whereas medivac consists of ambulances or patient transfer units (PTUs) which are loaded in choppers or fixed-wing aircraft with capabilities of on-road and in-flight patient management, in casevac, the general service vehicles/armoured carriers or aircraft are not equipped with man or material to handle any in-flight emergencies.

ATLS-OE (Operational Emphasis)

ATLS-OE (Figure 31.3) is a very important concept that is included in the ATLS, 10th edition.

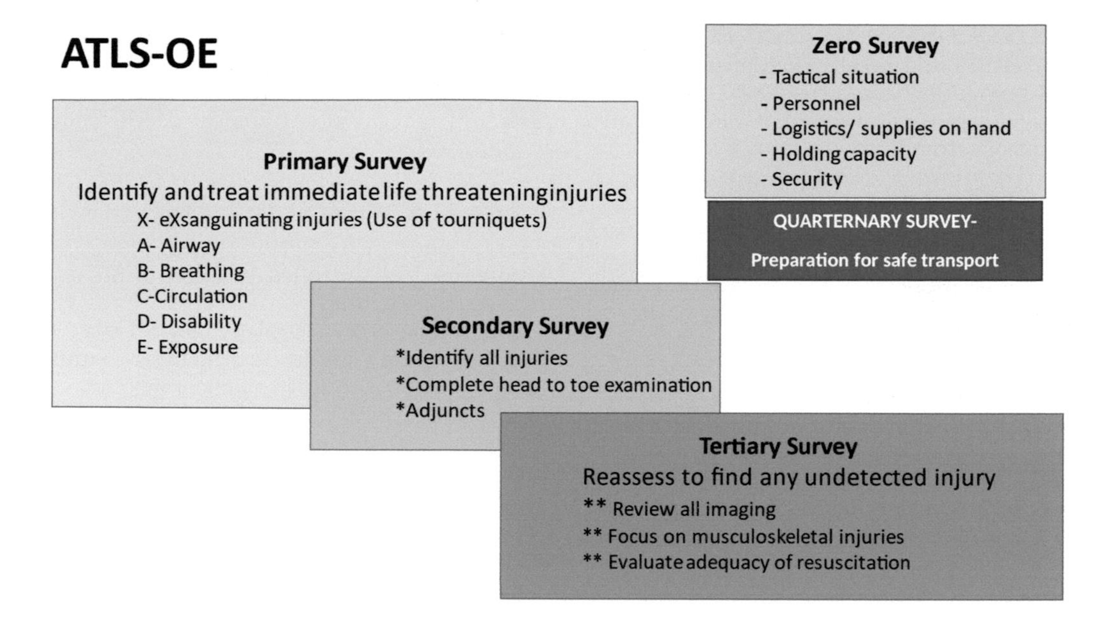

Figure 31.3 ATLS-OE (Operational Emphasis)

Just as TCCC is to Pre-Hospital Trauma Life Support, ATLS in the Operational Emphasis (ATLS-OE) is a course of instruction that emphasizes the importance of maintaining situational awareness while providing care in a potentially hostile, resource-constrained and manpower-limited environment.

Zero Survey

In an operational emphasis, the zero survey is critical as the first step in making appropriate triage decisions in the setting of multiple casualties. The zero survey identifies provider issues or system issues that may not have been identified till now and which will subsequently impact the overall outcome. The fluidity and chaos inherent to the austere environment dictate the importance of zero survey practice.

The evaluation of capabilities with an accurate inventory of resources is paramount.

1. Local resources (availability of oxygen, blood products, whole blood)
2. Staffing and surgical expertise available
3. Holding and critical care capacity
4. Environmental and operational conditions
5. Logistic and supply line considerations

This is followed by the primary survey, where identification and treatment of immediate life-threatening injuries are done. The never-changing concept of ABCDE of primary survey changes here for the first and only time to XABCDE, where X stands for control of exsanguinating haemorrhage. The control of exsanguinating haemorrhage is the only care that can be provided during CUF after returning fire.

As per the ATLS protocol, in the secondary survey the identification of all injuries in a head-to-toe examination is done. In tertiary survey, reassessment for the identification of any undetected injuries is performed.

Quaternary Survey

The quaternary survey formalizes the preparation of the patient for safe transportation, as the patient in an operational environment may require sequential transfer over prolonged distances while initial resuscitation is in progress. Assessing the patient's response to resuscitation is critical. It is desirable to have a stable patient before transfer, but that may not be the case in an operational environment. Blood products are usually not available. The considerations in the quaternary survey are en route care capabilities equipment (ventilator, suction), supplies (blood, IV fluids) and medication (inotropes), and expertise available en route (surgical airway).

The ATLS-OE is now the accepted norm for managing casualties in the austere and combat environment. It has shown great results on the ground in both Iraq (Operation Desert Storm) and Afghanistan (Operation Enduring Freedom).

CONTROL OF MASSIVE HAEMORRHAGE

Before TCCC and effective battlefield tourniquets, extremity haemorrhage was the most frequent cause of preventable battlefield deaths. For major extremity haemorrhage control, ATLS recommends direct pressure, packing with gauze and then tourniquet application, whereas in TCCC and the combat environment it is recommended to directly go for massive bleeding control by application of a tourniquet bypassing the other steps, especially in the CUF phase.

Tourniquets

It is recommended that tourniquets for all major extremity bleeds be tied above the clothes. If a clear bleed is not identified, it has to be tied high and tight till bleeding stops. If bleeding doesn't stop, a second tourniquet above or proximal to the previous tourniquet is applied. TCCC recommends a Combat Application Tourniquet (CAT), Special Operation Forces Tactical Tourniquet (SOFTT), and Emergency and Military Tourniquet (EMT) (Figure 31.4). They can be used with a single hand. Evidence has shown that tourniquets can be used for 2 hours straight. TCCC also advises the use of combat gauze in addition to tourniquets. The tourniquet is not to be used on the neck, axilla or groin; for these areas a SAM Junctional Tourniquet (SJT) is used. There are other efficient tourniquets available like Target Compression Devices (TCDs). Various types of haemostatic dressings are shown in Figure 31.5.

Damage Control Resuscitation (DCR)

The amount of fluid and blood required for resuscitation is difficult to predict on initial evaluation of the patient. The goal of resuscitation is to restore organ perfusion and tissue perfusion, which is accomplished by administering crystalloid solution and blood products to replace lost intravascular volume. Balancing the goal of organ perfusion and tissue oxygenation with the avoidance of rebleed by accepting a lower-than-normal blood pressure has

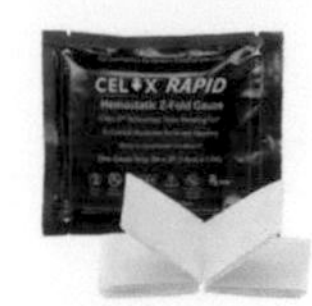

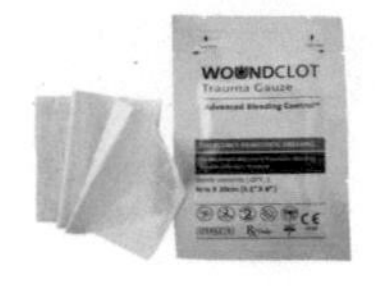

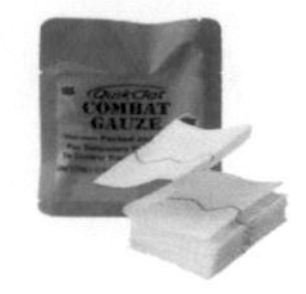

Figure 31.5 Haemostatic dressings

been termed as controlled, balanced or hypotensive resuscitation.

Such a resuscitative strategy may act as a bridge to, if not a substitute to, definitive surgical control of bleeding. In a patient with no head injury, the BP goal is 80–90 mm Hg systolic (50–65 mm Hg mean) or normal mentation and peripheral pulses. DCR in a pre-hospital setting is also called remote DCR.

PAIN MANAGEMENT

Injuries to the extremities are the most common combat injuries. The pain and suffering of a fellow soldier breaks the morale of the fighting troops. Adequate analgesia and critical care without worsening the disease state is vital. Depending upon the severity of pain and location of management, the options of analgesia administration can be by oneself, fellow paramedic or by trained anaesthesiologists.

A. Mild to moderate pain and when the casualty is conscious.
   1. Tab paracetamol 1 gm 8 hrly
   2. Tab tramadol 100 mg BD/TDS

B. Moderate to severe pain, casualty not in shock
   1. Oral transmucosal fentanyl citrate (OTFC) 800 mcg.
   2. Inj tramadol 50mg IV BD/TDS/SOS
   3. Inj morphine 10mg (IM autoinjector)

C. Moderate to severe pain, a casualty in shock.
   1. Inj ketamine 50 mg IM or 20 mg IV

D. Inj nalbuphine 10 mg IV is recommended due to its lesser side effect profile compared to morphine or fentanyl.

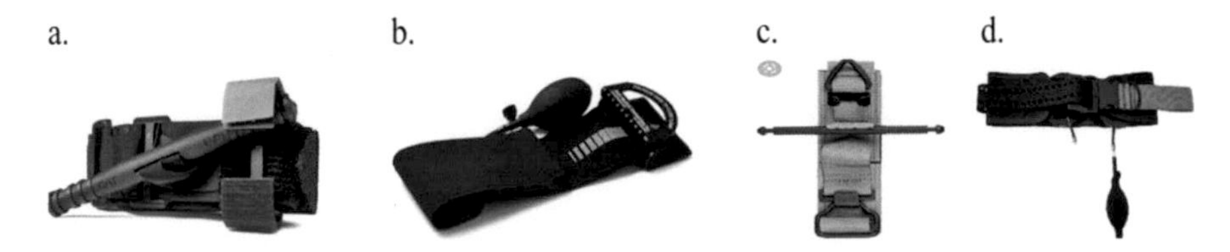

Figure 31.4 Tourniquets. (a) Combat Application Tourniquet (CAT); (b) Emergency and Military Tourniquet (EMT); (c) Special Operation Forces Tactical Tourniquet (SOFTT); (d) SAM Junctional Tourniquet (SJT).

E. Regional anaesthesia by trained anaesthesiologist at forward surgical centre.

CONCLUSION

Modifications in the ATLS algorithm to introduce the nuances of combat and austere environments are not just about saving lives but giving quality care at the very onset to provide quality life thereafter. This requires adequate training and implementation at all echelons.

SUGGESTED READING

1. Champion HR, Lawnick MM. *Wound Data and Munitions Effectiveness Team (WDMET) Study.* Annapolis, MD: Tech Med, Inc.; 2006.

2. Butler F. Tactical combat casualty care: combining good medicine with good tactics. *J Trauma.* 2003;54(5 Suppl):S2–3.

3. Bellamy RF. The causes of death in conventional land warfare: implications for casualty care research. *Mil Med.* 1984;149(2):55–62.

4. Kelly JF, Ritenour AE, McLaughlin DF, et al. Injury severity and causes of death from operation Iraqi freedom and operation enduring freedom: 2003–2004 versus 2006. *J Trauma.* 2008;64(2 Suppl):S21–27; discussion S26–27.

5. Tactical Combat Casualty Care Guidelines. 2009 Nov [cited 2010 May 31]. Available from: URL: http://www.usaisr.amedd.army.mil/tccc/TCCC%20Guidelines%20091104.pdf.

6. Tarpey M. Tactical combat casualty care in operation Iraqi freedom. *US Army Med Dep J.* 2005:38–41. PB 8-05-4/5/6 Apr/May/Jun.

7. Wedmore I, McManus JG, Pusateri AE, et al. A special report on the chitosan-based hemostatic dressing: experience in current combat operations. *J Trauma.* 2006;60(3):655–8.

8. Neuffer MC, McDivitt J, Rose D, et al. Hemostatic dressings for the first responder: a review. *Mil Med.* 2004;169(9):716–20.

9. Fowler R, Gallagher JV, Isaacs SM, et al. The role of intraosseous vascular access in the out-of-hospital environment (resource document to NAEMSP position statement). *Prehosp Emerg Care.* 2007;11(1):63–6.

10. Mabry RL, Edens JW, Pearse L, Kelly JF, Harke H. Fatal airway injuries during operation enduring freedom and operation Iraqi freedom. *Prehosp Emerg Care.* 2010;14 (2, Apr 6):272–7.

11. Arthurs Z, Cuadrado D, Beekley A, et al. The impact of hypothermia on trauma care at the 31st combat support hospital. *Am J Surg.* 2006;191(5):610–4.

12. De Lorenzo RA. Military and civilian emergency aeromedical services: common goals with different approaches. *Aviat Space Environ Med.* 1997;68(1):56–60.

Index

Note: Locators in *italics* represent figures and **bold** indicate tables in the text.